D1488546

Health Care Regulation in America

Robert I. Field

Health Care Regulation in America:

Complexity, Confrontation, and Compromise

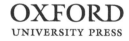

UNIVERSITY PRESS

2007

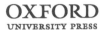

Oxford University Press, Inc., publishes works that further
Oxford University's objective of excellence
in research, scholarship, and education.

Oxford   New York
Auckland   Cape Town   Dar es Salaam   Hong Kong   Karachi
Kuala Lumpur   Madrid   Melbourne   Mexico City   Nairobi
New Delhi   Shanghai   Taipei   Toronto

With offices in
Argentina   Austria   Brazil   Chile   Czech Republic   France   Greece
Guatemala   Hungary   Italy   Japan   Poland   Portugal   Singapore
South Korea   Switzerland   Thailand   Turkey   Ukraine   Vietnam

Published by Oxford University Press, Inc.
198 Madison Avenue, New York, New York 10016

www.oup.com

Oxford is a registered trademark of Oxford University Press

Library of Congress Cataloging-in-Publication Data
Field, Robert I.
Health care regulation in America : complexity, confrontation, and
compromise / Robert I. Field.
     p. ; cm.
Includes bibliographical references and index.

ISBN-13 978-0-19-515968-4

1. Medical policy—United States.   I. Title.
[DNLM: 1. Delivery of Health Care—legislation & jurisprudence
—United States.   2. Government Regulation—United States.   3. Health
Care Sector—legislation & jurisprudence—United States.   W 32.5
AA1 F4566h 2006]
RA395.A3F535 2006
362.10973—dc22   2006006137

Printed in the United States of America
on acid-free paper

To the memory of my parents.

Preface

Virtually no aspect of American health care escapes regulatory oversight. Anyone who works anywhere in the health care system can attest to the overriding, and some might feel overbearing, influence of regulators. This is true for hospital administrators managing the delivery of health care services, physicians delivering those services, pharmaceutical executives planning the development of new drugs, pharmacists dispensing those drugs, medical directors making coverage decisions for health maintenance organizations, and even computer consultants planning a medical Web site. Outsiders, both in the government and in private accrediting and certifying organizations, have a major role in telling health care workers at all levels what to do.

The prominence of regulation in health care arises for a good reason. It would be difficult to identify another industry that is as directly involved in the health and well-being of its customers. While policy debates swirl around the proper role and extent of health care regulation, it is an area in which few would find no place for oversight of some sort. Despite the apparent need, however, health care regulation in America is neither uniform nor consistent. It encompasses a broad range of regulatory programs that apply in different ways to different aspects of the industry. Hospitals, physicians, insurance companies, pharmaceutical companies, and equipment manufacturers, to name just a few key players, each face distinct kinds of monitoring. Health care regulations are developed and implemented not only by all levels of government—federal, state, and local—but by private organizations as well.

American health care regulation has a diverse landscape. At the federal level there is the Department of Health and Human Services and its many components, including the Centers for Medicare & Medicaid Services, the Centers for Disease Control and Prevention, and the Food and Drug Administration, in addition to the Environmental Protection Agency, the Occupational Safety and Health Administration, and numerous other agencies. In each state there are departments of health, welfare, and insurance. In cities and counties there are municipal health departments. Turning to the private side, there is the Joint Commission on Accreditation of Healthcare Organization, the National Committee on Quality Assurance, and numerous professional boards and societies. These agencies and organizations, and the programs they administer, have arisen at different times but primarily over the course of the past century. New ones are often added with little consideration for those already in place, sometimes resulting in redundancy and conflict.

To some observers, this landscape indicates that there is not really a "system" of health care regulation in America, but rather a disjointed set of programs that often work at cross-purposes. Many states, for example, encourage the development of clinical service monopolies through certificate-of-need programs, while federal antitrust enforcers promote free-market competition. The Food and Drug Administration approves drugs for use only under narrowly circumscribed conditions, but licensed physicians can prescribe them for any purpose they see fit. For those who make up the health care industry, however, professional life requires dealing with this morass, no matter how frustrating the conflicts may be.

The goal of this book is to present an overview of health care regulation in America in its breadth and scope and to help develop an understanding of its most significant components. Each regulatory program's policy goals and conflicts are the focus, rather than the technical details, which tend to change frequently. Regulation is more than a set of laws and rules. It is a network of heterogeneous bureaucratic structures that fulfill distinct missions, sometimes complementary and sometimes conflicting, in response to public policy challenges that have emerged over many years and that continue to arise. The book is intended as a resource for students of the health care system, for professionals who work in America's health care enterprise, and for readers outside the field who have an interest in understanding an important set of forces that shape the health care that Americans receive.

Because of the tremendous breadth of the subject, it is impossible to cover every regulatory program that relates to health care. However, an attempt has been made to be as comprehensive as possible and to describe every significant kind of regulation that is directly targeted to the provision or financing of health care. It is hoped that the reader will gain not only a perspective on the enormous variety of ways in which health care is regulated but also an appreciation of the complexity of the system and of the policy conflicts that drive it.

Chapters 2 through 8 are organized around substantive areas of regulation. Since the spheres of regulatory responsibility cannot be divided with complete precision, chapters cross-reference one another. Chapter 1 sets the stage with a brief historical overview and discussion of central policy challenges that regulation presents, and chapter 9 brings together overriding themes and considers emerging regulatory challenges.

Each chapter begins with a historical overview of the evolution of regulatory programs and of related government policy in its area of focus. This offers the clearest perspective on the reasons that programs and policies developed in the ways that they did. Since historical events are often key catalysts for regulatory responses, the progression of government actions brings to light the conflicts and compromises that shaped the web of laws, rules, and bureaucratic structures that have emerged. With the historical overview as a base, the current structure of key programs, agencies, and organizations is then presented. Finally, there is a discussion of overriding policy issues, including some that are specific to each sphere of regulatory attention and some that policy makers perennially face in all health care policy. The persistence of these conflicts provides the best explanation for the lack of a cohesive system and the best window on the forces that one can expect to operate in the future as health care evolves and new challenges for oversight emerge.

Acknowledgments

This book, as most, would not have been possible without the assistance of many people. I am indebted to my research assistants, who gathered copious amounts of material. Michelle Sahl researched the regulation of clinical service delivery for chapters 2 and 3; Barbara Plager, the development and implementation of Medicare and Medicaid for chapter 4, as well as reviewing and commenting on several chapters; Nirav Shelat, the history of food and drug regulation and the evolution of the Food and Drug Administration for chapter 5, as well as extensive checking of references for the entire volume; Holly Unger, the regulation of public health for chapter 6; Jamie Howell, the development of medical privacy regulation for chapter 7; and Mona Fiorentini, the funding and regulation of medical research for chapter 8. I am also indebted to Professor Barry Furrow for his review of and comments on the entire manuscript. I owe special thanks to Catherine Gebauer for extensive editorial assistance, reference checking, and typing. Of course, the responsibility for any errors is mine alone. I would also like to express appreciation to my wife, Mary, and sons, David and William, for their patience, support, and encouragement along the way.

Contents

List of Tables

Health Care Regulation in America

1

Introduction: The History, Policies, and Structures That Shape Health Care Regulation

It is virtually impossible to find a social institution in the United States that does not affect the health-care enterprise or is not influenced by it.
—W. Kissick, *Medicine's Dilemmas*

Health care is among the most heavily regulated industries in America. Virtually every aspect of the system is subject to government oversight in one form or another, and often in several forms.[1] To take but a few examples, there are mechanisms to supervise the professionals who render care, the institutions in which care is provided, the drugs and devices that are used as tools of care, and the insurance coverage that finances it. Beyond directing actual elements of health care, government programs govern related activities as diverse as the business arrangements that are formed among providers, the biomedical research that scientists conduct, and the access of clinicians to computerized patient medical information. Regulatory authority over health care resides not only in the government at all levels but also in a set of private organizations that supplement public oversight. It would not be possible to fully comprehend the provision of health care in America without understanding the massive and pervasive regulatory machinery that guides it.

The Challenge Behind All Health Policy

Why does the government regulate health care? The simple answer is that it does so for the same reason it regulates most other industries. Impartial external oversight, rather than market forces, is seen as necessary to protect the public interest. Public protection is particularly important in health care because it directly affects the life

3

and health of its consumers.[2] Behind this simple answer, however, lies a set of more subtle and complex considerations.

The public interest in regulating health care derives from the need to control three basic features that in one form or another drive perennial policy attention. Policy makers want patients to receive care that meets standards of acceptable quality, that permits widespread access, and that is affordable. A well-functioning system balances all three. If any element is missing, the system is deficient in one way or another.

Unfortunately, maximizing quality, maintaining access, and controlling costs simultaneously is a daunting task that requires ingenuity and resourcefulness on the part of policy makers. Enhancing any one of the goals unavoidably challenges another. As described by Dr. William Kissick, one of the architects of the Medicare program, health policy represents a perpetual juggling act in which three balls remain in our control only if we keep them in balance.[3] Higher quality care, for example, is usually more expensive. Cutting costs tends to require either lower quality care or more restricted access. Wider access carries a significant price tag. If we pay too much attention to one of the balls, we will inevitably drop one or both of the others.

Every health care regulatory program can be seen as an effort to address one or another of these goals. Over time, however, the goals that were not addressed ultimately present new concerns in response. One result of this interplay is the development of a set of layers of regulation that has grown increasingly complex over time. Each new program generates the need for yet another one down the road. At the same time, scientific advances constantly reshape medicine's foundation. Health care regulation, as a result, has become a dynamic and vibrant field that continually seeks creative responses to this maze of conflicting influences.

The interplay of health policy goals and its formative effect on regulation is particularly apparent when viewed in historical context. The first significant health care regulatory programs were enacted in the late nineteenth century. Since then, the focus of policy has centered on each of the three goals in a progression over time. The evolution of health care regulation over the past century reflects the changing balance of the three core objectives as our society continually strives for the best overall solution. We see the result today in the intricate array of programs and policy conflicts that is described in the chapters that follow.

The First Steps in Health Care Regulation: Ensuring Basic Quality

The dawn of significant health care regulation in America can be traced to the late nineteenth century, when science developed the first tools to control the spread of disease on a broad scale.[4] (See chapter 6 for a discussion of the regulation of public health.) The discovery of the role of germs in causing illness led to an understanding of contagion, which in turn led government officials to develop programs to contain it. These included mandatory vaccinations, first in response to epidemics such as smallpox and later of schoolchildren to head off disease outbreaks, and mandatory quarantine of those who contracted or had been exposed to infectious agents. Other policies addressed causes of disease at their source in sewage and other forms of contamination. These were sanitation programs that improved sewer systems, provided clean drinking water, and inspected food.

The earliest drug safety law was enacted in the 1840s to control the sale of imported products.[5] (See chapter 5 for a discussion of the regulation of drugs.) The hazards of unsafe medications from domestic sources began to receive serious attention from federal regulators in the 1860s under the administration of President Abraham Lincoln. It eventually led to the first comprehensive national law, which was passed in 1906. Food safety laws date back to colonial times. The first national food law was also passed in 1906 to address unsanitary conditions in the meatpacking industry.

The late nineteenth and early twentieth centuries were also the time when regulators first considered the adequacy of the health care services that the public receives.[6] Prodded by the medical profession itself, every state implemented a licensing program for physicians that incorporated accreditation standards for medical schools. (See chapter 2 for a discussion of the licensure and regulation of professional practice.) Regulatory attention focused on hospitals and other health care institutions, as well. The result was a set of state laws that stopped untrained practitioners from laying claim to being healers and ill-equipped facilities from boasting that they were centers of care.

By 1920, a transformed health care system had emerged. In it, external regulatory standards were imposed on clinical education, professional practice, institutional administration, and the safety of food and drugs. Government authorities were also empowered to protect overall public health with forceful and coercive tools. American health care, at least in some respects, could actually be called a "system."

The unifying theme of regulatory interventions in this phase of health policy evolution was the assurance of quality. Poorly trained practitioners were vetted before they could provide services and were monitored by medical boards once they began to practice. Drugs could be ordered off the market if proved unsafe. Infectious disease outbreaks were halted or contained before they could jeopardize large segments of the population. American health care, which could be characterized as haphazard, inconsistent, and unscientific before this era began, took on respectability and enhanced clinical value.

Expanding Public Access to High-Quality Health Care

With the creation of a health care system that contained competent professionals, safe products, and qualified institutions, the ability of patients to gain access to care became a more important concern. America had created a health care system that people wanted and needed to use. Moreover, continual advances in medical science steadily bolstered its capabilities. (See chapter 8 for a discussion of the regulation and funding of research.) However, the best health care in the world is of little value to those with no means of access.

Health insurance as we know it today was born in 1929, when Baylor Hospital in Houston, Texas, developed a plan for unlimited access by schoolteachers in return for prepayment in the form of a set monthly sum.[7] (See chapter 4 for a discussion of the regulation of health care finance.) The concept spread to other hospitals across the country and was formally organized into nonprofit Blue Cross insurance plans that covered inpatient expenses. In 1939, a group of physicians in Sacramento, California, created the first Blue Shield plan to finance outpatient professional care in a similar fashion. With the combination of these two forms of coverage, a mechanism to fund widespread health care access had arrived.

Two federal regulatory initiatives during and immediately after World War II solidified the popularity of health insurance as a mechanism to finance care. A freeze on wages during the war left employers with few options to attract workers in a tight labor market. Regulations that implemented the freeze, however, exempted fringe benefits, such as employer-paid health insurance. Firms were free to entice prospective workers with prepaid medical care, a relatively low-cost benefit at the time, and many of them did. Subsequent tax regulations compounded the value of this new form of remuneration by excluding it from the calculation of wages that are subject to income tax. With this start, in the decade following the war health insurance spread as a common employee benefit, with for-profit commercial insurance companies joining Blue Cross and Blue Shield plans in the market.

Despite its widespread appeal, employer-based health insurance leaves many behind, including those who are unemployed, self-employed, or employed by companies that do not offer an insurance benefit, as well as their dependents. Proposals for universal national health insurance first became the focus of serious national policy debate immediately after World War II. Although none was enacted, a number of more limited solutions to fill gaps in access were. These included a massive federal program to fund hospital construction, the Hill-Burton Act of 1946, and regulatory programs to expand access to insurance coverage in many states. During this time, many veterans were able to access health care services through the expanding network of hospitals operated by the Veterans Administration. In 1965, national coverage was implemented for two broad segments of the population that lacked access to the employer-sponsored insurance market, the elderly and the poor. Medicare covered those age sixty-five and older, and Medicaid covered many of those whose incomes fell below the federally designated poverty level.

By the late 1960s, the combination of private employer-based insurance, Medicare, Medicaid, veterans care, and other federal programs had opened health care access to the majority of the population. While these programs still left substantial gaps in coverage that persist today, most Americans by this time could receive care in a system that equaled or surpassed the level of quality achieved in the early part of the century. Health care access and quality came to be widely expected as part of the fabric of our culture, with some advocates even proposing a legal and moral right to care.

Controlling Costs in a Growing System

With widespread access to a high-quality health care system, the third leg of the policy triangle had to give. Precipitous rises in the cost of care were first evident in the late 1960s and continue as an intractable challenge to this day. In response, regulatory policy shifted much of its focus to controlling costs with an array of programs that held great promise but seem to have had little long-term systemic effect. While quality and access continued to be underlying concerns for policy makers, it was the management of costs that took center stage.

The range of regulatory programs enacted to address rising health care costs was extensive. In 1973, Congress encouraged the spread of health maintenance organizations (HMOs) as a less costly alternative to traditional health insurance through passage of legislation to encourage their adoption in employer benefit plans. In 1976, Congress mandated that states implement health planning programs to rationalize the proliferation of expensive and duplicative services. A funding program enacted in the late 1960s took an opposite approach, encouraging the growth of medical school enrollments in the hope that competitive pressure within a larger pool of physician supply would reduce fees. A program of peer review of physician practice patterns under Medicare was enacted in 1972 to pressure heavy utilizers of hospital services to change their habits. Several states experimented with direct regulatory control of hospital rates. In 1983, the most aggressive regulatory cost-control initiative of all was implemented, when the Medicare program changed the method by which it reimbursed hospitals. The original system based on the actual costs of providing care was replaced with one based on prospectively set amounts determined by each patient's primary diagnosis.

Health care cost pressures abated in the mid-1990s but accelerated again at the end of the decade. Some attributed the hiatus to the success of managed care, which had become the predominant form of insurance coverage by then in many markets, but many decried accompanying restrictions on the freedom of patients to choose their providers and on overall access. Whatever the case, the growth of costs returned with renewed vigor. By the end of the twentieth century, some observers noted that America boasted a high quality health care system that the country could not actually afford.

The Regulatory Bind Today

The system of health care regulation that America has today is a complex web of programs that date from these different eras when each of the three foci of policy commanded attention in turn. Regulators now function at all levels of government and also in private organizations, often implementing policies that actually conflict with one another. The system has nurtured and guided the most comprehensive health care enterprise in the world but with a frequent lack of consistency and transparency. The result may be inevitable, and even appropriate, for the oversight of so complex an industry, but it can nevertheless be frustrating for those who must navigate it.

After a century of honing America's health care system and its regulatory oversight, all three policy imperatives seem to have returned to confront the country simultaneously. Quality is not as consistent as had been assumed. The Institute of Medicine of the National Academy of Sciences alerted America in 1999 that tens of thousands of patients, perhaps as many as 98,000 each year, die because of preventable mistakes made in hospitals.[8] Recent research on social aspects of medical care has revealed significant disparities in the quality and outcomes of care received by different racial, ethnic, and income groups.[9] Research on patterns of medical practice has demonstrated wide variations across geographic regions, with many best practices restricted in their dissemination.[10]

Access to care remains well short of universal, with about 15 percent of the population perennially lacking health insurance coverage.[11] Those without insurance can still obtain basic services at public clinics and in hospital emergency rooms; however, they receive little continuity of care, and treatment for routine conditions rendered in emergency rooms is extremely inefficient. These patients also have very limited access to specialists or specialty procedures, except in emergencies.

Costs continue to rise relentlessly.[12] Health care now consumes more than 15 percent of the nation's gross domestic product, and in most years, costs increase at a significantly faster pace than overall inflation.[13] The policy premise behind controlling costs, however, is a bit more complex than those behind enhancing quality and access. Higher costs in and of themselves are not necessarily harmful if patients get what they are paying for in an efficient system. The issue is whether the system is, in fact, efficient and, if it is, whether society is able and willing to pay for the quality of health care that it seeks. Studies of fraud and waste, however, indicate that overall efficiency is, indeed, lacking, and the demand for high-quality care based on technological advances seems to be outstripping the ability to pay for it.

In other words, health care regulation today faces considerable overall challenges. However, they are accompanied by significant opportunities. Medicine can do much more today than it could a hundred years ago. It saves many more lives and reduces much more human suffering. The conflicts in regulating this enterprise are large, but regulators can build on a history of tremendous success in enhancing quality, opening access, and occasionally moderating cost pressures. Regulation, with all its imperfections, has helped the health care system to achieve tremendous accomplishments, and it will likely continue to do so.

Pillars of the Regulatory System

The regulatory system that has evolved rests on pillars at the state, private, and federal levels.[14] Much of the remainder of the bureaucratic structure of regulation sits on this foundation. Some policy objectives rely on one, and some on a combination of them. Their variety and interplay are a legacy of the shifting policy foci of the past century mixed with various uniquely American political dynamics. A summary of all the significant health care regulatory agencies and organizations that are described in the chapters that follow is contained in appendix A.

The states were the original locus of regulatory activity, which they effectuated through departments of health and boards of medicine. Today, every state has a health department that oversees sanitation standards across a range of settings, conducts inspections, issues licenses, and gathers and disseminates data. Boards of medicine and of other health professions perform the basic functions of professional licensure and oversight of practice. Some are independent bodies, and some are contained within health departments or other larger agencies. This bureaucratic structure remains the first line of defense in addressing fundamental public health needs and assuring the quality of clinical services. Related state-level functions are performed by departments of welfare, which in many states administer Medicaid programs of public insurance coverage for the poor, departments of aging, which administer services for the elderly, and departments of insurance, which oversee much of the financing of care.

Private organizations arose in tandem with state bureaucracies to play key roles early in the development of regulation. The American Medical Association (AMA), which was founded in 1847, promoted and guided the development of physician licensure laws and accreditation standards for medical schools.[15] Those programs relied heavily on other private professional organizations that the AMA helped to create for coordination and implementation. A more direct regulatory role for nongovernmental organizations arose in the 1930s with the establishment of professional boards to certify physicians as qualified to practice in specialized fields. Similar groups were created over time to play analogous roles in several other clinical professions. In the 1950s, the Joint Commission on Accreditation of Hospitals (now the Joint Commission on Accreditation of Health Care Organizations [JCAHO]), a private organization controlled by member hospitals, established a process of accrediting facilities according to quality standards that were generally more stringent than those required for state licensure. In the 1990s, the National Committee for Quality Assurance (NCQA), which represents large employers and other major payers for care, began to accredit managed care plans.

This network of private organizations underpins much of the regulation of quality, and it functions in close coordination with the network of governmental bodies. As a result, America's health care regulatory system can be more accurately characterized as a public-private partnership than as a process of direct government oversight.[16] All major segments involved in delivering and financing health care services—professionals, hospitals, and payers—complement the policing functions of external overseers through their own regulatory efforts. Though this facet of the system has been criticized as rife with conflicts of interest, nonetheless it has become ingrained in the fabric of our regulatory infrastructure. It may actually reflect an inevitable consequence of the uniquely American ambivalence over the appropriate roles of government and of private industry in driving economic activity.

In contrast to the emerging regulatory system of the early twentieth century, which relied mostly on state and private interventions, the most significant player in health care regulation today is the federal government. Federal programs represent the largest source of payment for health care, their implementation effectuates the most aggressive cost-control strategies, and they are moving into more central roles in assuring quality. The provision of health care may be local, but it is now unquestionably a national concern.

The vast majority of federal health care regulatory activity is conducted through the component agencies of the Department of Health and Human Services (DHHS), which oversees every aspect of the health care system in one way or another.[17] Under its umbrella are such key agencies as the Food and Drug Administration (FDA), the Centers for Medicare & Medicaid Services (CMS), the Centers for Disease Control and Prevention (CDC), and the National Institutes of Health (NIH). The pervasive influence of DHHS can be seen in every area of regulation discussed in the chapters that follow.

DHHS is a behemoth organization. Its 2005 budget of $581 billion represented almost one-quarter of all federal spending and was second only to that of the Department of Defense among cabinet-level agencies.[18] The payroll included 67,444 employees. The agency manages more than 300 different programs and administers more grant funding than all other federal agencies combined.

DHHS was born as the Federal Security Agency under President Franklin Roosevelt in 1939. It brought together several existing federal agencies that had responsibilities for health, welfare, and social insurance. Among the agencies that were included were the Social Security Board (now the Social Security Administration [SSA]), which administers the Social Security program; the FDA, which oversees the safety of drugs; NIH, which conducts and funds biomedical research; and the Public Health Service (PHS), which operates public hospitals and provides physician staffing for public health clinics. In 1953, under President Dwight Eisenhower, the agency was elevated to cabinet-level status and renamed the Department of Health, Education, and Welfare (DHEW). In 1979, Congress created a separate cabinet-level Department of Education, which assumed DHEW's education-related programs, and in 1980, the agency's name was changed to its present form.

DHHS is headed by a secretary who is appointed by the president subject to Senate confirmation. Reporting to him or her are an array of assistant secretaries and a set of administrators, commissioners, and directors of the component agencies. DHHS's headquarters is located in Washington, D.C., but several of the components are based elsewhere, including Bethesda, Rockville, and Baltimore, Maryland, as well as Atlanta, Georgia. DHHS and its component agencies have field offices throughout the country.

There are currently ten major constituent agencies within DHHS. A list is contained in table 1.1. Seven of them grew out of the original PHS. These are NIH, FDA, CDC, the Indian Health Service (IHS), the Health Resources and Services Administration (HRSA), the Substance Abuse and Mental Health Services Administration (SAHSA), and the Agency for Healthcare Research and Quality (AHAQ). The others include CMS, the Administration for Children and Families, and the Administration on Aging. In addition, a network of physicians and other health care professionals serve as commissioned officers in public health clinics around the country and within DHHS and other federal agencies as part of the United States Public Health Service Commissioned Corps, headed by the surgeon general.

Since 1939, new policy challenges have expanded DHHS's range of responsibilities with an ever-growing list of new regulatory programs. More than half of the component agencies did not exist when the original Federal Security Agency was created. Through these new elements, the scope of influence continues to grow today unabated.

The Process of Regulation

The health care agencies and programs that developed over the past century grew against a backdrop of specific legal constraints.[19] Regulation holds an anomalous position in the American legal system. It has features of both the legislative and judicial processes but exists within a structure all its own. Rules issued by regulatory agencies have a force that is similar to that of statutes, but they are not enacted by legislators. Adjudications by regulators have an effect that is similar to that of court rulings, but they are not conducted by judges. This is a unique role in America's system of laws.[20]

Congress and state legislatures create regulatory agencies to develop and implement practical details of government programs that require specialized expertise and resources.[21] For example, when state legislatures enacted licensure requirements for physicians, they created a mechanism in the form of medical boards to

Table 1.1
Component Agencies of the Department of Health and Human Services

Agency	Major Functions	Employees (2005)	Budget (2005)
National Institutes of Health	Funding and conducting biomedical research	17,543	$28.6 billion
Food and Drug Administration	Assuring the safety of foods and cosmetics and the safety and efficacy of pharmaceuticals, biological products, and medical devices	10,446	$1.8 billion
Centers for Disease Control and Prevention	Public health surveillance and monitoring and disease prevention	8,837	$8 billion
Indian Health Service	Providing health services to 1.6 million Native Americans	16,251	$3.8 billion
Health Resources and Services Administration	Providing access to health care to vulnerable populations	2,034	$7.4 billion
Substance Abuse and Mental Health Services Administration	Funding to states for substance abuse and mental health services	558	$3.4 billion
Agency for Healthcare Research and Quality	Supporting research on health services	296	$319 million
Centers for Medicare & Medicaid Services	Administering the Medicare program and the federal portion of the Medicaid program	4,943	$489 billion
Administration for Children and Families	Administering 60 programs providing health and other services to children of needy families	1,382	$47 billion
Administration on Aging	Providing support services including meals and transportation for the elderly	126	$1.4 billion
DHHS Overall	Protecting the health of Americans and providing essential human services	67,444	$581 billion

Source: http://www.hhs.gov/about (3 August 2005).

devise standards for medical practice and procedures for enforcing them by granting or denying licenses. The statutes that enabled this arrangement contained overall policy guidance but left to the boards the tasks of formulating details of the standards and of applying them in individual cases. Legislators did not consider themselves competent to resolve such technical issues, nor did they have the time or resources to apply the outcomes in practice to every physician applicant. Similarly, when Congress created the Medicare program, it determined the outlines and procedures for providing insurance coverage to the elderly but left to DHEW the task of deciding on reimbursement for specific services.

Within this context, regulators perform functions that characterize each of the three branches of government.[22] They extend the legislative reach of Congress and state legislatures by filling in the practical details of policy initiatives. They act as executives in implementing the managerial and administrative aspects of government programs. They adjudicate disputes in a similar manner to the courts. Regulatory actions that create rules or standards to supplement legislative directives, for example, by setting discharge standards for pollutants under environmental protection laws, are known as "rule-making" proceedings. Those that resolve disputes in matters such as medical license revocations are known as "adjudicatory" proceedings. Regulators take "executive" actions when they administer government services, such as health care in a Veterans Administration hospital.

Regulatory bodies, whether they are characterized as boards, commissions, agencies, or departments, are headed by officials who are appointed by the president or, in the case of state-level programs, by the governor. They are commonly subject to confirmation by the Senate or the state legislature. Bodies with a single chief official generally change leadership with each change in government administration. Members of boards and commissions, however, are often appointed for fixed terms that extend beyond elections to ensure some continuity of leadership across administrations. Appointed officials provide overall policy guidance for the agencies that they lead. Most of the day-to-day work is conducted by staff who remain in place over time and facilitate institutional consistency.[23]

As components of the government, regulatory agencies are directly subject to restrictions contained in the Constitution. These include the prohibition on discrimination contained in the Fourteenth Amendment, and the proscription on limiting the right to free speech or religious practice contained in the First Amendment. The most significant operational effect of the Constitution on governmental agencies results from the requirement contained in the Fifth and Fourteenth Amendments that "due process" be provided before life, liberty, or property may be denied.[24]

Regulators routinely impinge on property interests in many ways. Denial or suspension of a medical license, for example, limits a physician's ability to earn a living. Rejection of a pharmaceutical company's request for approval of a new drug denies it the ability to make a profit. Disallowance of reimbursement for a medical procedure under Medicare or Medicaid limits the flow of funds to patients, providers, or both. Fines levied for antitrust or billing violations take money directly out of the hands of alleged violators. Due process protections dictate that no such action may be taken without full consideration of relevant facts and of the positions of all affected parties. They are implemented through a set of procedural safeguards that protect against arbitrary decision making.

To ensure that Constitutional due process is afforded in federal regulatory proceedings, in 1946 Congress enacted the Administrative Procedures Act (APA), which lays out a road map for administrative decision making.[25] Most states have similar laws governing their own regulatory programs. The application of the road map varies according to the kind of proceeding involved, but a few underlying elements always apply. The common touchstone under the act for judging an administrative decision is that it may not be "arbitrary, capricious, an abuse of discretion, or otherwise not in accordance with law."[26]

A regulatory proceeding that passes muster under the APA must first gather as much relevant information as possible. In a medical licensure revocation, as an example in a health care context, this would include all available facts bearing on the physician's conduct and delineation of the relevant standard of care. An FDA review of a new drug application would take account of all data from clinical trials of the drug and perhaps the assessment of an expert advisory committee. In deciding whether to reimburse the expense of a new medical treatment under Medicare, CMS would consider data on costs and effectiveness. This fact-finding phase of regulatory decision making is usually conducted by an agency's permanent staff.

Before the fact-finding can be considered complete, however, the agency must notify all affected parties and offer them an opportunity to be heard. A suspect physician, for instance, must be allowed to present evidence in his or her defense, a drug manufacturer to submit all favorable clinical findings that bear on approval for marketing, and an industrial manufacturer to put forward information on the burden of compliance with a new environmental emissions standard. When the proceeding applies to an individual, such as a physician, he or she is given notice directly. When it affects the broader public, as would be the case for a Medicare coverage rule or an environmental discharge limit, wider notice is required. Summaries of these kinds of proposed federal actions are published in the *Federal Register,* a daily publication containing official information from agencies throughout the government. Most states have a similar periodical. Regardless of the kind of proceeding, the notice must fully describe the nature of the proposed action, the law under which it is authorized, and the basic facts known to the agency.

Government agencies may accept responses from affected parties in written or oral form, or both, depending on the nature of the proceeding. A proposed environmental standard, for example, would be accompanied by a solicitation for written comments. If the impact is expected to be substantial, there may also be a hearing to receive oral statements. A physician charged with a license violation would have the chance to present his or her defense at a hearing. The presiding officer at a hearing is known as an administrative law judge (ALJ) and is usually a member of the agency's staff. Formal rules of procedure generally apply. To ensure that the rights of affected parties are fully protected, each is usually afforded the right to representation by an attorney. The evidence presented, combined with the other information collected by the agency in support of its proposed action, constitutes the formal record of the decision-making process.

Agency actions rely on the formal record. The procedures for making and reviewing the decision vary somewhat across agencies and types of proceedings, but the basic elements remain the same. An initial determination is usually made at the staff level, but it can be modified by the ruling of an ALJ or an internal reconsideration. The decision that emerges is subject to review by the agency's leadership, whether that is a single head or a board or commission, before it is considered final. If the proceeding involves a rule-making, the final decision is published with an accompanying preamble that explains the agency's consideration of the relevant information that had been submitted by affected parties. In the case of an adjudication, it is accompanied by a written decision similar to a judge's opinion. Affected parties have an avenue for appeal before another administrative body that may be either a component of the agency or an independent entity.

An affected party that remains unhappy with the result after this appeal may then challenge it in court. However, in reviewing decisions of regulatory bodies, judges generally consider only the validity of the process by which the determination was made, not its underlying substance.[27] Litigants may, for example, challenge the accuracy of the notice with which information about the proceeding was disseminated or the fairness of hearing procedures that were applied by an ALJ. However, courts are usually reluctant to second-guess the scientific or technical merits of the outcome when it lies within the agency's area of expertise. To prevail, the complaining party must establish that the procedures followed by an agency, rather than a specific technical judgment, were so defective as to bring the APA's touchstone phrase into play—that the action was "arbitrary, capricious, an abuse of discretion, or otherwise not in accordance with law."[28] A reviewing court can uphold the agency, overturn a decision, or send the matter back for further consideration.

Under this road map, regulatory proceedings can be long and complex. A major environmental rule can consume as many as ten years before all legal challenges are resolved. The intricacy of the system, which is intended to guarantee due process, reflects a commitment to protecting the rights of citizens against arbitrary government actions. In a typically American fashion, the process fosters a forum in which all affected interests can collide and from which a result can emerge that reflects either consensus or reasoned analysis. The system has its share of critics who contend that the process is too slow, too expensive, or too tilted toward those with the greatest access to legal and technical resources. However, whatever its merits or failings, it embodies an ingrained American bias toward protecting rights. The complexity of the process and the intricacy of the policy issues that surround health care may help explain the level of complication of the regulatory structure that has resulted.

Perennial Policy Conflicts

In more than 100 years of health care regulation in America, much has changed, but much remains the same. The greatest changes are in the science and technology of health care and the complexity of the economic arrangements that form its financial foundation. (See chapter 7 for a discussion of health care business relationships.) The greatest consistency is in the subtext of perennial conflicts and controversies that form the landscape for regulation as it seeks to balance concerns over quality, access, and cost.

The chapters that follow discuss each area of regulation as it is characterized by specific kinds of policy conflicts. These conflicts reflect clashing philosophies that have shaped health policy since it began. A few of them tend to arise in all contexts. The most basic is the clash between reliance on external regulation and on market discipline as the primary approach to public protection. It strikes at the fundamental rationale for regulatory oversight.[29] Market economies allocate goods and services according to the laws of supply and demand and let consumers determine what they will purchase and at what price. If a manufacturer's products are shoddy or a provider's services rendered carelessly, the flight of consumers will force them either to leave the market or to lower their price. The threat of lost revenue thereby enforces standards of acceptable quality and fair pricing.

In several regards, however, this model does not fit health care.[30] The effectiveness of market discipline depends on well-informed consumers who can judge quality and price. Health care services are highly technical, though, and most lay consumers lack the means to evaluate the proficiency with which they are rendered. Even when consumers are armed with technical knowledge, the measurement of quality is still an extremely inexact science, so accurate comparisons among providers are difficult. In addition, most patients do not even make health care purchasing decisions themselves. Managed care organizations that pay for their care decide which hospitals and physicians patients may use and what services they may receive. Moreover, in health care more than in almost any other industry, the consumer's life and health are at stake. A poor choice of provider could have fatal consequences, but reputations for poor quality spread only after the fact.

Replacing or supplementing market forces with regulatory oversight addresses these concerns but leaves open the question of how pervasive its role should be.[31] Consumer choice can still serve as a powerful tool to impose quality standards within a heavily regulated system. In fact, some regulatory programs are specifically designed to promote it. Antitrust enforcement seeks to enhance market competition in all segments of the industry. Recent federal legislation facilitates "health savings accounts" from which patients can pay providers directly without insurance company interference.[32] Several other existing and proposed government payment programs rely on market competition among payers to encourage them to offer the most fair and efficient coverage plans. The Federal Employee Health Benefit Plan (FEHBP) does so for federal government workers, and the health reform plan proposed by President Bill Clinton in the mid-1990s would have done so on a national scale.[33]

The advantage of market-based quality enforcement is that it places decision-making authority in the hands of patients themselves instead of those of distant regulators. Of course, whether patients desire or are able to excise this authority is a continually open question. Over the years since the first quality oversight programs began with physician licensure in the late nineteenth century, policy makers have repeatedly balanced the merits of each approach.

If regulation is to be imposed, the next question to decide is by whom. Health care is unusual in its extensive reliance on private regulatory mechanisms. Do private bodies that coordinate professional licensure, certify specialist physicians, accredit hospitals, and review managed care organizations effectively serve the goal of public protection, or are they tainted by professional self-interest? On the other hand, do they bring needed technical expertise to bear that government regulators would otherwise lack? The interplay between the public and private sectors affects almost every sphere of health care oversight.

When the government is involved, which level should take the lead? The United States has a complex federalist system in which powers are divided between state and federal authorities. For the most part, basic legal functions are assigned to the states under the Constitution, except when national concerns such as interstate commerce or defense are involved.[34] Health care is a local concern to the extent that it serves identified geographic communities, however many aspects of the industry are national in scope. For example, patients routinely travel out of state for specialty services, pharmaceutical products are sold nationwide, and infectious diseases spread without respect for state or national borders.

The earliest forms of health care regulation, such as sanitation standards, vaccination mandates, and physician licensure, were almost all effectuated at the state level. Food and drug regulation enacted in 1906 was the first significant federal effort. By the end of the twentieth century, the federal government had come to play a pervasive role in regulating health care that far outstripped the role of the states. The magnitude of DHHS attests to the size of federal influence. However, many states still advocate for greater authority in some aspects of health care oversight. For example, public health efforts, including new bioterrorism defense initiatives, must be coordinated nationally, but the logistics require local efforts through hospitals, clinics, and physicians' offices. Medicaid funding for health care for the poor is administered separately by each state within federal standards, and states routinely seek permission to experiment with new methods of administration. A few states, such as Pennsylvania, have taken the lead in confronting the problem of medical errors with initiatives to track them.[35] Each new regulatory program forces policy makers to consider which level of government is legally and strategically best suited for the job.

The Regulatory System Today

With a 100-year history of shifting policy imperatives and a set of interlocking public and private interests, it is not surprising that the regulation of health care in

America is extremely complex. In a sense, it is a system that is uniquely suited to the United States. As citizens of a nation that seems to thrive on competitive interplay between conflicting forces in many forms, Americans take great pride in the constitutional system of government but remain historically ambivalent about the role that the public sector should play.[36] The Constitution creates different branches of government but also checks and balances between them, and it assigns distinct but sometimes overlapping ambits to federal authority and to the states. Our economy relies heavily on both private and public initiatives. The balance between all these forces in regulating health care effectively creates a dynamic tension that works to prevent any one from gaining too much power. As a consequence, the industry receives regulatory input from every level, but no level operates unchecked.

The reviews of each sphere of regulatory attention that are contained in the chapters that follow trace the historical evolution of regulation, the major agencies and organizations that emerged to play significant roles today, and the policy conflicts that shaped the development of regulatory policy. The structure in each sphere reflects the continual juggling of the three basic policy goals and the continual balancing of competing interests. It is a system of complexity, confrontation, and, at least in most cases, compromise. Its story reflects the progress of American medicine in both its triumphs and shortcomings and offers hints of the shape of the health care regulatory system in the years to come.

2

Regulation of Physicians and
Other Health Care Professionals

State licensing of medical providers is the cornerstone of quality
health care.
—J. A. Snow, *American Health Care Delivery Systems*

Government regulation of health care has no more fundamental role than to determine who may and may not provide services. Government-sanctioned standards for medical practice go back at least as far as the first century A.D. in India and China and to the year 1140 in Italy.[1] In England, the Royal College of Physicians was created by Charter of King Henry VIII in 1518 to "grant licenses to those qualified to practice and to punish unqualified practitioners and those engaging in malpractice."[2] Long before insurance reimbursement, managed care, and electronic medical records were ever imagined, regulators were enforcing standards for the medical profession.

Regulation of health care delivery today, of course, involves much more than controlling access to medical practice. In addition to physicians, many other kinds of professionals provide clinical services, some independent of and others subject to physician supervision. The Bureau of Labor Statistics of the federal Department of Labor recognizes more than 100 different health professions.[3] There are also complex institutions in which the members of some of these professions provide services from hospitals to nursing homes to outpatient clinics. The work of physicians has expanded beyond the roles that most practitioners of just fifty years ago would be able to recognize, into an array of new specialties.

In the United States, the cornerstone for regulation of clinical service delivery is the government's licensing function. Under America's federalist system, this is an area primarily assigned to the states. For most health care professionals, no autonomous practice of any kind is permitted unless a license has been granted by the state in which services are rendered.

Beyond the basic level of state licenses, however, the web of regulation and oversight is extensive. The federal government plays an active role, mostly by imposing criteria for reimbursement under the Medicare and Medicaid programs. It also plays an indirect role in coordinating state licensure programs through a centralized data bank of disciplinary actions, and it directly regulates practice in federal health care facilities. Private insurance companies impose requirements of their own on professionals whose services are eligible for reimbursement. On top of these layers of oversight, most health care professions themselves add elements of self-policing. Among these are physician specialty societies that grant certification status to members who meet their standards and associations of allied health professionals that monitor the quality of care rendered by their members.

With such an extensive societal investment in regulating health care service delivery, the conceptual foundations for the process would seem to be long settled. However, significant policy disputes remain. For example, policy makers still debate whether regulation is best left to the states, to the federal government, or to the members of the health care professions themselves; whether discipline is best accomplished in public view or in private; and whether patients are best protected through government oversight or through market forces. With health care regulation involving so many layers, there is much room for dispute over the proper role and scope of each one.

The history of the regulation of health care service delivery is a fascinating story of competing interests and changing public needs. It is far more complex than the simple imposition of professional standards in response to the risks presented by unqualified clinicians. The system of regulation that exists in America today is the product of professional and political conflicts that played out over the past century and continue to operate today, with economics as much a factor as medical science.

Licensure of Physicians and Oversight of Training

Origins of Physician Regulation

In light of the long history of the medical profession and its oversight, universal governmental physician licensure is a surprisingly recent phenomenon. Until the end of the nineteenth century, American physicians did not need licenses to practice in most states. The first modern regulatory scheme was enacted in 1873 in Texas.[4] Entry into the profession before then was easy, and the supply of physicians was large.[5] With little regulatory oversight, many physicians had limited medical knowledge, and quality control was sporadic at best. The open nature of the profession brought important economic consequences as well, as the large supply of physicians diluted the incomes of all.

The medical profession itself took the first steps to change this situation.[6] The American Medical Association (AMA) was founded in 1847 primarily to strengthen the requirements for medical education and thereby to contain the number of practicing physicians. During the latter part of the nineteenth century, the AMA also supported the enactment of state licensing laws, which further restricted the number of people entering the profession. These efforts were extremely successful, resulting in the enactment of more than 400 statutes regulating medical practice between 1874 and 1915, including the promulgation of licensing requirements in all states.[7] In 1912, all the state licensing boards joined to form a coordinating organization, the Federation of State Medical Boards (FSMB).[8]

In promoting physician licensure laws, the AMA walked a fine line. Licensing at the state level accomplished the goals of driving many unqualified practitioners from the profession and raising its overall status. However, creating an opening for state regulation carried the risk of building momentum for a broader governmental role at the federal level, which the organized medical profession did not want. The AMA succeeded in walking this line, and to this day, the basic regulation of medical practice remains with the states.

Licensing of physicians, as well as that of other health care professionals, has two primary components. Prospective physicians must pass a state-administered examination, and they must graduate from a medical school that has been certified by the state in which it is located.[9] If the medical school is located in a foreign country, a separate set of examination requirements applies. The educational requirement brings with it state supervision of medical education, and of the curricula that medical schools teach. It is this prong of the licensing process that has had the greatest effect in narrowing the gates to the medical profession.

The movement to strengthen standards for medical education began in earnest in 1904, when the AMA established the Council on Medical Education to recommend uniform requirements.[10] Among its proposals were that physicians complete four years of high school, four years of medical training, a fifth year of training in basic sciences that later evolved into a set of undergraduate premedical courses, and a one-year hospital internship. The association set out to grade all American medical schools according to the pass rates of their graduates on state licensure examinations and found that it could fully approve only about half. Instead of publicly releasing the list, which could have generated political ill will, it asked a reputable outside organization to perform the task. This was the Carnegie Foundation for the Advancement of Teaching, which hired a young educator named Abraham Flexner to lead an investigation of medical education.

Even before the release of Flexner's report in 1910, the number of medical schools had begun to decline as licensing boards in several states adopted the AMA's curriculum recommendations. Few of the marginal school could afford to upgrade laboratories, libraries, and other facilities to meet new standards, and many potential students were unable to afford the additional years of training required by the schools that remained. When release of the Flexner report reinforced the momentum behind the movement for quality improvement in medical education, it pushed many more marginal schools over the edge.[11]

Flexner recommended closing more than half of the schools he visited for failing to meet the AMA's standards. The result over the next few years was a series of mergers and dissolutions that dramatically shrank the number of medical schools in America. Admission standards also rose, as most states began to require that schools impose at least one year, and later two years, of college as a prerequisite. When the FSMB was formed in 1912, the AMA's ratings of schools was accepted by the new organization as authoritative.[12]

The triumph of the AMA's Council on Medical Education in creating standards for physician training has been called "an extraordinary achievement for the organized profession."[13] In the late 1880s, few physicians saw national standards as feasible. Nevertheless, acting without the aid of centralized governmental coordination, the profession transformed itself. In the history of American government, there are few instances in which such nationwide regulatory uniformity has been achieved without federal involvement.

The enhanced standards for admission into the profession of medicine transformed its overall character, not just the qualifications of new entrants.[14] Consistent with recommendations of the Flexner report, the AMA encouraged reliance on research as the foundation of medical education, using Johns Hopkins University as the model. This focus enhanced the role of larger universities and promoted the status of scientists and researchers in the profession.[15] It also increased the influence of hospitals in defining the nature of medical practice. In 1904, about half of all medical school graduates completed subsequent training in hospitals, but by 1923 virtually all of them did.[16]

State Policing of the Medical Profession

For aspiring physicians who have obtained the necessary educational credentials, state medical boards serve as the gatekeeper into actual clinical practice.[17] They issue licenses to those who pass required tests, renew licenses at regular intervals, and, perhaps most important, enforce basic standards of practice. It is this last function that generates the most controversy.

Initial licensure is fairly straightforward. Applicants document their education, pass a set of examinations that are now nationally standardized, and provide the board with basic background information on themselves.[18] Renewal is based on the absence of disciplinary proceedings in the time since the last license review and, in most states, on completion of a minimum amount of continuing medical education each year. Granting and renewing licenses for physicians and other health care professionals falls within the administrative functions of regulation.

Discipline, however, is another matter. Medical boards devote a large portion of their resources to investigating and prosecuting deficiencies in physician behavior.[19] According to one estimate, in 2002 a total of 2,864 serious disciplinary actions were taken by state medical boards across the country.[20] The stakes are high, since personal reputations and professional livelihoods are on the line. As a result, the legal requirements for board actions are strict, and the consequent administrative burden to implement them is substantial.[21]

For a government agency to restrict the ability to earn a living as it does when it revokes or suspends a medical license, the Constitution requires that it provide due process for the individual involved. (See chapter 1 for a discussion of the process of regulation.) This essentially means the right to a fair proceeding in which the action can be contested. A doctor who is subject to discipline must be informed of the charges and the evidence that supports them, must have the opportunity to contest them at a hearing, and generally must have the option of representation by an attorney. Much of the work of medical boards is in documenting alleged violations of practice standards and conducting hearings at which physicians can defend themselves. When discipline is imposed, an appeal board is empowered to consider challenges to the way the procedure was conducted. If the discipline is upheld, a sanctioned physician may then appeal to the courts.

Disciplinary proceedings against health care professionals are usually kept confidential until a penalty is assessed and upheld on internal appeal. This protects the reputations of physicians against whom charges are ultimately dismissed. However, it leaves patients unaware that their health care provider is a focus of concern. Patient advocates argue that disciplinary proceedings should be public matters from the start, since receiving care from a substandard practitioner could be a matter of life and death. Physicians counter that careers could be ruined by false charges.

Although final disciplinary actions are publicly disclosed, historically they have not been widely publicized. In response to complaints that patients should have access to information about sanctions that have actually been imposed, several states have recently begun to post the names of disciplined physicians on Web sites.[22] Some consumer organizations publish lists, as well.[23]

In one area, however, secrecy is commonly maintained even after proceedings have concluded. Most states have special procedures for physicians and other practitioners who are impaired by abuse of drugs or alcohol.[24] Practitioners can be recommended for these proceedings by colleagues or by officials at institutions where they work. In return for successful completion of addiction treatment, no discipline is imposed and the proceedings are sealed. The goal of these procedures is to induce health care providers to enter treatment voluntarily so that they can regain the ability to function professionally.

Issues in State Licensure

Despite the presence of this well-established system based on constitutional safeguards, some aspects of the oversight of physician practice remain controversial. In particular, although it is the backbone of the regulation of clinical practice, state licensure of physicians is marked by unevenness.[25] States vary in the rigor with which they police physician misconduct and in the standards for medical practice that they impose.[26] More important, despite the many mechanisms that have developed over the years to facilitate communication between state licensing bodies, including the National Practitioner Data Bank (NPDB) discussed later, coordination is often elusive. Regulators continue to have imperfect information about physicians under their jurisdiction who have practiced in other states, and as a result, physicians with discipline records can still sometimes slip past enforcement by applying for licensure in a different state.

Licensure of physicians and other health care professionals is conducted by boards composed of members of the regulated profession, sometimes with the addition of a few consumer representatives.[27] In some states, the boards function independently, while in others they are components of the department of health. The composition of boards with members of the regulated profession is a point of considerable contention. On the one hand, who would be a better judge of the qualifications needed to practice than those who do so themselves? However, reliance on professional peers raises the concern that state licensure is actually a form of self-regulation, and as such, the objectivity of the regulators could be compromised.[28] Critics fear that their primary interest may be in maintaining the reputation of the profession or that they could administer professional entry requirements as a means of stifling competition from newcomers.

Consumer advocates often point to a seemingly low frequency of enforcement actions in many states as evidence that licensure by peers serves the profession more than the public.[29] Those who defend the boards counter that their mission is to maintain standards, not simply to punish physicians, and that effective quality control is not necessarily a punitive process. Moreover, licensure boards operate under a range of legal and political safeguards that private organizations do not face. Their activities are directly governed by statutes and regulations, they must adhere to rules of evidence and procedure, and they are subject to legislative oversight. At least some safeguards of regulatory vigilance, therefore, are in place.

Private Oversight of Physician Practice

In addition to state licensure, private organizations, including professional societies, represent an integral part of the oversight of clinical practice. Their role often involves a form of explicit self-regulation, but it can be quite thorough. The inclusion of this component in the landscape of medical practice oversight makes the regulatory enterprise truly a public-private partnership, a reminder of its origins as an initiative of professionals themselves.

Private Coordination of Physician Discipline

While primary legal authority to license physicians resides in state governments, they rely on an assortment of nongovernmental and quasi-governmental organizations that have evolved to coordinate the process. In 1912, the National Confederation of State Medical Examining and Licensing Boards, which had been founded in 1891, and the American Confederation of Reciprocating Examining and Licensing Boards, which had been founded in 1902, merged to form the FSMB.[30] The two original groups had issued similar recommendations for medical school entrance examinations and for a standardized curriculum, which were adopted by the new organization.

Under the leadership of Dr. Walter Bierring, who headed the FSMB from 1915 to 1961, the organization directed its focus to developing standards for licensure over and above the minimum needed to demonstrate competent training. Dr. Bierring sought improved "methods of determining fitness for licensure and the practice of medicine as distinguished from those required for graduation from an approved school or college of medicine."[31] Under his leadership, the FSMB looked to continually improve "the quality, safety, and integrity of health care."[32]

With this mission, the FSMB took on a number of coordinating roles over the years, but its actual effectiveness in enhancing physician quality is unclear. Most of its functions have been largely administrative.[33] Initially, its primary activity was to collect information on disciplinary actions and report them in a monthly bulletin. Beginning in the 1960s, it published a journal devoted exclusively to that purpose. In the early 1980s, a computerized Board Action Data Bank was created, which formed the precursor to the NPDB, a federal initiative that was enacted in 1986. In 1996, it established a service to centrally verify physician credentials for state medical boards and private organizations. Today, much of its role stems from its status as the parent agency for the Accreditation Council for Graduate Medical Education (ACGME) and the Educational Commission for Foreign Medical Graduates (ECFMG), which are discussed later in this chapter. Undoubtedly, the FSMB has helped state medical boards with many of their data management needs. However, coordination of physician discipline information has been the subject of perennial criticism, and it remains so today.

Another private organization, the National Board of Medical Examiners (NBME), has played a more active role.[34] The NBME was formed in 1915 to administer a single uniform national examination that each state could accept as the basis for physician licensure. The test, known as the United States Medical Licensing Examination, is cosponsored and co-owned with the FSMB. Each state uses it but sets its own standards for passing. The NBME also consults to several medical specialty boards, which administer proficiency examinations in individual fields of practice.

While state licensure requires that physicians complete an approved educational curriculum, direct oversight of the institutions providing this training has remained mostly in private hands. The Liaison Committee on Medical Education (LCME), a nonprofit organization jointly sponsored by the Association of American Medical Colleges (AAMC) and the AMA, accredits medical schools in the United States and Canada.[35] Two other private nonprofit groups that are housed within the FSMB accredit postgraduate training programs. ACGME accredits the nearly 7,800 medical residency programs in the United States.[36] ECFMG certifies graduates of foreign medical schools to enter ACGME-accredited residency and fellowship programs.[37]

Although it has no explicit certifying or oversight responsibilities, historically the AMA has been the most influential private organization of all.[38] It has been the driving force behind almost every significant regulatory program for the medical profession, including the system of state licensure, the standardization of medical school curricula, and the system of private specialty certification. The AMA continues to promote the medical profession in a number of ways. Its primary publication, the *Journal of the American Medical Association,* is among the most respected medical research journals. The association's rules of ethics, while often a source of controversy, serve to highlight critical issues on a national level. The AMA also exerts an extremely strong lobbying presence at the federal and state levels on almost every issue of importance to physicians.

Specialty Certification
In addition to their role in coordinating physician oversight, private regulators directly oversee some aspects of clinical practice. Of most significance, the trend toward specialization of physicians was standardized not by state regulators but by professional organizations. State licensure legally permits a physician to work in any specialty and to perform any service or procedure that is part of accepted medical practice.[39] Private certification is not a legal requirement for a physician to claim a field of specialization, but it is necessary for recognition within the profession and in the larger health care industry.

The transformation of American medicine into a predominantly specialty-oriented profession can be traced to the 1930s, when the AMA first established a formal structure to recognize a tier of training and expertise beyond general medicine.[40] Specialization reshaped the practice of medicine during the 1950s. A study of medical students during that decade found a decline from 60 percent to 16 percent in the number planning to become general practitioners and a rise from 35 percent to 74 percent in the number planning to specialize.[41] Public acceptance of the legitimacy of a specialist designation depended on a system that could authoritatively recognize the superior specialized knowledge involved.[42]

The system that developed in the 1930s to recognize specialized medical expertise was the certification process of specialty boards composed of members of the disciplines themselves. Today, there are twenty-four such boards, ranging from the

American Board of Internal Medicine, which was founded in 1936, to the American Board of Medical Genetics, which dates from 1991.[43] (Medical specialty boards are listed in table 2.1.) Their activities are coordinated by the American Board of Medical Specialties (ABMS), which was founded by the AMA in 1933 to coordinate the four boards in existence at that time.[44]

Board certification is an essential credential for physicians holding themselves out as having expertise in a specialty. Boards certify physicians with examinations that combine written answers and demonstrations of clinical skills. Regular recertification is now required in most fields. Although certification is not legally required for specialty practice, it is necessary for membership as a specialist on most hospital staffs and for inclusion as a specialist in the provider networks of most managed care organizations. Although a small number of physicians continue to practice as specialists without board certification, they are a dwindling minority.

Much of the draw of specialization for physicians stems from advances in science and technology that have given specialists an array of powerful clinical tools. It

Table 2.1
Member Boards of the American Board of Medical Specialties

Specialty Board	Headquarters Location
Allergy and Immunology	Philadelphia, PA
Anesthesiology	Raleigh, NC
Colon and Rectal Surgery	Taylor, MI
Dermatology	Detroit, MI
Emergency Medicine	East Lansing, MI
Family Practice	Lexington, KY
Internal Medicine	Philadelphia, PA
Medical Geriatrics	Bethesda, MD
Neurological Surgery	Houston, TX
Nuclear Medicine	Los Angeles, CA
Obstetrics and Gynecology	Dallas, TX
Ophthalmology	Bala Cynwyd, PA
Orthopedic Surgery	Chapel Hill, NC
Otolaryngology	Houston, TX
Pathology	Tampa, FL
Pediatrics	Chapel Hill, NC
Physical Medicine and Rehabilitation	Rochester, MN
Plastic Surgery	Philadelphia, PA
Preventive Medicine	Chicago, IL
Psychiatry and Neurology	Deerfield, IL
Radiology	Tucson, AZ
Surgery	Philadelphia, PA
Thoracic Surgery	Evanston, IL
Urology	Charlottesville, VA

Source: http://www.abms.org/member.asp (25 May 2006).

also stems from reimbursement rates paid by public and private payers that have historically rewarded this form of practice more generously than generalist medicine. In response to recent government initiatives to reverse this trend, such as the use of a resource-based value scale to reimburse physicians under Medicare, which is discussed later, associations of specialists have become more politically active to lobby to maintain the differential.

Oversight through Managed Care

The most direct form of private regulation of physician practice is relatively new and comes not from the profession itself but from an industry segment that often has interests that are adverse to it. The insurance industry now exerts considerable influence over clinical conduct through managed care arrangements. Most notably, these include health maintenance organizations (HMOs), but other kinds of managed care mechanisms, such as preferred provider organizations (PPOs) and point-of-service (POS) plans, can also direct activities of participating physicians. Through managed care, the entities that pay for health care actively oversee the services that they fund.[45] (The regulation of managed care is discussed in chapter 4 on health care finance.)

HMOs, as the most aggressive form of managed care, seek to control costs by reducing the provision of unnecessary services.[46] They use several tools toward this end. Primary care physicians are paid based on capitation, a set fee for each patient assigned to the physician that is remitted each month regardless of the amount of care actually rendered. This is intended to discourage overtreatment. Patients may see specialists for more intensive services only with a referral from their primary care physician, and the specialists to whom they are referred must participate in the HMO's provider network. The number of referrals that each physician provides is tracked, and those who refer excessively may be financially penalized with a lower capitation rate in subsequent years. Procedures and diagnostic tests, whether performed by primary care physicians or specialists, may be subject to prior review before reimbursement is authorized. The same may apply to admissions to hospitals and procedures performed in them. Physicians who perform excessive numbers of procedures and tests may be "deselected" from the HMO's network. In other words, their participation may be terminated.

In addition to controlling costs, HMOs also seek to assure the quality of care rendered by their providers. The initial tool that they use is to screen prospective physicians according to a number of measures. In addition to verifying basic attributes, such as medical school graduation, residency training, and licensure, HMOs also examine more direct reflections of quality, such as prior malpractice judgments and settlements, prior licensure-related discipline, and board certification. This process, known as "credentialing," is mandated by regulations governing HMOs in many states.[47] It is also called for by rules of the National Committee for Quality Assurance (NCQA), which accredits many HMOs. NCQA further requires recredentialing every three years. (The role of NCQA is discussed in more detail in chapter 4.) Once physicians are part of an HMO network, their practices may be regularly monitored for features such as hours of operation, promptness of answering office telephones, and maintenance of thorough and legible medical records. Recent HMO initiatives have examined actual clinical behavior by reviewing patient charts for key indicators of quality, such as administration of recommended childhood vaccines, provision of screening tests for adults, and counseling of smoking cessation where indicated.[48] HMOs may also require physicians to document attendance at continuing medical education sessions.

The most aggressive form of HMO quality oversight is through a mechanism known as "disease management," a process through which protocols containing recommended procedures for the treatment of specific conditions are disseminated to guide physician decision making. It places the HMO in a position to assist the physician in the medical management of patients.[49] The protocols may, for example, direct which diagnostic tests to perform or drugs to prescribe based on a patient's symptoms and responses to previous treatments. Most protocols developed to date address the care of patients with chronic diseases, such as diabetes, asthma, and hypertension, although the range of conditions for which protocols have been devised is constantly growing. Physician compliance with protocol recommendations can be monitored by HMOs through review of patient charts, and it is increasingly facilitated by the use of electronic medical records. Mandates to follow protocols are new and still infrequent, but disease management represents a potentially substantial expansion of HMO oversight of physician behavior.

The performance of physicians on any of these measures can lead to counseling by an HMO or, in extreme cases, to deselection. Some HMOs are also trying a new tack to bring pressure to bear on physicians to excel on quality measures by posting performance scores on publicly available Web sites.[50] The hope is that patients will act as informed consumers in selecting the best performing physicians in response, thereby encouraging all physicians to strive to meet standards. (Emerging forms of information-based quality oversight are discussed in chapter 9.)

HMOs have no direct legal authority to impose quality standards on physicians and other participating clinicians. Their power derives from their position in holding the purse strings for a large portion of health care finance. As with the government's role in administering Medicare and Medicaid, which is discussed later, the power to pay inevitably brings with it the power to direct the uses to which payment will be put. The spread of managed care reflects the realization by private payers that they have a stake in the cost and quality of the care that they finance and that they also have the ability to exert control over these factors. As the cost of health care continues to rise, the assertiveness of HMOs is likely to increase. The result may be that private payers come to play a central role in regulating health care quality that rivals that of governmental and professional organizations.

Private Oversight through Hospital Credentialing

Physicians are also regulated by the hospitals in which they practice.[51] In order to admit patients to or provide services in a hospital, physicians must be granted membership on the medical staff.[52] This is accompanied by the granting of clinical privileges to render designated kinds of care. This system dates from the early part of the twentieth century, when hospitals achieved the organizational structure that they maintain today.[53] (The history and structure of hospitals are discussed in chapter 3.) Medical staff membership is achieved through a credentialing process conducted by a staff committee that is dedicated to this purpose. Prospective members must verify basic qualifications such as medical school graduation, residency training, and licensure and must report any prior adverse licensure actions and any sanctions at other institutions. Hospitals must also check for listings of such actions with the NPDB, as discussed later. Accreditation rules governing hospitals require that physicians be recredentialed with a similar process every three years.

Once on a hospital's staff, physicians may be subject to review for quality lapses. Individual incidents that result in patient harm are investigated by quality review committees, and patterns of substandard care may be examined by the credentialing committee or by the department in which the physician has clinical privileges. Physicians who are found to lack competence may be subject to a range of disciplinary actions. These can include measures that impose required medical education, supervision by other medical staff members, suspension of clinical privileges for a period of time, and complete revocation of privileges with expulsion from the medical staff. Hospitals have a strong incentive to oversee the quality of physicians who practice under their auspices, as they are legally liable for malpractice committed by physicians whose poor quality could have been detected upon initial credentialing or through ongoing supervision.[54] In addition to credentialing procedures, most hospitals maintain risk management programs to advise physicians on ways to avoid lawsuits.[55]

Hospital oversight of physician practice is limited to services rendered in the institution or in an affiliated facility. However, it is an important supplement to other regulatory mechanisms, such as licensure, in that it represents a direct form of monitoring of ongoing practice. A hospital is likely to discover quality lapses before outside government regulators, since any harm to patients often occurs within its walls. Hospital credentialing, therefore, represents another important piece of the web of private regulation that is intertwined with government oversight.

The Federal Role

In many important respects, the market for health care services is national, and it affects the country as a whole. Physicians and patients move across state lines, and accepted standards of practice are, for the most part, uniform nationwide. While continuing to respect the primacy of the states in the responsibility for basic licensure, Congress has over the years added several layers of federal oversight to address perceived regulatory gaps.

National Coordination of Physician Discipline

In 1986, Congress addressed concerns about a lack of coordination between states in physician discipline. Over the years, press accounts had told familiar stories of physicians disciplined in one state moving to another to regain their license.[56] State medical boards operated largely in isolation and in ignorance of the actions of others. The FSMB's reports of discipline were often ignored, and there were no laws formally requiring coordination among licensure agencies.

Another factor pushing Congress to act was a Supreme Court decision in the mid-1980s that brought the confusing state of physician discipline to a head. Hospitals, which discipline staff physicians in much the same manner as licensure boards, had been increasingly subject to lawsuits challenging disciplinary actions. In 1985, an Oregon physician received a jury award of $2.2 million for a claim that sanctions imposed on him by a hospital represented a conspiracy to undermine his practice, and the award was eventually upheld by the Supreme Court.[57] This ruling put hospitals in a difficult position. Disciplining an errant physician could bring antitrust liability, but failing to impose discipline could jeopardize patient care and perhaps spawn a lawsuit for malpractice.

Congress responded in 1986 by passing the Health Care Quality Improvement Act (HCQIA).[58] That law granted hospitals immunity from physician lawsuits stemming from good-faith disciplinary proceedings. However, this immunity was conditioned on the hospital's compliance with reporting requirements of a new national physician discipline database, the NPDB. The HCQIA required that all significant disciplinary actions be reported to the NPDB and that all physician applications for staff privileges be checked against its records for prior sanctions. In addition to reporting of hospital discipline, the law also required state medical boards to report physician sanctions and required malpractice insurers to report verdicts and settlements. The NPDB is maintained by the Health Resources and Services Administration (HRSA), a component of the Department of Health and Human Services (DHHS).

The NPDB represented a technological quantum leap beyond the early efforts of the FSMB, which had used index cards to track physicians. However, it has its critics. Recent research indicates that despite the law, many disciplinary actions still go unreported.[59] In particular, HMOs, which, as discussed earlier, can play a significant role in overseeing physician practice, regularly fail to report sanctions, and malpractice cases are often settled with the physician removed as a named defendant to avoid the reporting obligation. Without complete data, the databank's value is limited.

The NPDB's structure has also raised controversy over access to the information that it maintains. Reporting entities such as hospitals may see reports for their own physicians, and physicians may review their own data and add short comments or corrections. Consumer advocates believe that patients should also have the right to see the databank's contents to evaluate their own physicians.[60] Opponents counter that misinterpretation of data may result and careers may be unfairly jeopardized. So far, the NPDB's data remain protected from public view.

Management of the National Physician Workforce

The federal government also plays a central role in shaping America's overall physician workforce. It is ironic that after policy initiatives in the early 1900s sought to limit the supply of physicians through licensure requirements in order to enhance the quality of care, federal efforts later in the century sought to dramatically expand it to enhance access to care. Federal policy determines the total number of physicians who practice in the United States and the specialties in which they work. It exerts this control in much the same way as the states did when licensure was first introduced, by regulating the education and training needed to enter the profession.

Federal policy makers have several tools for determining the size and shape of the physician workforce. The most direct is through the funding of medical schools. Physician training is extremely expensive, and most schools rely extensively on external support. Grants and loans for medical training are administered by HRSA. (The role of HRSA in regulating the health care workforce is also discussed in chapter 6 on public health.) Another important tool is funding of hospital-based residency and fellowship programs, which provide physicians with clinical training after medical school and form their gateways into specialties. This is accomplished largely through reimbursement of the cost of this training under the Medicare program. Finally, reimbursement rates for different medical specialties under federal coverage programs, most notably Medicare, can determine their relative attractiveness.

The 1960s and 1970s were a period of rapidly rising medical costs, which some policy makers attributed to a shortage of physicians. They predicted that the law of supply and demand would bring down costs if the physician supply increased. Beginning in 1965, federal funding increased for the creation of new medical schools and the expansion of existing ones.[61] The effort was extremely successful in its immediate goal, as the number of medical schools grew from 88 in 1965 to 126 in 1980 and the number of graduates from 7,409 to 15,135.[62] As a result, the number of physicians per 100,000 population increased from 148 in 1960 to 202 in 1980, so that today the United States has one of the highest proportions of physicians to population in the world. In 2004, there were almost 780,000 physicians in the United States, of whom 81 percent were in clinical practice. About two-thirds of these were specialists.[63]

Unfortunately, the laws of supply and demand did not work as expected, and medical cost inflation continued unabated even with this dramatic growth in the physician supply. The focus of cost-control policy during the 1980s and 1990s shifted to the proportion of specialists, who tend to provide more costly services than physicians who practice in primary care. In 1986, Congress created the Council on Graduate Medical Education (COGME) to advise DHHS on physician workforce trends, training issues, and financial policies.[64] The council has seventeen members, including representatives of primary care, specialty, and other segments of the medical profession, medical schools, teaching hospitals, and several government agencies. While the council's role is only advisory, its creation reflected the first formal policy review of the specialty–primary care balance.

Another powerful tool for shaping the physician workforce is reimbursement policy. Through Medicare, the federal government administers the largest single health care reimbursement program in the country. In addition to directing 19 percent of national spending for personal health, Medicare influences the way that private insurance and other government programs are administered.[65] In the 1980s, Medicare developed a new way to pay for physician services that permitted a larger role for explicit policy oversight. Instead of paying based on a percentage of usual and customary charges in each region, Medicare began paying based on the relative amount of resources that were required for the physician to perform the service involved. (For a fuller discussion of Medicare, see chapter 4 on health care finance.) The Resource Based Relative Value Scale (RBRVS) sets a relative value for each physician service that is reimbursable by Medicare.[66] Services are evaluated in terms of the training needed, the resources required, and the malpractice cost, and then they are ranked in order. Procedures are valued as multiples of an index service, which is a primary care office visit of intermediate complexity.

The rankings were intended to rationalize pricing, but they had an important side effect. Complex medical procedures were priced at much lower multiples of primary care visits than under the old system, and more cognitively oriented services of primary care doctors consequently rose in value in relation to them.[67] A narrowing of the gap between the incomes of specialists and of primary care physicians was predicted to result, which could influence the career direction of future doctors and change the overall direction of the profession. This new reimbursement mechanism was intended to replace the old system's inefficient rewards for specialty practice with a mechanism that more accurately reflected the expenditure of health care resources. In practice, however, it has so far had little effect.

Congress again tried to use Medicare reimbursement to change the primary care–specialist physician balance in the Balanced Budget Act (BBA) of 1997.[68] That law dramatically cut reimbursement to hospitals and physicians under Medicare, with especially severe cuts in funding for hospital-based training of medical students, residents, and fellows. Much of the funding that remained was redirected to increase slots for primary care at the expense of those for specialists. Specialty residencies became more difficult to obtain as a result. However, the effect on the overall practice of medicine in America and on the rate of growth of health care costs has not been evident.

The final tool of federal policy to control the physician workforce is by regulating the entry of foreign medical graduates into the American market. Each year, approximately 25,000 graduates of foreign medical schools enter residency programs in American hospitals, accounting for about one-fourth of all American hospital residents.[69] Many are Americans who attended medical schools abroad. Of those foreign medical graduates training in the United States, approximately 75 percent ultimately remain in the country for their clinical practice.[70] Federal regulations affect the entry of foreign medical graduates by setting standards for their licensure and by controlling the number of visas granted to non-American physicians.[71]

The Educational Commission for Foreign Medical Graduates (ECFMG), a component of the FSMB, assesses the readiness of graduates of foreign medical schools to enter accredited medical residencies and fellowships in the United States.[72] Certification by ECFMG is required before an applicant is permitted to take the third component of the United States Medical Licensing Examination and for medical licensure in most states. This is conferred based on a series of examinations of medical proficiency, a test of English proficiency, and verification of credentials.

Clinical Oversight through Medicare

Although licensure and certification, the mainstays of clinical practice oversight, reside in state-level and private bodies, the federal government also has a powerful tool for overseeing the qualifications of physicians. More than 30 percent of all physician services rendered in the United States are reimbursed through the Medicare program of public insurance for the elderly.[73] Many physicians, particularly those in specialties with large proportions of geriatric patients, could not maintain economically viable practices without Medicare reimbursement. To qualify to receive payment, physicians must enroll in the Medicare program by demonstrating basic qualifications. This requires that they verify some of the same information that is needed for licensure, such as medical school graduation and residency status, and some in addition, such as any adverse legal history and any past Medicare overpayments that they may have received.[74] The Medicare program also has the authority to revoke enrollment and exclude physicians from participation as a sanction for misconduct.[75] This authority effectively makes Medicare another arbiter of physician quality through the Centers for Medicare & Medicaid Services (CMS), the agency that administers it.

The Parallel World of Osteopathy

What we know today as traditional medical practice, commonly referred to as "allopathic medicine," competed with an array of alternative approaches to healing during the nineteenth century. One of the most prominent continues to be practiced today as a closely allied and parallel profession known as "osteopathy." In 1891, Dr. Andrew Still, a Missouri physician, developed a set of medical techniques based on the notion that the human body is like a machine and that when people become ill, they are best treated by fixing the relationships between their body parts.[76] It relies on the underlying philosophy that understanding the patient, rather than the disease, is the key to treatment. Dr. Still called his approach "osteopathic medicine."

Today, there are twenty-three osteopathic medical schools in the United States that grant the Doctor of Osteopathy (DO) degree.[77] They teach a curriculum that is almost identical to that taught in allopathic schools, except for the addition of training in osteopathic manipulation, a technique of spinal massage that is designed to properly align body parts. More than 11,000 students are enrolled in these schools, which include more than 1,400 full-time faculty members.[78] The schools are represented by the American Association of Colleges of Osteopathic Medicine (AACOM), which also collects statistical data on training in the profession and centralizes applications for admission. In terms of postgraduate clinical training, 500 hospitals offer training programs for 6,700 osteopathic residents. The American Osteopathic Association (AOA), founded in 1897, represents the overall profession.

Vermont was the first state to license doctors of osteopathy starting in 1896.[79] Dr. Still's home state of Missouri followed the next year. In 1947, the AOA approved the first hospital residency program. Most states today regulate osteopathic physicians through a system that is separate from but parallel to that for allopathic physicians. Applicants for licensure must graduate from an accredited school and pass a licensure examination. Standards for renewal of osteopathic medical licenses include completion of continuing medical education and other requirements that are similar to those for allopathic physicians. The process is overseen in most states by a board of osteopathic medicine that is similar in composition and function to the allopathic medical board.

Increasingly, osteopathic medical graduates complete conventional allopathic residencies alongside graduates of conventional medical schools. As a result of litigation during the 1980s, osteopathic physicians are now eligible for full medical staff privileges at all allopathic hospitals.[80] Osteopathic specialty societies certify specialists in twenty-three fields, paralleling the certification process for the same disciplines in allopathic practice.[81] Certification is coordinated by the Bureau of Osteopathic Specialists, which was organized in 1939 by the AOA. As a result of these trends, the number of hospitals and postgraduate training programs devoted specifically to osteopathic practice has declined dramatically over time, and other distinctions between osteopathic and allopathic physicians are beginning to fade.

Allied Health Professions

In addition to allopathic and osteopathic physicians, many other kinds of health care practitioners also render services.[82] The fields in which they work, known as "allied health professions," actually have a larger total number of members.[83] Some of these professions, such as dentistry and pharmacy, date back hundreds of years. Others, such as nursing, developed at the same time as the medical profession was adopting its formal structure during the nineteenth century. Many others, including physical therapy, occupational therapy, and psychology, developed during the twentieth century and in some respects are still working to solidify their professional standing.

The model of state-based licensure that evolved to regulate physicians forms the basis for government regulation of most allied health professions.[84] As with the AMA's efforts on behalf of physicians, it has generally been the professions themselves that have pushed to be licensed. The pattern has been to standardize education, including curricula and practical training, through private professional organizations, with a state board verifying an applicant's training and administering a licensing examination as a prerequisite to clinical practice.

The movement to license allied health professionals began in earnest at about the same time as that for physicians. During the first two decades of the twentieth century, most states implemented licensing programs for dentists, pharmacists, nurses, optometrists, and podiatrists. By 1960, dental hygienists, practical nurses, physical therapists, psychologists, nursing home administrators, and emergency medical technicians were subject to licensure as well. Licensing boards for allied health professions are usually composed primarily of members of the regulated profession, as they are for physicians.[85]

Each profession has a national organization that represents its interests. Often, they also certify the clinical qualifications of members.[86] Examples include the American Psychological Association (APA), the American Nurses Association (ANA), the American Physical Therapy Association (APTA), the American Occupational Therapy Association (AOTA), and the American Pharmacists Association (APhA). In some instances, a profession has more than one.[87] There are also private organizations in many fields that coordinate licensure activities of the states and of certifying activities of professional boards.[88] Many of them work in conjunction with government agencies, and some were created through federal legislation. The regulation of allied professionals, as of physicians, therefore, also functions as a type of public-private partnership. Table 2.2 lists several of the major organizations that serve this coordinating role.

The federal government began to play a supporting role in encouraging allied health professional training in the 1960s. In 1966, Congress passed the Allied Health Professions Personnel Training Act to promote and fund education in these fields.[89] This law supported creation of the Association of Schools of Allied Health Professions (ASAHP), which coordinates the certification of training programs. The federal government is also involved in promoting and managing the allied health professional workforce through the Bureau of Health Professions in HRSA, which conducts policy evaluations and gathers statistics. In addition, Medicare maintains standards for allied health professionals who provide services, as it does for physicians.

Structure of Regulatory Agencies and Organizations

State Medical Boards

State medical boards, the oldest and most fundamental component of the regulation of clinical practice, differ to some extent across states, but some features are consistent. The underlying legislation directing the operations of these boards is known in most states as the medical practice act. Similar laws and regulatory structures apply to allopathic and to osteopathic physicians and to most allied health professions that are subject to licensure. Of the different kinds of health care profes-

Table 2.2
Organizations Coordinating Regulation of Allied Health Professionals

Organization	Role/Government Relationship
Association of Schools of Allied Health Professions	Provides resources for professional schools; facilitated by the Allied Health Professions Personnel Training Act of 1967
National Commission for Certifying Agencies	Sets standards for organizations that certify allied health professionals; supported by federal Bureau of Health Professions in HRSA
Commission on Accreditation of Allied Health Education Programs	Accredits programs representing 18 allied health professions
Association of Regulatory Boards of Optometry	Provides resources to state boards
American Registry of Radiologic Technologists	Administers a voluntary certification examination that is required in some states
American Board of Podiatric Surgeons	Certifies podiatric surgeons
American Association of Medical Assistants	Provides certification examination of the American Association of Medical Assistants
National Council of State Boards of Nursing	Develops nursing licensing examinations
Federation of Chiropractic Licensing Boards	Provides centralized support for state chiropractic examination boards
Association of Social Work Boards	Develops and maintains social work licensing examination and serves as central resource for state boards
Federation of State Boards of Physical Therapy	Develops, maintains, and administers national physical therapy examinations
National Association of Boards of Pharmacy	Coordinates activities of all state pharmacy boards
National Commission on Certification of Physician Assistants	Sets certification standards that are required in all states
National Certification Commission for Acupuncture and Oriental Medicine	Sets certification standards in acupuncture

sionals, oversight of physicians tends to generate the most public attention and is described here as illustrative.

Medical boards are generally composed of physicians with occasional non-physician members, all of whom serve as volunteers appointed by the governor.[90] Some boards are independent, whereas others are part of larger departments of health or of consumer affairs. Their funding comes primarily from fees for licensing and registration of physicians. Although board members themselves are usually unpaid, these bodies employ administrative staffs, including an executive officer, attorneys, and investigators. The process of disciplining physicians can be extremely labor intensive, requiring considerable staff work. Investigators must gather facts, and attorneys must defend charges before hearing officers if a physician challenges an action.

Investigations of physician misconduct can be initiated in several ways. Agency staff often conduct random audits of medical charts at physician offices. In response to suspicious findings that arise from these audits or from outside information, they may covertly visit practices posing as patients. Investigations may also result from specific complaints by patients, professional colleagues, or other health care providers, such as nurses, with whom a suspect physician works.

If evidence of a violation is found, the agency staff is responsible for collecting sufficient information to bring charges. The offending practitioner is then informed of the allegations and offered the opportunity to contest them at a hearing. After considering the evidence, a hearing officer determines whether a violation has, in fact occurred and, if so, the kind of discipline that should be imposed. Sanctions can include required medical education, license suspension, restrictions on practice activities, for example, on prescribing privileges on either a permanent or temporary basis, and, in extreme cases, license revocation. The board itself can accept the hearing officer's recommendation, reject it, or modify it to impose a different penalty. An administrative appeal board is then available to hear a final appeal. Any subsequent challenge by the physician must be to the courts. Disciplinary sanctions imposed by a state board are reported to several national nongovernmental organizations, including the FSMB, state and local medical or osteopathic societies, the AMA or the AOA, and the NPDB.

The medical boards of two large states reflect the range of board structures. In California, the medical board was founded in 1876.[91] It and the board of osteopathic medicine are contained in the Department of Consumer Affairs. In addition to administering licensure and discipline, both boards operate programs to rehabilitate physicians who are impaired by drug or alcohol abuse. The boards also maintain information for consumers on the credentials of licensed physicians. In New Jersey, the State Board of Medical Examiners licenses and regulates a range of health care professionals from physicians to podiatrists to bioanalytical laboratory directors.[92] The board is part of the Division of Consumer Affairs of the Department of Law and Public Safety. Other boards within the division regulate a range of other health care professionals, including acupuncturists, athletic trainers, nurse-midwives, hearing aid dispensers, physician assistants, electrologists, and perfusionists.

State departments of health, within which many medical boards are located, have broader responsibilities for a range of health issues. (State departments of health are also discussed in chapter 6 on public health.) These include environmental health, vital statistics, oversight of county health departments, facility licensure, and emergency preparedness. Most state health departments are headed by a commissioner appointed by the governor. Many have councils or boards composed of health care professionals and members of the public to which the commissioner reports and which have ultimate authority to issue rules and regulations.

Federal Agencies

The basic structures of the federal agencies involved in regulating clinical practice are discussed elsewhere, since all have other primary functions. CMS is described in chapter 4 on health care finance, and HRSA in chapter 6 on regulation of public health. Significant components of CHS that directly affect the functioning of health care institutions are also discussed in chapter 3.

Health Resources and Services Administration (HRSA)

HRSA, a component of DHHS, is charged with increasing access to health care services for the nation's most vulnerable populations in rural and urban regions.[93] To this end, it administers programs to manage the nation's supply of health care professionals. The agency operates through four main bureaus. The Bureau of Primary Health Care (BPHC) funds and administers a network of primary care clinics.[94] The Bureau of Health Professions (BHPr) supports the National Health Service Corps of primary care clinicians who serve populations designated by its Health Professionals Shortage Areas criteria. BHPr also contains the National Center for Health Workforce Analysis, which regularly evaluates regions across the country for medical shortages to assist in the planning process for medical resource allocation.[95] The Maternal and Child Health Bureau administers block grant programs to states and communities to promote quality and access to care for underserved mothers and children.[96] The HIV/AIDS Bureau, which was established in 1997, administers grants to improve the quality and availability of care for people with HIV/AIDS.[97]

Private Organizations: Medical Specialty Boards

Each of the twenty-four boards that certify medical specialists operates as an independent nonprofit organization. They are governed by boards of directors composed of members of the specialty that they oversee. A fairly typical example is the American Board of Internal Medicine (ABIM), which certifies internists. It has a thirty-three-member governing board of directors that includes experts in medical education, clinical practice, and research.[98] This body selects the board that oversees actual development and implementation of certification standards, including the initial and recertification examinations. Physicians who have received basic certification in internal medicine can also apply for subspecialty designation in one of nine fields, including cardiology, hematology, and rheumatology. ABIM also maintains a nonprofit subsidiary, the ABIM Foundation, which sponsors research and other activities to improve the quality of physician care.

Perennial Policy Conflicts: Regulation versus the Market

During the time since medical licensure was first implemented, medicine has produced dramatic advances in curing disease and prolonging life. Debates rage over whether licensure hurt or helped that progress. Licensing restrictions that are too heavy-handed may impede innovation by restricting entry into the market by new practitioners, who can create competitive pressures for improvement.[99] A market with restricted entry can thereby permit those already providing services a measure of complacency. Perhaps physicians and hospitals would adhere to higher standards if potential competitors were more abundant. On the other hand, restrictions that are too lax could permit unqualified clinicians to practice.

Advocates of a strong central role for licensing see it as the public's best protection against unqualified practitioners and unsafe institutions. They point to the pervasiveness of poorly trained physicians in the late nineteenth century, many of whom made more of their incomes selling ineffective patent medicines than treating patients. Qualified physicians may have benefited financially from licensing laws, but the public surely gained, as well. Even if a more market-based approach to physician quality were theoretically desirable, could it work in practice? Consumers would have to evaluate a tremendous amount of technical information in order to judge physician performance, and they would need an impartial source to provide the information.

On the other hand, recent advances in information technology have made data on physicians much more accessible.[100] Perhaps patients finally have the tools to begin to take greater responsibility for assessing the quality of their own care. This might enforce standards for physician behavior more effectively than the cumbersome process of external oversight.

The tension between reliance on market forces and on government regulation for public protection is a perennial one in many fields. Licensure is widely accepted in health care and is commonly seen as essential to maintaining minimal levels of quality. Skepticism over its effects on competition and innovation, however, will always raise questions.

3

Regulation of Hospitals and
Other Health Care Institutions

In the public eye, the hospital symbolizes modern life.
—J. T. H. O'Connor, *Doing Good: The Life
of Toronto's General Hospital*

Medical care has been rendered in institutions dedicated to patient care for centuries. The first ones date at least as far back as the Romans. Records from between 27 B.C. and 14 A.D. document the establishment of army hospitals to treat soldiers. During the Middle Ages, isolation houses for patients with leprosy were maintained throughout Europe. With the Renaissance, institutional medical care became more widespread to serve a broader range of needs, as access to printed texts improved medical training. The development of hospitals in Europe, however, was no match for that in the Islamic world. By the twelfth century, institutions similar to hospitals operated in Cairo, Damascus, and several cities in Islamic Spain. The city of Baghdad had sixty of them. These facilities included separate wards for different diseases, training areas, convalescent rooms, and stores of medications. Most of them also served as training sites for medical students and were regularly inspected by government regulators.[1]

The Western-style hospitals that we know today began as wards for the sick in the 1700s.[2] Most were founded by religious orders. Patients with financial means hired physicians for treatment at home, so these early hospitals primarily served the poor, and many began as almshouses. Since few medical treatments were available at the time, hospital patients were provided mostly comfort and palliative care. In fact, medical care was so primitive that patients were often as likely to acquire new diseases in a hospital as to be cured of the one that brought them there. The first hospital in the United States was Pennsylvania Hospital, founded in Philadelphia in

1751 by Benjamin Franklin and Dr. Thomas Bond.[3] Others followed in major cities, mostly along the model of wards for indigent patients. This tradition is still felt today in the predominance of hospitals that operate on a nonprofit basis.

The number of hospitals increased dramatically in the aftermath of the Civil War with the need to treat wounded soldiers. Soon after the war ended, a transformation began that turned hospitals into the prototype for modern institutions.[4] Promoting this change was the rise of nursing as a profession in the 1870s, which provided a more rigorously trained workforce to staff the institutions, and the development of antiseptics and anesthesia, which permitted wider use of surgery. As hospital treatments became more scientifically based, physicians become more active in running the institutions.[5] By the early twentieth century, the standardization of medical education based on hospital training had solidified the central role of physicians in hospital care and of hospitals in physician practice.[6] Today, the hospitals that provide the most sophisticated training, which are those that form the hubs of academic medical centers affiliated with medical schools, continue to hold special status among health care institutions.[7]

As American hospitals emerged in their modern form, similar changes were occurring in Great Britain, led largely by the efforts of Florence Nightingale. In 1854, as the Crimean War was raging, she transformed the British military hospital in Scutari, Turkey, by adding trained nurses and improved sanitation. The value of these innovations was readily apparent in improved care, and it formed the basis for the emergence of nursing as a profession.[8]

Hospitals that treat patients with acute illnesses and injuries are, of course, not the only providers of institutional health care.[9] Among other important health care institutions are long-term care facilities and hospitals that treat chronic diseases, which have a long history as well. Psychiatric hospitals date back at least as far as the "Bedlam" hospital founded in England in 1377.[10] The first such institution in the United States was established in 1841 as part of Pennsylvania Hospital.[11] Nursing homes were first created in the mid-1800s.[12] Some evolved from poorhouses in a similar manner to that of hospitals, and others evolved from old-age homes. They were commonly established by charitable and benevolent societies to house the poor and chronically ill elderly who could no longer live on their own.[13]

Regulation of the Quality of Hospital Care

The medical profession's model of regulation by the states with national coordination is mirrored on the institutional side.[14] Hospitals and other health care institutions are licensed by the state in which they are located. Many of the standards on which licensure authorities rely were originally developed by physician organizations. As the importance of physicians in hospitals increased during the early years of the twentieth century, organized medicine took a more active role in defining hospital operations. In 1917, the American College of Surgeons (ACS) established standards for approving those hospitals at which its members could practice.[15] These included a requirement that the institutions maintain formal medical staffs. The same year, the AMA adopted rules for hospital internships for physician training. As medical specialty societies grew over the next several decades, they developed further standards for hospital functions in their areas of expertise.

Today, state licensure is the primary oversight mechanism, but hospitals are also regulated in other ways. A variety of mechanisms both public and private developed over the course of the twentieth century, so that hospitals now face a wide range of compliance requirements. Of particular importance is a form of self-regulation known as "accreditation" that hospitals collectively impose on themselves.

Private Oversight of Hospitals: The Joint Commission on Accreditation of Healthcare Organizations

As with the regulation of physicians, the oversight of hospitals can best be characterized more as a public-private partnership than as a purely governmental function. Hospitals in most states actually face more rigorous and far-reaching oversight from industry self-regulation than from government licensure. The self-regulation takes the form of accreditation by the Joint Commission on Accreditation of Healthcare Organizations (JCAHO). This private nonprofit organization, whose membership is composed of virtually every hospital in the country, sends auditors to survey facilities for compliance with quality standards and grants them "accredited" status if they pass. While in most states hospitals may legally operate with a license but without accreditation, JCAHO approval is needed for reimbursement under Medicare and Medicaid and under most insurance plans. Moreover, many states accept JCAHO accreditation as a substitute for the formal licensure inspection process. Therefore, while not legally required, accreditation is a functional necessity for most American hospitals to do business.[16]

JCAHO traces its origins to 1910 and the work of Dr. Ernest Codman, who proposed an "end result system" under which hospitals would track all patients to assess outcomes and evaluate reasons for ineffective treatments. The ACS was founded in 1913 in part to implement this approach to quality enhancement. In 1917, it devised a five-point "minimum standard" for hospitals, the Hospital Standardization Program, which formed the basis for all subsequent accreditation review efforts. It was a demanding standard. In the first survey that ACS conducted using it in 1918, only 89 of 692 hospitals passed.[17]

JCAHO was created in 1952 as the Joint Commission on Accreditation of Hospitals to carry on the ACS's quality review work.[18] The ACS transferred the Hospital Standardization Program to the new entity, which initiated its accreditation program the next year. In 1965, the newly created Medicare program incorporated the organization's accreditation process into its operational structure by accepting accredited status as evidence of compliance with its hospital participation requirements. In 1966, the Joint Commission took the first step of many to expand the scope of its mission by adding long-term care facilities to its accreditation program.

Over the years since then, the JCAHO has expanded its scope several times to include a range of other kinds of facilities. In 1970, it established the Accreditation Council for Psychiatric Facilities; in 1971, the Accreditation Council for Long Term Care; and in 1975, the Accreditation Council for Ambulatory Health Care. These councils were replaced in 1982 by Professional and Technical Advisory Committees for each kind of facility. In recognition of the range of institutions involved, the name of the organization was officially changed in 1987, with the word "Hospitals" changed to "Healthcare Organizations." Since then, it has branched out beyond institutions to add accreditation programs for managed care plans and health care networks.[19]

JCAHO accreditation is based on regular surveys conducted at almost 17,000 facilities at intervals of every three years. In hospitals, a broad range of operational details are examined, including the completeness of medical charts, the minutes of medical staff committees, the structure of the medical staff bylaws, the process of quality assurance, and the implementation of operating room procedures. Most surveys result in at least some recommendations for improvement before accreditation is granted or renewed. Previously unaccredited institutions receive provisional accreditation, which remains in effect until a survey can be completed and an official accreditation category can be assigned.[20]

Policy Debates over JCAHO Accreditation

Although it stands at the core of the hospital regulatory process, private accreditation remains controversial.[21] JCAHO is a membership organizations controlled by the institutions it oversees. The purpose of regulation by the government is to place a disinterested outside party in a position to enforce standards that protect public welfare. Consumer advocates have long criticized the JCAHO for being too lenient with its members.[22]

Those in the hospital industry see it differently. JCAHO surveys are extremely thorough, and audited facilities take them very seriously. Preparations for the visit of the survey team can consume administrators for a year or more prior to the actual arrival. Most surveys recommend at least some corrective measures and often a re-review for compliance. With a three-year audit cycle, this means that many hospitals are constantly either preparing for the Joint Commission or dealing with the consequences of its last visit.

The debate over the role of JCAHO accreditation mirrors similar debates over physician self-regulation, and indeed over the regulation of many other industries, as well. Who is best suited to oversee a technical field that impacts public health and safety? Is it outsiders who tend to be disinterested in the outcome but perhaps less knowledgeable, or is it those who are regulated and have the deepest understanding of how the industry operates? Perhaps because of unresolved policy debates such as this, the health care regulatory system assigns roles to both public and private regulators in many spheres, including hospital oversight, which contributes to its tremendous complexity.

Aside from critiques of its objectivity, JCAHO faces an even more fundamental policy challenge. What is the best way to oversee hospital care and to measure quality? There are different approaches and no clear answer.[23]

The easiest way to measure the adequacy of a health facility is by examining physical features of the institution itself. In its early years, Joint Commission surveys focused on factors such as cleanliness, construction, and equipment. They considered criteria such as whether rooms and corridors were kept clean, whether hallways were of adequate width and rooms of appropriate size, and whether necessary machinery was available and in operating condition. A facility survey is relatively easy to conduct and provides basic information on whether the institution is capable of providing quality care. However, it does not say whether the hospital actually does so. The best facility is useless if it does not function properly. A more thorough approach is to examine the operational processes that are actually in effect. This approach looks at such factors as whether appropriate protocols are in place for nursing tasks, whether the procedures for surgical preparation of patients are proper, and whether medical charts fully document the care that is provided. The answers to these questions are necessary to determine whether the quality of facilities translates into quality of care.

Adequate facilities and appropriate processes, however, still do not guarantee quality care. Errors can, and often do, occur.[24] The best procedures do not ensure that clinical judgments will not be flawed. The next step in the evolution of hospital accreditation, therefore, is to measure actual clinical outcomes. This is the most accurate way to determine whether the institution is performing as it should, but it is also by far the most difficult. Outcomes measurement is a science that is still in its infancy, and researchers continue to debate what outcomes should be assessed. For each medical procedure, there are a range of factors to consider, such as patient survival, the need for follow-up procedures, and the return of patients to functional status. When outcomes are applied as a measure of an individual clinician's or institution's quality of care, there is also the more difficult question of how to take into account the level of severity of the cases that are treated. For example, surgeons who treat sicker patients will likely have poorer outcomes than their colleagues by any measure, but they may actually be providing better quality care than practitioners whose patients recover well but were not very ill to begin with.

Although comprehensive outcome measurement is the truest reflection of health care quality, it will likely be some time before it is ready to be fully applied. In the meantime, the JCAHO is hoping to introduce some outcome indicators into its standards as they become available and reliable.[25] The results could eventually transform the oversight of hospital performance, and much of the functioning of hospitals as well.

Confronting Medical Errors: Oversight through Data

Public confidence in the quality of care in American hospitals received a shock in 2000. The Institute of Medicine (IOM), the health policy research arm of the National Academy of Sciences, reported that serious preventable errors are far more common than had previously been suspected. The IOM asserted that they are so widespread that as many as 98,000 patients may die from them each year.[26] The report documented a range of mishaps that occur with alarming frequency, including administration of incorrect medications and of erroneous doses, errors in diagnosis, flawed laboratory results, failure to protect against hospital-acquired infections, and performance of the wrong surgery. In addition to the toll in human suffering, the total national cost was estimated at between $17 and $29 billion a year. In some respects, it appeared that hospitals had not advanced as far from the quality of their early days as most people had thought.

The IOM recommended a set of changes to hospital procedures to address the problem. The focus of the suggestions was to reshape the culture of institutional health care into a more collaborative enterprise among clinicians in which errors could be freely discussed. The existing environment, the IOM found, responded to shortcomings by blaming those responsible, as did the legal mechanisms for compensating victims of errors with its reliance on lawsuits. This approach discourages openness and full discussion of possible solutions. The IOM proposed that the answer lies in correcting the operation of the overall system, rather than in threatening individuals who perform poorly.

In a subsequent report issued in 2001, the IOM elaborated on ways in which hospitals could improve their systems to reduce the frequency of errors.[27] The starting point was better accumulation and sharing of data. This would enable hospitals, and those who regulate them, to learn from past mistakes. The challenge was to devise a mechanism that would facilitate data sharing without threatening hospitals with public disclosures that could damage their reputations or provide fodder for lawsuits.

The first government regulatory response to the rising public concern that followed on the heels of the IOM reports was implemented by a state. In 2002, Pennsylvania established a mandatory hospital error reporting system under the Medical Care Availability and Reduction of Error Act.[28] That law required hospitals to report incidents that could have caused harm to patients and events that actually did cause harm to the eleven-member Patient Safety Authority, which can issue recommendations for improvement. The institution must also notify patients in cases of serious injuries.

In 2005, Congress added a federal role in overseeing medical error reduction when it passed the Patient Safety and Quality Improvement Act, which authorized the creation of patient safety organizations (PSOs) within hospitals to examine possible dangers to patients.[29] PSOs are certified by the Agency for Healthcare Research and Quality (AHRQ), a body whose other responsibilities include funding of health services research. (AHRQ's role in funding research is discussed in chapter 8.) They report information that has been submitted voluntarily by individual providers, and which is then included in patient safety databases that facilitate investigation of systemic solutions. To encourage reporting to PSOs, the act protects the confidentiality of information that is submitted and exempts it from use in government proceedings, including lawsuits.

Other regulatory responses to concerns about medical errors include requirements that hospitals conduct patient safety initiatives as a condition of participating in Medicare.[30] These efforts are formally known as quality assessment and performance improvement (QAPI) programs, and they must include mechanisms to identify and correct quality lapses. Other aspects of quality oversight of hospitals through Medicare are discussed later in this chapter. Error reduction is also scrutinized by JCAHO, which, in response to the IOM reports, added it as a criterion that is assessed in accreditation audits.

The use of data as a regulatory tool raises many issues.[31] Mandatory reporting of errors is the most direct approach, but providers may resist complying out of concern that information will be used against them in legal proceedings. Statutory provisions that prohibit the use of reported data as evidence in court, such as those included in the federal Patient Safety and Quality Improvement Act, offer some reassurance, but hospitals may still fear that public disclosure will engender bad publicity. Even the strongest confidentiality protections are rarely absolute in practice. Moreover, assurances of confidentiality raise issues of their own. They deny patients information about medical mishaps that have caused them harm. Voluntary reporting encourages hospitals to be more forthright and comprehensive but permits serious problems to go undisclosed. Regulation by private watchdogs, such as JCAHO, brings the greatest expertise to bear but risks the conflicts of interest that are inherent in any form of self-oversight.

The use of statistical data analysis as the foundation of regulatory oversight is relatively new. Its application to patient safety responds to the IOM's call for solutions on a system-wide basis. While regulators have long collected information on individual health care providers, they have not previously used aggregated data across an entire industry segment to analyze and address systemic failings. This newer approach has been facilitated by advances in information technology that permit the collection and manipulation of large amounts of data. (Other recent and emerging regulatory initiatives that rely on information technology are discussed in chapter 9.) The approach represents a new paradigm for health care regulation, although it has been applied in the oversight of other industries, such as aviation.[32] It is a significant development, because as regulators at the federal, state, and private levels struggle with their respective roles and approaches in implementing information-based oversight, many of their functions may be transformed.

Private Coordination of Hospital Activities:
The United Network for Organ Sharing

The public-private partnership that characterizes much of American health care regulation is also evident in the coordination of some functions across hospitals. In no activity is this more apparent than in the intricate process of securing organs for transplants. There are few aspects of medicine as technologically complex as organ transplantation or as effective in saving lives. Organ transplants can give patients who face death or severe disability from the failure of a vital organ the chance for a full life. However, the replacement must come from a donor whose tissues match those of the patient according to various biological markers. Organs that do not match may be rejected by the recipient's immune system, leading to renewed organ failure and often death. Moreover, the replacement organ must be transplanted quickly lest it deteriorate. The process of matching donor and recipient and of doing so in a timely manner, therefore, is crucial.

Identifying a suitable organ donor for a patient in need could be daunting without an effective management system. The process requires coordination across institutions and often across geographic regions, and it must rely on a major administrative apparatus on a national scale. Rather than using a governmental mechanism, however, the apparatus that takes the lead in the United States operates through a private nonprofit organization, the United Network for Organ Sharing (UNOS), which functions under government supervision.

The first successful organ transplant was of a kidney in 1954. Healthy people have two of them but can function with only one; thus organs can be harvested from living donors. Over the next several decades, techniques were perfected for transplanting other organs that are not found in duplicate, so cadavers were required for donations. Surgeons performed the first transplant of a pancreas in 1966, liver in 1967, heart in 1968, heart and lung combination in 1981, single lung in 1983, double lung in 1986, and intestines in 1987. Procedures for transplantation from living donors have also recently advanced, with the first liver procedure performed in 1989 and lung in 1990. In 2001, the total number of living organ donors, 6,528, first surpassed the number of deceased donors, 6,081.[33]

The first coordinating organization for organ donations, the Southeast Organ Procurement Foundation (SEOPF), was founded in 1968 as a professional association of transplant professionals.[34] SEOPF implemented the first computer-based organ matching system in 1977 and called it the United Network for Organ Sharing. In 1982, SEOPF established the Kidney Center to provide hospitals with twenty-four-hour-a-day assistance in placing donated organs. In 1984, Congress passed the National Organ Transplant Act, which created the Organ Procurement and Transplantation Network (OPTN) as the framework for a national organ sharing system to be operated under private auspices.[35] The Kidney Center and the United Network for Organ Sharing were spun off from SEOPF the same year as a single nonprofit organization to create UNOS as it exists today. In 1986, UNOS formally received its initial contract from the Department of Health and Human Services (DHHS) to operate the OPTN.

Under its contract with DHHS, UNOS sets central policies that are administered by local organ procurement organizations around the country. However, a study of the OPTN system conducted in 1993 by the General Accounting Office (GAO, now the Government Accountability Office), a federal watchdog agency, found that almost every organ procurement organizations failed to comply with UNOS allocation policies to at least some extent.[36] In response, in 1999 DHHS issued new regulations governing the system under which it took a more active role in setting policies and supervising UNOS operations through the Health Resources and Services Administration (HRSA), which is one of its component agencies.[37] This body also oversees the National Marrow Donor Program, a private nonprofit organization that coordinates bone marrow transplants.[38] The new rules standardized criteria for prioritizing transplant waiting lists and for distributing organs. Among the most significant changes that they effectuated was to replace a policy of retaining organs within geographic regions with one that allocates organs, other than hearts and lungs, based primarily on medical need regardless of location.

Administration of the organ sharing system today relies on an Internet-based database, which UNOS launched in 1999. When an organ becomes available for transplantation, generally through the death of a potential organ donor, the local organ procurement organizations either accesses the database directly or works through UNOS's Organ Center to try to find a suitable match.[39] Potential recipients who are identified are ranked according to criteria that include blood type, tissue type, size of the organ, medical urgency, and time already spent on the waiting list, as well as geographic distance between donor and recipient. The criteria and their weightings vary somewhat between types of organs. An organ procurement coordinator or organ placement specialist then contacts the transplant center of the highest ranked patient. If the organ is turned down, the next person on the list is contacted until the organ is placed.

Organ transplantation has transformed treatment for many serious medical conditions and saved many lives, but it raises a host of ethical issues. Of perennial concern is the process for determining organ allocation, since the supply of available organs is consistently lower than the demand. Although the 1999 regulations reduced the unfairness of relying on geographic proximity, which had permitted waiting lists to vary considerably between regions, other issues remain.[40] For example, using medical necessity as the primary criterion ignores behavioral factors that may bear on the transplant's likelihood of success. A transplant may be wasted on a patient who is noncompliant with medical directives, for example, by failing to adhere to a regimen of antirejection medications. Lifestyle factors can also determine long-term outcomes, as might be the case for an alcoholic who returns to drinking after a liver transplant or a smoker to cigarettes after receiving a new lung. Some critics of the present system wonder whether scarce organs would best be allocated to those patients who seem the least likely to engage in self-destructive behavior. On the other hand, behavioral considerations can be subjective, and their use risks creating an allocation system beholden to personal biases.

As long as the demand for organs for transplantation exceeds the supply, ethical and policy concerns will continue to permeate this aspect of medical practice. However, the present system of partnership between federal oversight and private implementation offers avenues for policy input from many sources, which may facilitate further regulatory adjustments as technologies advance. This is an area in which public policy is likely to remain controversial for the foreseeable future.

The Web of Oversight and Funding for Emergency Services

Another aspect of hospital operations that is guided by a combination of public and private oversight is the provision of emergency services to treat traumatic injuries. In a medical emergency, access to an acute care hospital may not be enough to meet a patient's needs. Because time is of the essence in an urgent situation, rapid transportation and initiation of care even before the patient reaches the hospital may be crucial to survival. Moreover, arrival at the hospital may not, in and of itself, be sufficient to guarantee that needed care is provided. Facilities differ considerably in their ability to treat medical emergencies, and the variation is particularly strong with regard to trauma. Those facilities that are specially skilled in treating traumatic injuries tend to produce better outcomes than those that are not.[41]

The basic clinical structure of trauma care was developed by the U.S. military beginning at the start of the twentieth century.[42] Lessons from World War I, World II, the Korean War, and the Vietnam War led to refinements in protocols for initiating treatment on site, transporting wounded soldiers rapidly to hospitals, and providing specialized trauma expertise once they arrived. Government and professional efforts to improve trauma care in civilian settings began in the 1960s with a focus on automobile accidents. The focus was prompted by a National Academy of Sciences report issued in 1966 that recommended government action to address an "epidemic" of trauma that had aroused surprisingly little public concern up to that time.[43] Among the report's recommendations were the establishment of standards for ambulances to compel them to carry fully trained attendants, the creation of a new medical specialty of "emergency medicine," and the categorization of hospitals into four groupings according to their capabilities for treating trauma. It also suggested better data reporting of outcomes and greater funding for research.

Later that year, Congress passed the National Highway Safety Act of 1966, which allocated funding to states to improve ambulance services and overall trauma care.[44] Three states in particular, Florida, Illinois, and Maryland, used the newly available support to develop innovative emergency services and trauma treatment programs. Additional federal funding was provided by the Emergency Medical Services Systems Act of 1973 and by amendments to it passed in 1976 that encouraged states to develop statewide emergency medical services (EMS) systems.[45] With federal funding beginning to flow and public attention starting to focus on the area, private professional organizations added their voice to the nation's new concern over trauma services. The AMA proposed a plan for categorizing hospitals according to their emergency care capabilities in 1971, and in 1976, the ACS issued a report outlining the essential features of effective trauma centers and of larger trauma systems.[46]

The ACS report has retained considerable influence in the development of trauma systems as officials in most states have adopted it as authoritative guidance. On an ongoing basis, the ACS's Committee on Trauma updates the report's guidelines for operating trauma centers, including standards for physician coverage and hospital resources. The guidelines also classify trauma facilities into three levels.[47] Those with a level I designation care for the most seriously injured patients and often provide education and conduct research in trauma care. Level II centers treat injuries of comparable severity but do not generally offer education and research. Level III centers provide a lesser level of care. They stabilize patients, treat less complex injuries, and prepare those requiring the most intensive care for transport to level I or level II facilities. The classification of individual facilities according to these criteria is conducted in most states by state and regional authorities.

The system of classifying trauma facilities limits the number of hospitals that can lay claim to specialized treatment expertise. Trauma researchers feel that this can have several beneficial effects. In addition to directing patients and ambulances to the most appropriate facility, it ensures that those facilities designated as trauma centers generate sufficient volume to maintain the proficiency of their surgeons and staff.[48] It may also effectuate cost savings by concentrating resources in a limited number of locations.

After almost two decades of growing financial support for the development of state-level emergency and trauma systems, federal funding declined substantially in the 1980s. Much of the funding that remained was turned into block grants, which are allocations that combine several objectives and permit states considerable flexibility in assigning spending priorities. This shift also marked the end of the federal government's involvement as the principal facilitator of the development and implementation of emergency and trauma care systems. From this time forward, states took primary responsibility for designing and funding their own services, including the regulation of EMS professionals and of institutional trauma care. While this change afforded states enhanced flexibility, it also produced substantial variation in the programs that developed. In response to the block grants, some states eliminated or substantially reduced funding for EMS, whereas others sought to maintain extensive systems.[49]

Although it is indirect and of a lesser financial magnitude, federal participation in the oversight of trauma care has, nevertheless, continued through three agencies that support research, planning, and coordination of state efforts. In the mid-1980s, the Centers for Disease Control and Prevention (CDC), a component of DHHS, added the Center for Injury Control, which funds research into injury prevention, prehospital care, acute trauma care, and rehabilitation. The National Highway Traffic Safety Administration (NHTSA), a component of the Department of Transportation, has remained active since its initial role in the 1960s in encouraging states to develop trauma care systems. It publishes and updates a document known as "EMS Agenda for the Future," which identifies features of effective systems.[50] Another of its initiatives is to fund development of a Model National Scope of Practice Act that states can adopt on their own as the basis for regulation of EMS providers.

HRSA is the federal agency that has remained the most active in encouraging states to develop substantial emergency and trauma services systems. In the early 1990s, it offered planning support to states that adopted a model system plan under the Trauma Care Systems and Development Act, but lack of funding hindered this effort, and in 1995, Congress decided not to reauthorize it.[51] Today, HRSA operates the Trauma-Emergency Medical Services Systems Program, which affords less prescriptive support for the development of statewide trauma systems.[52] The program conducts assessments of systems, provides strategic planning, and funds state infrastructure development. HRSA also encourages states to create trauma registries containing data on trauma care.[53] These databases have proved to be effective resources for improving systems, comparing outcomes across providers, and identifying injury trends. Because its role is only advisory, however, HRSA does not have the authority to require states to use this tool. About two-thirds of states do, but the content is not standardized across them, limiting the value for nationwide assessments.[54]

The combination of regulation at the state level and loose federal coordination has produced a national pattern of extreme variability. As of 1999, only about half of all states even had systems with statewide coverage, meaning that many areas of the country lacked organized EMS and trauma center access.[55] An even smaller number had dedicated funding streams for the systems that were in place.[56] Existing state systems also differed considerably in their compliance with ACS criteria for measuring effective operation.[57] In 1995, fewer than half of all states had regulatory bodies with actual legal authority to designate trauma centers according to the ACS categorization scheme.[58]

Overall, the oversight of emergency and trauma services holds an anomalous position in the American system of health care regulation. Despite the participation of three federal agencies, state and local regulators, and private organizations, effective oversight seems to have fallen through the cracks. There is no coordinated national system or even comprehensive statewide system in many states. Regulation of EMS personnel and of trauma facilities is inconsistent between states and even, in many instances, within states. Conventional regulatory mechanisms that oversee the professionals and institutions involved, such as licensure of physicians and accreditation of hospitals, do not give distinct consideration to the provision of emergency and trauma services.

Renewed policy attention to medical response capabilities has arisen from concern over vulnerability to terrorist threats since the attacks of 11 September 2001. The Department of Homeland Security (DHS), which was created in 2002, includes among its responsibilities coordinating the activities of first responders. (For a discussion of DHS's health care role, see chapter 6.) Americans are also becoming increasingly aware of their susceptibility to naturally engendered health crises that could be caused by infectious diseases, such as severe acute respiratory syndrome (SARS), West Nile virus, and influenza. Perhaps this heightened sensitivity will promote greater interest in a more comprehensive approach to ensuring consistent access to specialized emergency care.

Federal Oversight through Medicare

General Quality Supervision

Like physicians, hospitals must be certified to participate in the Medicare and Medicaid programs.[59] While such certification is not legally required in order to operate, it is a practical requirement for financial viability for most acute care hospitals, since these programs usually represent a major portion of their revenues. Moreover, the vast majority of American hospitals have no choice about participating in Medicare and Medicaid, since under the Hill-Burton Act, which is discussed later, those that received federal construction subsidies in the decades following World War II are obligated to take part. The Internal Revenue Service (IRS) also requires acceptance of Medicare and Medicaid as a condition of granting charitable status. (See chapter 7 for a discussion of the IRS's role in regulating health care business relationships.)

Medicare certification can be met with JCAHO accreditation, which is the route taken by 80 percent of hospitals.[60] The other 20 percent are certified through other means, generally through state surveys, which tend to be lax.[61] Because of the ease of obtaining certification, Medicare and Medicaid participation requirements do not present a significant additional bureaucratic burden. However, they permit another set of federal and state regulators to concern themselves with hospital operations.

Regulation of Access to Emergency Rooms

In one regard, Medicare's regulation of hospital operations is direct. Under the Emergency Medical Treatment and Active Labor Act (EMTALA),[62] passed in 1986 as part of the Comprehensive Omnibus Budget Reconciliation Act (COBRA),[63] hospitals that participate in Medicare must provide an "appropriate" medical screening to all patients entering the emergency room regardless of their ability to pay. They must also stabilize these patients before transferring or discharging them. Similarly, women in active labor who present themselves in an emergency room must receive obstetrical care to the conclusion of childbirth, unless their condition stabilizes enough to permit transfer. Penalties for violations can include fines and exclusion from Medicare, and patients who are injured by a hospital's failure to comply with the law can sue for any resulting damages.

Congress passed EMTALA in the wake of repeated reports that private hospitals were refusing to examine indigent emergency room patients and were transferring them to public facilities before they were medically stable. One study found that the number of transfers from private to public hospitals increased from 1,295 in 1980 to 6,769 in 1983 in Chicago, with almost one-quarter of the patients unstable and 87 percent reportedly transferred because of lack of insurance.[64] In one incident that resulted in a prominent court case, an indigent Texas woman in active labor was told at an emergency room to drive herself to another hospital, and she delivered a stillborn child on the way.[65] To many observers, this did not seem appropriate behavior for institutions that receive substantial public funding.

EMTALA has had a tremendous impact in improving access to emergency care by indigent patients. The requirement that they be screened usually results in a full examination of their medical complaint and in treatment when it is in the emergency room's capability. If a serious problem is found and transfer is not possible, liability rules generally induce hospitals to provide needed care on an inpatient basis to the completion of the course of treatment.

However, EMTALA has also created significant economic inefficiencies. Knowing that a nearby hospital emergency room must screen them regardless of the seriousness of the complaint, many indigent uninsured patients visit emergency rooms for routine care. While they are technically responsible for the resulting bill in the absence of insurance, their indigent status usually makes hospital collection efforts futile. As a result, many emergency rooms now serve, in effect, as primary care clinics that treat sore throats, earaches, and a range of nonemergency conditions. In an emergency room, the cost of providing this care is many times what it would be in a doctor's office.[66]

Hospital operations, like most business activities, are customarily regulated at the state level in the United States. Federal regulation of emergency room access, therefore, presents a legal anomaly. As discussed in more detail in chapter 4 on the regulation of health care finance, the authority under which the federal government involves itself in this aspect of clinical oversight stems from its role in paying the bills. The federal spending power carries with it the ability to decide what will be spent and how funds will be disbursed. As the largest single financer of health care through Medicare and Medicaid, the federal government has become a significant regulator by setting conditions on the receipt of funding, a role that can eclipse the regulatory authority of the states in its influence on clinical operations.

In all respects aside from access, however, emergency room regulation remains with the states. Direct oversight of the quality of care in emergency rooms beyond the obligation to assess patients remains the province of state regulators and private accreditors. EMTALA does not require that hospitals maintain this service, only that if they do, it be open to all regardless of ability to pay. Nevertheless, mandates to maintain emergency rooms are imposed by some states.[67]

Regulation of Clinical Laboratories

Medicare's administrative structure also provides the mechanism for regulatory oversight of clinical laboratories. Congress passed the Clinical Laboratory Improvement Amendments (CLIA) in 1988 to create quality standards for laboratories, and it gave primary responsibility for implementation to the Health Care Finance Administration (HCFA, now the CMS), a component of DHHS, which administers Medicare and Medicaid.[68] While CLIA's reach extends beyond Medicare and Medicaid, applying regardless of who pays for the service, certification under the law is specifically required for reimbursement under these programs. The law applies not only to laboratories located in hospitals but also to those in physicians' offices and clinics and to those that operate as freestanding facilities.

CLIA regulatory standards, which were issued by HCFA in 1992, classify laboratory tests into three categories according to their complexity.[69] To perform the lowest level, "waived tests," a lab must enroll in CLIA and pay a fee but need only follow the manufacturer's instructions. Performance of "high complexity tests," on the other hand, requires compliance with stringent quality rules. While the law designated HCFA as the lead agency in implementation, enforcement is actually achieved in collaboration with two other federal bodies. CDC conducts studies on laboratory improvement, and the Food and Drug Administration (FDA), a component of DHHS that regulates the safety of food and drugs, regulates in vitro diagnostic tests. CLIA's implementation is funded by user fees imposed on laboratories seeking certification. About half of the states also impose their own licensure requirements. In two states, New York and Washington, this replaces

CLIA certification. For some kinds of tests, laboratories may substitute accreditation by various private organizations, including the College of American Pathologists, the American Society for Histocompatibility, and the JCAHO. CLIA requirements of one kind or another govern almost 200,000 laboratories across the United States.[70]

The enactment of CLIA added needed oversight for the laboratory industry, which had historically experienced variable quality. Enforcement of laboratory standards is vital to patient protection because errors can have fatal consequences. However, the combination of compliance costs and user fees has driven many smaller operations out of business. In particular, many physicians' offices abandoned or limited laboratory functions once the law went into effect. One result was inconvenience for some patients. Another was a business opportunity for large centralized freestanding laboratories to which many tests were sent, instead. Hospitals must maintain their own laboratories, so for them CLIA compliance is another essential part of the regulatory web.

Economic Regulation of Hospital Supply and Rates

Regulating the safety of hospitals has a fairly straightforward purpose—to protect the public against deficient care and to enhance and maintain the quality of care. Over the past fifty years, hospitals have also faced another form of regulation with less clear, and often conflicting, goals in the form of economic oversight. The federal government and several states have sought to achieve the financial objectives of enhancing access and controlling costs through a variety of direct and indirect regulatory approaches.

Hill-Burton Construction Funding

In the years immediately following World War II, the American health care industry expanded tremendously with new sources of funding. Budgets of the National Institutes of Health (NIH) grew dramatically, and the relatively new financial mechanism of health insurance began to spread. The benefits of this growth, however, were distributed unevenly, and remain so today. In particular, geography created a substantial barrier for many who lived in inner cities and for those outside of cities where the major medical centers were located.

To remedy the disparity in access to hospital care, the Hospital Survey and Construction Act of 1946, popularly known as the Hill-Burton Act, approved major new spending to fund the creation of new hospitals and the expansion of existing ones.[71] By 1971, the aggregate amount of funding under this law had reached $3.7 billion.[72] In return for receiving this money, hospitals were required to provide minimum amounts of indigent care, to operate emergency rooms, and to decline from discriminating against patients based on race.[73] In the 1970s, participation in Medicare and Medicaid was added as a retroactive requirement.

Creating a funding program to remedy geographic impediments to care raises the obvious question of where the funds will be used. To answer this question, Congress approved the creation of local planning boards in each state to recommend spending priorities.[74] They, in turn, drafted statewide health plans. Initially, these boards were advisory, but this advice became extremely influential in shaping health care at the state level because of the large amounts of money involved.[75] The boards also laid the groundwork for a more comprehensive health planning system that was implemented beginning in the 1960s.

Health Planning and Certificate-of-Need

In 1966, Congress gave the health planning process a major boost by enacting the Comprehensive Health Planning and Services Act.[76] That law funded state public health services and encouraged states to use health planning to coordinate their programs to achieve comprehensive geographic coverage. For the first time, state-level health planning was used for a purpose other than allocation of construction funding. In 1974, the act was amended to further promote health planning by establishing a national network of Health Systems Agencies (HSAs) to conduct planning at the local level.[77] Congress charged these organizations with developing annual plans to improve health services in their regions, making grants for needed resources, approving proposed federal funding, evaluating the necessity for new facilities, and conducting five-year evaluations of facility requirements. The boundaries of the regions for which each HSA planned were determined at the federal level by the Department of Health, Education, and Welfare (DHEW, now DHHS).

The newly created network of HSAs also took on an important regulatory role. Congress directed that their plans form the basis for state regulation of the construction and expansion of health care facilities. Each state was required to implement a certificate-of-need (CON) program under which hospitals were permitted to spend funds for new health care services, facilities, and equipment only if a need had been identified in the HSA plan for their region. For example, if a plan foresaw the need for additional hospital beds in a region, then a hospital could add them. If it did not, then no addition of beds by any hospital would be permitted. If the plan identified a need and more than one hospital wished to fill it, then a competitive adjudication by the state would determine which institution could proceed.

CON programs were intended to reduce hospital costs, a goal that may seem paradoxical given their approach. Classical economics teaches that costs decrease when supply expands, yet CON programs seek to reduce, not expand, the supply of hospital services. The answer to the paradox lies in the ability of health care providers to generate demand for their own services. As observed by economist Milton Roemer in the 1960s, when a third party pays the bill, hospital beds will be filled as long as they are available.[78] By imposing limits on the quantity of health care services in the market, Congress hoped that CON regulation would reduce provider-induced demand and thus lower overall health care spending.

The federal requirement for state implementation of CON programs was also ironic in its direct contradiction of the thrust of the Hill-Burton Act, which preceded it and initiated the use of health planning. Billions of dollars of Hill-Burton funds were spent over a thirty-year period to expand hospital services, but starting in 1974, millions more were spent administering the CON process to limit the ability of hospitals to expand further. The irony may be explained by a lesson that was learned. Improvements in health care access inevitably lead to higher costs.

Health planning to control the supply of services has been controversial from the start. The biggest concern of critics has been the effect on access and quality. CON programs may reduce unnecessary utilization of health care services, but they can also make care more difficult to obtain by limiting services to fewer locations. Moreover, administering these programs involves considerable cost, which can outweigh any savings to the overall health care system. CON programs also raise questions of equity across health care providers. Some state programs apply only to hospitals, others include freestanding outpatient facilities, and others also apply to physicians' offices. Programs that are limited to hospitals may give an unfair advantage to other kinds of facilities that can add new services or expand without the need to obtain state approval. Programs that regulate all facilities, on the other hand, may become overly expensive to administer and may impose compliance costs that smaller facilities, such as physician offices, are not able to afford.

In 1986, Congress allowed the federal health planning mandate to lapse, which returned to the states discretion to decide whether or not to maintain CON programs. In response, several states abandoned theirs, and most of them soon experienced large increases in hospital construction.[79] Today, thirty-six states and the District of Columbia continue to require CON approval in some form for the expansion of health care facilities.[80] The programs vary widely in the scope of services to which they apply, the types of facilities affected, and the financial threshold above which review is triggered.[81]

Indirect Cost Control through Medicare Reimbursement

A significant form of economic regulation of hospitals is imposed through the Medicare payment structure. This is accomplished through a system of reimbursement for acute care hospital services based on "diagnosis-related groups," commonly known as DRGs. While this system was developed specifically to govern payments for patients covered by Medicare and Medicaid, its perceived success at controlling costs and promoting efficiency has prompted many private insurance plans to adopt DRG-based reimbursement as well. (DRG-based reimbursement is discussed in more detail in chapter 4 on the regulation of health care finance.)

The DRG approach was pioneered in 1980 in the New Jersey Medicaid program.[82] Regulators developed it to replace a system of cost-based reimbursement under which hospitals were paid for the actual expenses they incurred in treating patients. With expenses fully covered, hospitals had no incentive to control them. The new system was designed to pay a set amount prospectively for each patient based on medical need and regardless of actual expenditures.[83] The DRG approach rewards efficiency and penalizes waste, since hospitals reap the rewards of holding down costs and pay the price of providing excessive care. It was adopted by the federal government for the Medicare program starting in 1983 and subsequently by many state Medicaid programs.

DRG reimbursement bases payments to hospitals on the patient's medical condition. All diagnoses that are eligible for Medicare reimbursement are grouped into 540 categories. Originally, there were 465, but they are periodically reevaluated, and the number has increased over time. Each has a payment assigned that is based on the cost to treat a typical case at an efficient hospital. Other than a few limited exceptions described later in this chapter, the payment is uniform for patients regardless of the resources that are actually used. Excess spending, therefore, provides the hospital with no reward.

The structure of DRG categories and payments is regulated by the Centers for Medicare & Medicaid Services (CMS). Payment rates are subject to adjustment over time as costs change, and diagnostic categories are regularly reevaluated based on clinical criteria. CMS also administers supplemental payments under the DRG program to teaching hospitals for the cost of training medical residents and fellows and to inner-city and rural hospitals that treat a "disproportionate share" of indigent patients. Additional supplements can be made on a case-by-case basis for "outlier" patients who are particularly ill and generate excessive expenses.

Implementation of the DRG program taught hospitals three operational lessons. The first was the one anticipated by policy makers—the importance of financial efficiency. The other two were unintended. One was a technique to game the system by switching procedures from inpatient to outpatient settings, where cost-based reimbursement still prevailed. Many ambulatory surgery centers and diagnostic clinics were opened as a result. The other was to focus on providing those health care services for which DRG-based payments provided the highest financial margins. Hospitals increasingly emphasized such services, often at the expense of other needed but less profitable activities.[84]

While it represents a payment rather than a regulatory program, the DRG reimbursement system has exerted a profound effect on the functioning of most hospitals. The groupings of diagnoses, the criteria for adding outlier payments for particularly ill patients, and the rate set for each DRG can influence day-to-day hospital operational decisions as much as any explicit regulatory scheme. Similar prospective payment systems have recently been implemented for services other than acute inpatient hospital care, including resource utilization groups (RUGs) for long-term care and ambulatory payment classification groups (APCs) for outpatient hospital services.[85] Their operational effects are likely to be as significant as those of DRGs.

Hospital Rate Regulation

CON programs represent an indirect approach to regulating hospital costs. In the 1970s and 1980s, some states tried a direct assault through regulation of rates. These efforts had mixed results.[86] They succeeded to a limited extent in controlling inpatient hospital costs, but spending for other kinds of health care services grew commensurately as many hospitals learned to shift services to ambulatory settings.[87] Moreover, as with CON programs, hospital rate regulation is extremely expensive to administer.

The original impetus for state-based hospital rate setting was legislation passed by Congress in 1972 and in 1983 that encouraged states to develop and implement health care cost containment measures.[88] More than thirty states created some form of rate setting in response. These programs took different forms. Some states employed "per diem" rate controls on the amount charged for each day of an inpatient stay; others developed "per case" rates based on the amount charged for a course of treatment. The latter approach evolved into systems of setting reimbursement rates based on DRGs, which, as discussed, are used today by Medicare and Medicaid. States also differed with regard to whether their programs were voluntary, mandatory, or broad-based to apply to rates charged to both private and governmental payers.[89]

Massachusetts, New Jersey, New York, and Maryland implemented the most aggressive programs, which are representative of "all-payer" mandatory rate-setting systems. To develop programs that applied across all sources of health care reimbursement, waivers of federal rules that applied to payment under Medicare and Medicaid were required.[90] The effects of the programs were inconsistent, and with the exception of Maryland, all of the states have since abandoned them, with New York being the last to do so in 1996.[91]

Each state had its own timeline and rationale for eliminating rate setting. Health care reform legislation enacted in Massachusetts in 1992 replaced rate setting with privately negotiated rate arrangements.[92] New Jersey's experience with rate setting also ended in 1992. Ironically, by 1997, 20 percent of New Jersey's hospitals were reporting negative margins, particularly inner-city hospitals that provide the largest share of health care for the poor and uninsured.[93] New York concluded that most of its hospitals were fiscally sound in 1996 and that market forces could produce greater efficiencies than government rate controls.[94]

Maryland's program, which remains in operation, is overseen by the state's Health Services Cost Review Commission (HSCRC). It sets identical rates for care for all payers, including private insurance companies, individuals, and government programs. Maryland's rate-setting policies and methodologies have evolved considerably since their original adoption, and they underwent a significant redesign in 2000. This program has experienced more success than the others. The state's hospital costs tend to be lower than national averages, while its hospitals have continued to provide substantial amounts of uncompensated care.[95]

Additional Regulation of Hospital Access

Most hospital regulation seeks either to improve quality or to controls costs. Licensure, accreditation, and Medicare oversight are quality enhancement programs. Medicare prospective payment, rate regulation, and certificate of need restrictions focus on cost control. The access programs that are in force today are more limited. The Hill-Burton Act funded tremendous amounts of hospital construction in the decades after World War II in order to expand access in underserved regions, but it was phased out in the 1970s after its mission was perceived as having been completed. EMTALA ensures access to emergency rooms by those lacking insurance coverage, but it applies only to emergency services.

Nevertheless, several specific deficiencies in access to hospital care are addressed by a set of targeted legal directives. Although there is no universal right to nonemergency care in American health care institutions, patients are protected from some kinds of possible abuse. For the most part, these protections take the form of laws that can be enforced through lawsuits by affected patients, rather than direct regulatory programs; however, they have had a significant effect on hospital behavior.

When care is elective or nonemergency and EMTALA does not apply, private hospitals may decline to schedule admissions for patients who do not have insurance or cannot otherwise demonstrate the ability to pay. With few exceptions, there is no legal prohibition on financial discrimination in access to hospital services, other than those rendered in an emergency room. This is one of the reasons that America's high rate of uninsurance is of concern to many policy analysts.

However, the ability to discriminate in patient admissions based on economics does not include the right to do so based on other kinds of patient characteristics. In particular, hospitals may not pick and choose their patients according to disabilities that they may have or according to their race, color, or national origin. Two federal statutes directly protect patients who are denied care on these grounds, the Americans with Disabilities Act, which was passed in 1991, and the Civil Rights

Act, which became law in 1964. A number of other enactments also afford indirect protection.

Access to Care for Those Who Face Physical Barriers: The Americans with Disabilities Act

Those with impairments that limit their physical and mental abilities can face a range of obstacles to obtaining publicly available services. An obvious example would be a person confined to a wheelchair who seeks to enter a restaurant that has a flight of stairs in front of its door. A disabled person may face further challenges once inside a facility. For example, restrooms might not accommodate wheelchairs, or corridors might be too narrow for wheelchair navigation. Many less evident impairments can also limit access, such as visual limitations or deficiencies in hearing. While limits on access to many kinds of services can be extremely frustrating, those that prevent use of health care can be life-threatening.

People with disabilities may also encounter barriers to obtaining services even when their impairments do not create actual obstacles. This is because of discrimination based on a perception that they are unable to function normally. In particular, many who suffer from serious diseases such as AIDS have been denied hospital and physician services that they are physically capable of obtaining. They can also face discrimination in employment even when they are fully capable of performing a job. Disability status, in other words, can affect the ability to enjoy the benefits of society in many ways, both direct and indirect.

To address this perceived injustice, in 1991 Congress passed the Americans with Disabilities Act (ADA), which prohibits discrimination based on disability absent a compelling justification.[96] The act defines most publicly available services as "public accommodations" and requires that they be made accessible to those with disabilities of any sort. There is an exception if creating accessibility would present an "unreasonable burden," generally in the form of an exorbitant cost. For example, an older building might not have to be retrofitted with ramps for wheelchairs or wider restrooms under the ADA because of the expense of renovation, but a new structure would have to incorporate these features into its initial design. The kinds of general public accommodations that are covered by this requirement include hotels, restaurants, transportation services, and schools. With regard to health care, they include hospitals, clinics, and physicians' offices. The ADA also prohibits proprietors of public accommodations from discriminating in the provision of their services based on disability, on a perception of disability, or even on a record of a person's having had a disability. Additional provisions prohibit disability-based discrimination in employment, unless the applicant is unable to perform the "essential functions" of a job, in the availability of state and local government services, and to a limited extent in the sale of insurance.

The ADA's protections extend similar safeguards that are contained in the federal Rehabilitation Act of 1973.[97] Section 504 of that law prohibits discrimination based on disability in services and programs that receive federal funding. Because most American hospitals receive federal support in one form or another through Medicare, Medicaid, the Hill-Burton Act, or other programs, the ADA's provisions were not entirely new. However, they are more far-reaching than the provisions that had previously applied.

The ADA applies to hospitals and other health care institutions in many ways. They must maintain facilities that are accessible to those with disabilities, unless this would pose an unreasonable burden. They may not refuse admission or services to patients on the grounds that they suffer from a particular disease or condition, whether or not it is related to the treatment involved. This protection has been called into play a number of times with regard to patients who have AIDS or are HIV-positive.[98] Similarly, they may not deny employment to physicians or other health care workers on these grounds. There is an exception when the prospective patient or employee poses a direct threat to the health and safety of himself or others, but the hospital bears the burden of proving that this is the case.[99] Physicians face the same restrictions in the operation of their practices.

The ADA's prohibition against discrimination in rendering health care services is enforced by the Office for Civil Rights (OCR) within DHHS as it applies to hospitals that participate in Medicare and Medicaid.[100] (For a description of OCR's role in enforcing patient privacy protections, see chapter 7.) OCR handles complaints and initiates investigations. Enforcement of the ADA's prohibitions against discrimination in employment is the responsibility of the Equal Employment Opportunity Commission (EEOC). This independent federal agency, governed by a five-member commission that is appointed by the president subject to confirmation by the Senate, enforces several nondiscrimination statutes by investigating complaints and initiating lawsuits when violations that are found are not corrected after attempts at mediation.[101] It also issues regulations to guide compliance with the antidiscrimination laws that it enforces.[102] Patients and employees who feel they have been subjected to discrimination can also bring lawsuits on their own.

Enforcing Nondiscrimination Protections: The Civil Rights Act

Before the United States began to struggle with the rights of the disabled, the country had already grappled with discrimination based on a number of other personal characteristics. The Constitution prevents the government from discriminating among its citizens on the basis of race, color, religion, creed, or national origin. In 1964, Congress passed the Civil Rights Act to impose many of these restrictions on a range of private enterprises.[103] Title VI of that law applies to discrimination based on race, color, or national origin by any program that receives federal assistance. Title VII applies to discrimination in employment.

Although this law protects access to care by potential patients based on a set of protected personal characteristics, it does not apply to strictly economic concerns.

A patient can still be denied hospital admission based on an inability, or even a perceived inability, to pay. However, among those who do have insurance or other means of payment, it bars a kind of access limitation that was prevalent in parts of the United States before the middle of the twentieth century.

Like the ADA, the Civil Rights Act is enforced by OCR with regard to discrimination in the provision of services and by the EEOC with regard to employment.[104] Violations of requirements that hospitals provide equal access to care can result in penalties up to exclusion from participation in Medicare and Medicaid. As with the ADA, individuals who feel they have been harmed by discrimination may bring their own lawsuits, as well.

Other Access Protections

In addition to these two broad federal enactments, a number of other laws bar discrimination in rendering health care services. As discussed, the Hill-Burton Act barred discrimination based on race by hospitals that received its funds. Hospitals that participate in Medicare and Medicaid, which includes the vast majority, are subject to a similar restriction. Most states have their own statutes that serve a similar end. There are, as a result, an array of legal tools that prevent the use of race as a criterion for denying access to health care services.

An even more powerful mechanism applies to hospitals that operate on a nonprofit basis and are recognized as tax-exempt by the federal IRS. Despite the recent proliferation of for-profit hospitals, the majority still fall into this category.[105] Under the federal Internal Revenue Code, in return for exemption from an assortment of federal taxes, hospitals must fulfill a "charitable mission."[106] IRS regulations define this mission as involving the provision of health care services in a nondiscriminatory manner.[107] Institutions that are found to limit care according to race, religion, or national origin may be subject to fines or loss of their tax-exempt status. (For a more detailed discussion of IRS regulation of tax-exempt hospitals, see chapter 7.)

What is more, the IRS requires that charitable hospitals provide significant amounts of uncompensated care each year to indigent patients.[108] This role applies in the aggregate and does not prevent these institutions from discriminating based on financial resources in individual cases. They may still, as a routine business practice, require evidence of ability to pay for nonemergency care. However, in a substantial number of instances, care must be provided for free as a service to the hospital's community.

Government-Run Hospitals

The regulation of hospital care includes not only the oversight of more than 4,000 private facilities throughout the country but also the direct operation of institutions by various levels of government.[109] Three federal agencies and an array of state and local governments maintain hospitals. These include more than 1,500 facilities that represent a crucial resource for large segments of the population.[110]

Federal Hospital Care

On the federal level, the Department of Veterans Affairs (VA) operates a network of 157 medical centers, including at least one in each state. (For a description of the VA's structure and its role in research, see chapter 8.) Its health system also includes more than 800 ambulatory care clinics, more than 130 nursing homes, more than 40 residential rehabilitation treatment programs, more than 200 veterans centers, and more than 80 home-care programs. These facilities provide services to more than 5 million patients a year. VA hospitals serve as a major site for medical training through affiliations with 107 medical schools, 55 dental schools, and more than 1,200 training programs for other kinds of health care professionals. The agency boasts that more than half of all physicians practicing in the United States received at least some of their training in the VA health system.[111]

Use of the VA health system has grown substantially in recent years. The number of patients treated grew by 22 percent between 2001 and 2004. As of October 2004, 7.4 million veterans were formally enrolled to be eligible to use its services. In 2005, the agency had a total of more than 235,000 employees, second only to the Department of Defense among cabinet-level departments. Of these, more than 214,000 worked in the Veterans Health Administration, the component that runs the health system.[112]

The VA was created in 1930 during the administration of President Herbert Hoover. At that time, it operated a network of fifty-four hospitals. A separate division to administer health services was created in 1946 as the Department of Medicine and Surgery. In 1991, that component became the Veterans Health Administration. The agency achieved cabinet-level status in 1989.[113]

The Department of Defense (DOD) operates an extensive health care network that covers about 9 million active-duty military personnel, their dependents, and retirees. The military health system is comprehensive and includes a substantial preventive medicine component.[114] Military hospitals are located throughout the United States and around the world. They include several highly reputed institutions that provide considerable amounts of teaching and conduct significant amounts of research, including the Walter Reed Army Medical Center and the Bethesda Naval Hospital, both located in the Washington, D.C., area. About 60 percent of all military care is rendered in DOD facilities, with the remainder obtained from private providers.[115]

The hospital and other health care benefits that DOD provides are administered through a coverage arrangement known as "TRICARE," which functions as a huge managed care plan. In seeking nonemergency care, beneficiaries must first visit a primary care provider, who can then refer them for specialty services. Nonreferred care is subject to a charge. Most care is rendered in military treatment facilities, but administration of the plan is performed by private contractors. A fee-for-service option is also available that does not require referrals for specialty care but compels patients to pay deductibles and copayments for most care.[116]

A network of hospitals is also maintained by the Indian Health Service (IHS), a component of DHHS, for care of Native Americans. It includes 36 hospitals in addition to 110 outpatient facilities and five residential treatment centers. Most are located on or near reservations. In addition, 13 hospitals, more than 400 outpatient facilities, and 28 residential treatment centers are operated by American Indian tribes under contracts with IHS.[117]

IHS services are available to members of federally recognized Indian tribes, of which there are more than 560, and their descendants.[118] This includes 1.6 million people out of the estimated total of 2.6 million Native Americans and Alaska natives. Federal funds were first appropriated for health care services for this population in 1921. The IHS was created to administer them in 1955. Under the Indian Self-Determination and Education Assistance Act, passed in 1975, tribes have the option of operating health services themselves or remaining in the IHS-administered system.[119]

The combination of these three federal programs guarantees hospital care to almost 20 million Americans. While the quality of care may vary across institutions, at least a minimum level of institutional care is legally guaranteed. However, the benefits are narrowly targeted. Only those who fit into the three covered groups—veterans, military personnel and their dependents, and Native Americans—are eligible. Therefore, government-run hospitals fill only a small hole in the safety net.

Nevertheless, the federal hospital programs can influence the larger health care system by example. In the late 1990s, the VA began a major initiative to improve quality that includes enhanced use of electronic medical records and outcomes monitoring.[120] It may form a prototype for private sector efforts. VA hospitals also conduct a considerable amount of health services research, with results that may lead to improved care management nationwide. Research is also conducted in military facilities. As a result, the potential exists for government-run hospital care to have a wide effect on broader regulatory policy.

State and Local Public Hospitals

State and local governments operate more than 1,300 hospitals across the United States. These facilities represent a substantial proportion of the nation's institutional care, accounting for about a quarter of all community hospitals and about a fifth of all community hospital beds, admissions, and outpatient visits. Many are part of larger hospital systems operated by municipalities. Smaller public hospitals are maintained by many cities and towns that function in a similar manner to private nonprofit community facilities. Some larger cities such as New York, Los Angeles, and Chicago operate major public institutions that train medical students and residents and conduct research. Many of them offer advanced high-technology services, such as trauma care and burn treatment, and represent crucial parts of the local health care infrastructure.[121]

Public hospitals accept reimbursement from private and governmental insurance programs. Those in underserved areas also receive supplemental payments as "disproportionate share hospitals" under Medicare and Medicaid. (For a discussion of Medicare and Medicaid reimbursement, see chapter 4 on the regulation of health care finance.) However, much of the care they render is uncompensated, since they must treat all patients and cannot turn away those who lack insurance or other financial resources. As a result, their budgets are supplemented with allocations from tax revenues.

Public hospitals form a significant part of the safety net that provides care to indigent patients. Unlike private institutions, they may not discriminate in the admission of patients based on the ability to pay. As with federally run hospitals, the quality of care may be variable, but the guarantee of access to care is important to millions of Americans who lack the means to afford it. They also relieve private hospitals of some of the burden of uncompensated care that might otherwise result from the obligation to provide emergency services. The primary limitation of the public hospital safety net is its geographic variability. Many regions lack facilities, as do some major cities.

The National Association of Public Hospitals and Health Systems (NAPH) represents the interests of public hospitals and health systems. This organization, which was established in 1980, has more than 100 members. It promotes their concerns before Congress and state legislatures, and it conducts research on issues related to management of the health services that they provide.[122]

Long-Term Care Oversight and the Federal-State Approach to Regulating Nursing Homes

Acute care hospitals provide treatments that usually have a time-limited course. Most patients enter these facilities for a specific therapeutic or diagnostic procedure and are discharged once it has been completed. Those who are not ready to function independently or whose conditions require longer courses of care are generally transferred to a long-term care facility. Some of these institutions are structured as hospitals and are regulated in a similar manner, with state licensure, JCAHO accreditation, and Medicare oversight through rules of participation. These institutions include rehabilitation and psychiatric hospitals. Others are organized to emphasize residential care over extended periods of time with varying levels of medical intervention. These facilities are known as "nursing homes."[123]

There are two broad categories of nursing homes. Skilled nursing facilities (SNFs) offer sophisticated medical capabilities for extremely frail or ill patients. Although they do not have the resources of hospitals, they are equipped to oversee serious medical needs. Intermediate care facilities (ICFs) provide a lesser level of medical expertise. They primarily serve patients who do not need constant clinical oversight but who are too frail or ill to function independently. After admission, many ICF residents remain for the rest of their lives.[124]

In addition to nursing homes, assisted-living facilities (ALFs) serve as homes for elderly residents who are healthy enough to function independently but whose risk of illness or injury is substantial enough to require that medical services, such as on-call nurses, be readily available.[125] These facilities provide housing with medical personnel accessible on site to render basic services if needed. Because of the minimal amount of clinical care that they provide, ALFs are subject to almost no regulatory oversight, other than regulation of the health care professionals whose services they retain.[126] However, they can receive JCAHO accreditation.

Long-term care is also provided in a number of noninstitutional settings.[127] Home care agencies send nursing and other medical professionals to the homes of patients. This arrangement provides care and monitoring at a lower cost than residence in a nursing home. It serves the needs of patients who require regular medical attention but not around-the-clock surveillance and who can manage daily living needs. Visiting nurse services also provide care to patients in their homes and to many in institutions who have special needs. Hospices provide palliative care for patients with serious conditions for whom additional treatment appears futile. These services can be rendered in a patient's home or in a hospice facility. All these long-term care arrangements are subject to state licensure and can receive accreditation from the JCAHO. Since all are eligible for reimbursement under Medicare and Medicaid, they must also be certified by CMS, a process that includes additional quality oversight.

Most of the care rendered in nursing homes and other long-term care arrangements is financed by government programs.[128] Medicare pays for up to 100 days of care in a SNF but only if it immediately follows a hospitalization.[129] It does not cover stays in an ICF. Medicaid provides full coverage for intermediate nursing home care of indefinite duration for beneficiaries who are over age sixty-five or in need of care for a mental condition, but its benefits are only available for those who are extremely poor.[130] As a result, many elderly patients who need such care devise plans to spend down or transfer their financial assets to spouses or others in order to qualify. The availability of this benefit and the growing number of elderly in America has made long-term care the single largest financial cost for state Medicaid programs.[131] (For a fuller discussion of Medicare and Medicaid, see chapter 4.)

The quality of care in the nation's 17,000 nursing homes is jointly monitored by the federal and state governments. Basic oversight is accomplished through state licensure, but scandals over the years have revealed that its effectiveness in maintaining quality standards, and humane treatment of residents, is seriously deficient in many states. To address perceived shortcomings in state-based oversight, Congress in 1987 formalized an interconnected yet separate set of federal and state roles in regulating quality through the Nursing Home Reform Act.[132] This law identified quality standards that facilities must meet in order to participate in Medicare and Medicaid. Regulations implemented by HCFA (now CMS) under the act established a system of contracts between Medicare, Medicaid, and each state through which annual inspections are conducted and compliance of facilities with regulatory standards is certified.[133]

In 1997, reports reaching Congress suggested widespread problems in California's nursing homes, which prompted an investigation by the GAO.[134] The resulting GAO report to Congress described widespread lapses in enforcement of the Nursing Home Reform Act, and it suggested that substandard care was common across the country. In response, the Clinton administration, in collaboration with the Senate Committee on Aging, established the Nursing Home Initiative in 1998 to reenergize enforcement.[135] This effort promoted measures to strengthen state enforcement of the original mandates, which included developing protocols that required more frequent facility inspections, enhancing federal review of state survey programs, expediting state action on applicable facility sanctions, and terminating federal funding for states with poorly performing survey procedures.[136]

To bolster federal oversight, comparative federal surveys are now conducted as a follow-up to state surveys. Federal survey teams also periodically accompany state surveyors to review their performance.[137] In addition, CMS has established a publicly accessible database that provides the results of every state survey conducted on Medicare- and Medicaid-certified facilities through its On-Line Survey, Certification, and Reporting (OSCAR) system.[138]

Along with CMS oversight, individual states may impose additional quality initiatives. For example, in January 2001, North Carolina permitted its state Department of Justice to provide nursing homes with criminal history records, if requested, for facility employees.[139] Several states also have regulatory requirements that go beyond the federal mandates, for example, by imposing higher minimum staffing levels. In addition, many facilities obtain private accreditation through one of two private bodies—the JCAHO or the Commission on Accreditation of Rehabilitation Facilities (CARF).[140]

The large federal role in nursing home regulation raises familiar issues about the division of power between the federal government and the states in health care regulation. States are the primary enforcers of public safety under the Constitution, except when interstate commerce is involved, and federal programs are generally designed to support them. However, experience has shown that states can fall short. By financing care that is subject to lax state oversight, the federal government might effectively endorse substandard services. Many private insurers impose standards on providers whose services are eligible for their reimbursement, and federal payment programs can be seen as having a responsibility to do no less.

Structure of Regulatory Agencies and Organizations

Federal Agencies: Centers for Medicare Medicaid Services (CMS)

Although it is primarily a financing agency, CMS is the most significant regulator of health care quality at the federal level. It is described in detail in chapter 4 in terms of its role in administering funding through Medicare and Medicaid. Major components that oversee the quality of the institutions to which it provides reimbursement are discussed in this chapter.

As discussed earlier, CMS is a component of DHHS. In addition to enforcing rules of participation in Medicare and Medicaid, it administers several quality improvement programs and pilot projects in areas such as nursing home care, home health care, inpatient hospital care, managed care, and community-based services.[141] The quality initiatives tend to have a specific programmatic goal, such as improving consumer information availability, encouraging knowledge and resource sharing among providers, or enforcing quality standards through state-level surveys.[142]

CMS also oversees a network of independent nonprofit organizations that investigate quality concerns under Medicare and Medicare. These are quality improvement organizations (QIOs), which review hospital performance and physician practice patterns on a regional level. Prior to 2001, they were known as professional review organizations (PROs); they are discussed in chapter 4 on health care finance. QIOs have no direct enforcement authority, but they can recommend changes and bring serious deficiencies to the attention of CMS. They also perform reviews under contract for private health care payers.[143]

Private Regulators: Joint Commission on Accreditation of Healthcare Organizations (JCAHO)

As its name implies, JCAHO is a joint endeavor of several professional organizations. Five corporate members direct its governance, ACS, AMA, the American Dental Association, the American Hospital Association, and the American College of Physicians, which represents practitioners in the specialty of internal medicine. They appoint a twenty-nine-member board of commissioners, which serves as the actual governing body to oversee operations. The board contains a broad spectrum of professions and perspectives, including nurses, physicians, consumers, medical directors, administrators, employers, labor unions, health plans, quality experts, ethicists, health insurance companies, and educators. Its members serve three-year renewable terms. Outside experts are occasionally invited to participate in board meetings when it ventures into new areas. This was done for home care in 2002 and for long-term care in 2004. The Joint Commission's ongoing work is conducted by a staff of more than 1,000 based at its main office in Oakbrook Terrace, Illinois, and at a satellite office in Washington, D.C. In addition to issuing and implementing accreditation standards, the Joint Commission operates a subsidiary that consults with health care organizations on compliance, Joint Commission Resources, Inc.[144]

Much of JCAHO's development and refinement of accreditation standards is accomplished through advisory groups.[145] These enable it to access a wide range of expertise and to receive input from a spectrum of interests. The accreditation program for each kind of health care organization subject to Joint Commission review receives input from the Professional and Technical Advisory Committee that includes representatives of national professional organizations and of consumer advocates, with two members of the board serving as liaisons. The Public Advisory Group on Health Care Quality provides counsel on emerging health care quality issues. It includes similar representation from professional organizations and consumer advocates and also from disease prevention associations, with liaisons from the board. The input from these two bodies is supplemented by recommendations of advisory councils composed of representatives of organizations that are actually subject to accreditation. There are two councils for ambulatory care, three for behavioral health care, four for home care, and one each for hospitals, laboratories, and long-term care.

An additional collection of advisory groups and councils composed of outside professionals in an assortment of fields offers further expertise. These include the Advisory Council on Performance Measurement, which assesses evaluation techniques for health care outcomes; the Business Advisory Group, which surveys the attitudes of employers and other large health care purchasers; the Committee on Health Care Safety, which focuses on the physical environment of patient care; several Core Measures Advisory Panels, which identify measures to be used in accreditation surveys; the Liaison Network for communication with more than 170 health care professional groups; the Nursing Advisory Council, which focuses on issues such as nurse staffing shortages; the Sentinel Event Advisory Group, which identifies significant adverse occurrences for inclusion in safety goals; and the Work Group on Accreditation Issues for Small/Rural Hospitals. With this range of advisory bodies providing input, the JCAHO is able to represent a broad base of private interests throughout the health care industry. This may help it to diffuse some of the criticism of a perceived conflict of interest in its status as a regulatory organization governed by those whom it regulates.[146]

Perennial Policy Conflicts

Government versus Private Oversight

Despite the active regulatory role of government in licensing health care institutions, there are few American industries in which those subject to regulation have as much say over their own oversight as in health care. On the professional side, it was the medical profession, not consumer advocates or government reformers, that initiated its own licensure, as have most allied health professions. Most state medical boards include exclusive or predominant representation from practitioners. Medical specialty societies confer certification within their own fields of practice. For institutions, it is an association of hospitals and other kinds of facilities, the JCAHO, that confers accreditation on its own members.

Self-regulation raises concerns over self-interest, but oversight of health care requires the expertise of those actively involved in the field.[147] The involvement of professional societies is an effective way of obtaining it. The result is an ongoing conflict between the need for expertise on the one hand and for impartiality on the other. Pursuit of these conflicting goals has produced a large and highly complex assortment of regulatory mechanisms to oversee clinical practice at the state, federal, and private levels. This complexity, however, has a positive side. It has engendered wide-ranging oversight that a single regulatory body would have difficulty accomplishing. What the arrangement lacks in efficiency it makes up for in breadth.

Access to Regulatory Data

As information takes on an increasingly central role in health care regulation, longstanding conflicts that simmered in the past over public access to regulatory data on providers take on greater urgency. The JCAHO and other regulators maintain troves of information on which patients could rely in choosing between providers. State medical boards, for example, have data on licensure examination pass rates, on physician training, and on disciplinary actions. Specialty societies have results of certification examinations. The Joint Commission has detailed survey data on many aspects of hospital operations. Releasing this information to the public, however, presents risks. Health care is a complex technical field, and considerable training is required to evaluate raw data. Unwarranted conclusions can easily be drawn.

Of particular concern to many providers in the release of regulatory data is the confounding effect of a factor known as "case mix." Doctors who treat sicker patients are likely to experience worse clinical outcomes regardless of their clinical skills. They may even face more malpractice claims. However, it is often the best doctors who treat the sickest patients because these doctors possess superior abilities. Hospitals in which they practice could appear to provide poor-quality care when, in fact, they are actually the most proficient. Outcomes data that are used in quality analyses are usually adjusted to account for severity of illness, but many critics feel that these adjustments are not sufficient to accurately reflect the full range of variation.

Despite the controversy, the trend seems to be moving toward greater public disclosure of at least some regulatory information. The state of Pennsylvania has taken a leadership role in this movement by maintaining data on patient outcomes and costs related to open-heart surgery and other procedures in the state's hospitals. This is done through an agency known as the Pennsylvania Health Care Cost Containment Council (PHC4).[148] All hospitals in the state must report information on mortality rates and costs of care, which is then compared to rates that would be expected based on the severity of illness of the patients treated and to statewide costs. The PHC4's comparisons are released to the public each year and are reported widely in the press.[149] The results of the comparisons have at times been unexpected, with highly reputed hospitals scoring poorly. Hospitals identified as poor performers commonly respond that the statistical analyses do not fully account for the actual level of illness of their patients, but critics reply that members of the public have the right to make their own judgments.[150]

The issue of public access to regulatory information on health care providers, whether of individual practitioners or institutions, goes to the heart of the debate over market-based approaches to health care. Markets work only if consumers have adequate information, but in a field as complex as health care, public release of information can have many unintended consequences. Disclosure of provider regulatory data and oversight of its use, therefore, present a looming policy challenge.

4

Regulation and Administration of Health Care Finance

The most prominent feature of American health insurance coverage is its slow erosion.
—R. Kuttner, *New England Journal of Medicine*

One of the ironies of American health care is that in our market-based system, the largest single purchaser of health care services is the government. Almost half of all insured Americans are covered by state or federal government programs.[1] Medicare provides coverage for more than 40 million elderly and disabled Americans, Medicaid for more than another 50 million who are indigent or disabled, and the Federal Employee Health Benefit Plan (FEHBP) another 9 million who are federal employees.[2] This is in addition to almost 20 million for whom care is provided directly by the government through the Veterans Administration, the Department of Defense, and the Indian Health Service.[3] By one estimate, the combined spending of all public health care funding programs dwarfs that of the private sector, representing almost 60 percent of the total American health care budget.[4]

The remaining portion of insured Americans are covered by private insurance that is heavily regulated. Traditional indemnity insurance arrangements that reimburse for the cost of medical services are supervised by state insurance departments. Managed care plans in most states are also subject to oversight by departments of health and insurance. Federal regulation applies to health coverage that is funded by employers under a complex set of legal rules stemming from the Employee Retirement Income Security Act (ERISA) of 1974.[5]

The government roles of funding health insurance on the one hand and of regulating private insurance on the other are not as separate as they might seem. As the largest payer for health care services, the government can exert tremendous influence over what it pays for without resorting to direct regulation. To see what really influences any industry, it helps to follow the money. As discussed in chapter 3 on the regulation of health care institutions, government payment programs have grown to include substantial regulatory powers that in many instances were not originally anticipated.

The regulation and administration of health care finance represents one of the broadest and most pervasive aspects of health care regulation.[6] In addition to paying for health care, the Medicare program enforces clinical standards for hospitals, physicians, and other health care professionals, sets standards for physician training, and determines what products and procedures are eligible for reimbursement. The Medicaid program alleviates part of the burden of uncompensated care that many hospitals would otherwise face. The FEHBP sets standards for federal employee health insurance that also influence policies sold in the private market. State insurance regulations help to determine the availability of insurance that employers can offer to their workers. Regulation of funding, therefore, is as important as any factor in determining the overall shape of American health care.

The History and Structure of Private Insurance Regulation

Regulatory attention to the financing of health care is a fairly recent phenomenon. Before the start of the twentieth century, few hospitals charged for their services because few provided much that they could charge for. Hospital operations were financed primarily through voluntary donations. That situation changed with the emergence of scientifically based procedures beginning in the late nineteenth century, including antiseptic surgery and radiology. Physicians charged fees to patients, but generally in a range that patients could afford to pay out of pocket. Early efforts to create prepaid financing arrangements included union and railroad brotherhood funds in the late nineteenth and early twentieth centuries; however, the norm for most patients was self-payment.[7] Some European countries initiated public health insurance at about this time, but the United States did not.

Workers' Compensation

An exception to America's early resistance to publicly supported health insurance was workers' compensation. While it is offered primarily through private companies, this form of coverage responds largely to government mandates. Workers' compensation was instituted in the early decades of the twentieth century on a state-by-state basis and follows a model of similar programs in Europe.[8] It requires employers to purchase insurance to cover the expenses of medical treatment and lost wages for employees who are injured or become ill from their work. The coverage is provided in most states by private insurers but is subject to regulation of rates and of coverage terms.

The regulatory apparatus that implements workers' compensation remains today in much the same form as when it was created. A board in each state determines the amount of coverage that employers must maintain according to the level of hazard that workers in their industry face. The board also determines the amount of reimbursement that will apply for each component of coverage. Legislative fee schedules in most states set the payments to hospitals, physicians, and other health care providers. Similarly, limits apply to the amount that workers receive for each day of work that is missed from a work-related injury or illness, and predetermined formulas set the rates of payment to compensate for permanent disabilities. The board also controls the prices that insurers may charge employers for coverage and adjudicates coverage and reimbursement disputes.[9]

The effect of workers' compensation programs on health care providers has been mixed. It guarantees payment for a range of patients who might not otherwise have been able to afford treatment, but the payments have historically been set at fairly low rates. Nevertheless, it set an example for a broader private health insurance mechanism and for active government intervention to encourage and to regulate it.

The Origins of General Health Insurance

The predominantly self-pay basis of American health care survived until the Great Depression. With the rate of unemployment running as high as 30 percent, the Depression robbed many Americans of the means to pay for numerous essential needs, including health care services. Hospitals and physicians, therefore, faced the prospect of fewer patients and more unpaid bills. Some of them chose to intervene proactively before the unemployment of their patients dragged them down financially, as well.

The First Health Insurance Pioneers:
Blue Cross and Blue Shield

General insurance to cover medical expenses first came into being with an experiment in 1929, just as the Depression was beginning.[10] Baylor University Hospital in Dallas, Texas, offered to provide up to twenty-one days of hospital care each year to a group of 1,500 schoolteachers for the prepaid sum of six dollars each.[11] The concept worked, and it quickly spread to other hospitals.[12] In the early 1930s, the first plans were developed in California and New Jersey to cover multiple institutions. The organizational model on which they were based came to be known as "Blue Cross."

These early plans were structured on a nonprofit basis.[13] Their goal was to guarantee a steady source of revenue for hospitals at a time when relying on out-of-pocket payment by patients had become precarious. The early Blue Cross plans were not designed as profit centers but rather as a secure financing mechanism for the hospitals that controlled them.

In 1934, New York became the first state to grant special regulatory status to "hospital service plans" that followed the Blue Cross model.[14] The plans were required to maintain nonprofit status and to remain under the control of member nonprofit hospitals. In return they were exempted from financial reserve requirements that applied to traditional insurance companies. The reserve exemption eliminated the burden of maintaining large sums of money to guarantee funds for paying claims, which greatly eased the task of setting up and operating the plans. Member hospitals did not need the reserves of insurance companies because they could guarantee coverage with services rather than financial reimbursement to policyholders.

Enabling statutes similar to New York's were enacted in twenty-five states over the next five years.[15] In most of these states, Blue Cross plans were subject to rate regulation by state insurance departments but were freed of most or all reserve requirements. The plans also reached agreement among themselves that each would operate in an exclusive territory and they would not compete with one another.

The introduction of prepaid plans offering reimbursement for physician services followed about ten years after the first hospital plans.[16] In 1939, the first Blue Shield program was introduced in Sacramento, California, as California Physician Services.[17] The concept spread to several other states over the next few years. Like Blue Cross, Blue Shield plans were organized on a nonprofit basis and controlled primarily by providers who served on their boards of directors. However, with physician bills less of a burden for patients than hospital bills and with more resistance from organized medicine than Blue Cross plans had experienced, Blue Shield plans grew more slowly.

The Legacy of World War II
The years following the inception of Blue Cross and Blue Shield plans provided a new impetus for their growth. During World War II, the federal government imposed a freeze on wages and prices to control the threat of rampant inflation in a wartime economy. However, in 1942, the federal War Labor Board, which administered the freeze, ruled fringe benefits exempt from limits on wages.[18] This meant that employers competing for workers in a scarce labor pool could offer health insurance as an enticement. The number of people covered by Blue Cross plans increased almost fourfold during World War II, from 7 million to 26 million.[19]

The popularity of health insurance as an employee benefit that grew with the help of the World War II wage freeze drove its continued expansion after the war. Employers found that health insurance was an effective recruiting tool, and workers increasingly saw it as an important part of their compensation. These historical circumstances first linked private health insurance with employment in America, a pattern that remains in place today. A consequence is that coverage is expensive and difficult to obtain outside of employer groups. The growing problem of uninsurance for those without access to employer-sponsored plans, therefore, stems in part from the structure engendered by federal wartime economic policy in the 1940s.

Some incarnations of private health coverage that developed during World War II took the form of prepaid plans, formally known as "direct service plans." Rather than reimbursing patients or providers for medical expenses once they were incurred, these plans directly offered the services of designated providers for specified groups of employees.[20] They were the precursors of today's health maintenance organizations (HMOs). In 1942, the Kaiser Aluminum Company initiated such a plan for employees in its steel mills in Portland, Oregon, and Oakland, California, that offered comprehensive medical care through employed physicians and owned hospitals. In 1945, the plan was opened to the general public and grew under the name Kaiser-Permanente. In 1943, the city of New York began to investigate ways to help municipal workers bear the increasingly common financial burden of illness. Its response was to open the Health Insurance Plan (HIP) in 1947 to provide physician services to municipal workers through organized practices of employed physicians.

Direct service plans remained the exception in health coverage arrangements for the next several decades. Most insurance policies offered financial reimbursement for the cost of medical services, rather than direct provision of care by designated providers. Starting in the 1980s, however, HMOs and other managed care mechanisms inspired by the direct service plans began to spread widely. This new form of coverage, which is discussed later, laid the foundation for a dramatic change in the relationship between employers, insurers, providers, and patients.

The Federal Tax Subsidy

The most important element of all in the spread of employment-based health insurance after World War II was not the original wage freeze exception or a natural reservoir of market demand, but rather a different government decision. In 1954, Congress clarified and reaffirmed a position taken by the Internal Revenue Service (IRS) that the premiums paid by employers for their workers' health insurance benefits were not considered "wages" and so were not subject to income tax.[21] In other words, employees received this benefit tax-free.

The amount of tax revenue lost to the federal government by exempting health benefits from taxation is known as a "tax subsidy." In terms of economic effect, the foregone revenue is, in essence, the equivalent of a government spending program to promote employment-based health insurance. Since most states that impose an income tax use the federal structure as a base, state tax subsidies automatically followed as well. In 1998, the annual value of the combined federal and state tax subsidy for health insurance reached $125 billion.[22] This made it the third-largest government health care finance program after Medicare and Medicaid.

While the tax subsidy encouraged the spread of health insurance to many in the workforce, it also had a powerful effect on the shape of the market for coverage. Favorable tax laws made employment-based coverage attractive to workers, and insurers realized administrative savings from selling policies that covered groups with many employees. At the same time, insurance companies became increasingly reluctant to process individual coverage, which was more expensive to administer and offered no tax benefits. Those individual policies that were available generally came with higher premiums than group plans. In 1986, Congress added a limited tax benefit for health insurance obtained by self-employed workers, but it was no match for the subsidy afforded to participants in employee groups.[23] Recent legislative changes have brought the tax benefit for health insurance obtained by self-employed workers closer to that available for employee groups, but there has been a gradual phase-in. As a result, during the decades after World War II, a gap in access to coverage opened between those who worked for companies that provided health care benefits and those who did not. In 2003, the United States had almost 45 million citizens with no health insurance, many of whom fall into the latter group.[24]

The tax subsidy also suffers from an inherent unfairness in the distribution of its benefits. Under America's progressive income tax structure, the value of a deduction increases with the taxpayer's marginal tax bracket, which rises with income. In other words, those who earn more pay a higher percentage of their income in taxes, and thereby realize a greater benefit from a tax deduction. The tax subsidy for employment-based health insurance is, therefore, considered regressive in its disproportionately greater value with increasing wealth. Those with the lowest incomes, who presumably need the most financial help, actually receive the least assistance.

The tax subsidy for insurance premiums is today supplemented by other health care tax benefits directed to workers. Federal law enables employers to establish health care spending accounts into which employees can set aside a portion of their income for health-related expenses that are not covered by insurance.[25] The money allocated to these accounts is not subject to income tax. For workers and any other taxpayers who incur medical expenses that are large enough to exceed 7.5 percent of their annual income, outlays above this threshold are tax-deductible.

Private Commercial Health Insurance

With the help of the tax subsidy, the health insurance market experienced robust growth during the years after World War II and through the 1950s. As the market expanded, its structure was shaped by an important new player. Traditional commercial insurance companies discovered that the concept of prepaid financing for health care services that had been pioneered by Blue Cross and Blue Shield could represent a profit center by itself, not just a payment mechanism to protect providers. While they did not come close to eclipsing the market share of Blue Cross and Blue Shield, by end of the 1950s, commercial insurers had become a major force in the health insurance market.[26]

Commercial insurance companies thrived in large part by using a different approach to pricing and underwriting their coverage. Blue Cross and Blue Shield set rates according to claims experience across entire communities, a process known as "community rating." In contrast, commercial insurers set rates according to the experience of each employer whose workers they covered, which is known as "experience rating." This allowed them to offer lower prices to companies with healthier workers, skimming this part of the market from Blue Cross and Blue Shield. The market niche that they captured was much smaller but also highly profitable. Commercial insurers offering health coverage continued to be regulated by the states as traditional insurance companies without the benefit of the special enabling statutes that Blue Cross and Blue Shield enjoyed. However, the ability to focus on less risky policyholders overcame much of the advantage from the regulatory exceptions that these statutes conferred.

The rise of an insurance mechanism based on experience rating raises deeper policy issues. By offering lower rates to lower risk employers, private insurers left the rest of the market to Blue Cross and Blue Shield plans. One result is that these plans must charge higher premiums to those companies that remain with it, which makes coverage through private companies even more attractive to those firms that qualify. This is an example of a phenomenon that economists call "adverse selection." It occurs in an insurance market when the riskiest policyholders are increasingly concentrated under one insurer. Adverse selection is a hazard lurking in most health insurance arrangements and is an ongoing source of policy tension. Those who are healthiest do not want to pay premiums that effectively subsidize those who are ill. However, without the participation of healthier members in the risk pool, the insurance arrangement can become economically infeasible.

The Rise of Managed Care

America's private health insurance market underwent another revolution in the 1980s and 1990s as a new paradigm for providing coverage took hold. A growing segment of the market offered a mechanism that combined the financing of care with the management of care in an effort to control costs. The mechanism, known as "managed care," was an outgrowth of the direct service plans developed during the 1940s. The market demand for this new kind of coverage arose from draconian increases in health insurance premiums in the late 1980s and early 1990s. However, the seeds for this demand were planted by a government regulatory program that had been enacted over a decade earlier.

Managed care can take several forms.[27] The original form, and the one most commonly associated with the managed care insurance mechanism, is that of the

HMO. This model was first conceived in the late 1960s by a Minneapolis physician, Dr. Paul Elwood, based on the existing prepaid, direct service plans such as Kaiser-Permanente.[28] HMOs use several tools to manage health care to control costs. The most radical is a change in the form of physician reimbursement. Rather than paying for each service performed, HMOs compensate physicians with a set monthly fee for each patient assigned to them for care, regardless of the amount of services actually rendered. These "capitation" payments are designed to mimic the salary that staff physicians receive in prepaid plans. The resulting financial incentive is intended to discourage overuse and favor efficient provision of services.

Under Dr. Elwood's scheme, the capitated payment structure is reserved for primary care physicians. All patients in the plan are assigned to one, and that physician initiates all care. Visits to specialists must follow a referral from the primary care physician, which may be only to specialists within the HMO's network. While specialist physicians continue to be paid under the traditional fee-for-service arrangement, costs for their services are controlled by imposing discounted negotiated fees and by central monitoring of the number of referrals that primary care physicians make to them. Other HMO cost-control techniques include prior review before reimbursement may be approved for many diagnostic tests, specialty procedures, hospitalizations, and other expensive services.

The HMO payment structure was originally designed to implement more than just a series of blunt limits on the use of health care services. It was intended to create a new paradigm of health care based on the primacy of preventive care and concern for population health. With capitated payments, it was hoped that physicians would try to keep their panel of patients as healthy as possible to limit the demand for services. Unlike traditional indemnity insurers of the time, HMOs paid in full for preventive services, such as checkups and immunizations. Dr. Elwood envisioned a transformation of American medicine from a focus on caring for the sick to one of preventing sickness before it occurred.

The theory of HMOs held a short-term promise of lower insurance premiums and a long-term promise of better health. However, without an external impetus, the market in the early 1970s was not yet ready to embrace this new concept. Congress responded in 1973 by passing the federal Health Maintenance Organization Act, which was intended to give HMOs an initial toehold in the market.[29] It required employers that offered health insurance to include an HMO among the options if the HMO met specified standards and if it requested inclusion. The standards, administered by the Department of Labor (DOL), covered features such as the size of the physician and hospital network available to members, the coverage of preventive services, the ease of the enrollment process, and the nature of the grievance policy for patient complaints. They also required the use of community rating in setting premiums. HMOs that met the standards were classified as "federally qualified," and the law also provided them with subsidies and loan guarantees for start-up costs.

Employers that did not offer health insurance were not required to do so in order to accommodate an HMO, but HMOs were guaranteed the opportunity to compete against traditional indemnity plans where the market for those plans was already in place.

Although DOL could grant "federally qualified" certification, the underlying regulation of HMOs, which are essentially insurance companies, remained with the states. In most states, the insurance department oversees the financial aspects of HMO operations, and the department of health oversees the clinical care that they provide. Federal qualification was designed to supplement, rather than replace, these state functions.

In two respects, however, the HMO Act specifically overruled traditional state law. As hybrids that both finance and deliver health care, HMOs could run afoul of two kinds of common state restrictions. One, known as the prohibition against the "corporate practice of medicine," prohibits private for-profit corporations from directly employing physicians to practice medicine.[30] This rule is intended to prevent profit-making financial interests from trumping physicians' clinical judgments. It would prevent for-profit HMOs from hiring physicians to work in their provider networks. The other restriction prohibits health insurers from directing patients to specific providers. This is intended to guarantee patient freedom of choice. It would prevent HMOs from requiring that patients use only physicians and hospitals within their networks. The HMO Act required that states, as a condition of receiving HMO funding, enact laws exempting HMOs from these restrictions. The laws permit HMOs to operate with a measure of flexibility that other insurers do not enjoy. Some states, however, have also enacted laws known as "any willing provider" laws that require HMOs to include in their networks any providers that meet their qualifications and are willing to accept their terms.[31]

The HMO Act's effect on the health insurance market was limited during the decade after its enactment as the national market share of HMOs remained below 10 percent into the early 1980s.[32] However, by the late 1980s, the dynamics of health insurance had begun to change. Premiums rose dramatically at this time, and many smaller companies found the financial burden of providing health benefits to be unsustainable. Largely overlooked as an eccentricity up until then, HMOs with their lower premiums increasingly seemed a viable alternative to traditional health insurance plans.[33] As a result, during the late 1980s and early 1990s, the market share of HMOs in several regions of the country reached 50 percent. Along with looser forms of managed care, such as preferred provider organizations (PPOs) and point-of-service (POS) plans, managed care of one type or another came to predominate nationwide.[34] It took twenty years, but the small toehold created in 1973 through a limited government regulatory program blossomed into a commanding market position. Today, few HMOs accept the regulatory constraints of obtaining federal qualification because strong market demand for their kind of coverage has made it largely unnecessary.

Looking back, the regulatory intervention that initially facilitated the managed care revolution, the HMO Act, may have been fairly modest in scope, but it marked a transition in health care regulation that was far more significant than the substance of its actual provisions. The HMO Act marked the first time that Congress created a direct federal role in the regulation of health insurance. Although Congress had assigned primary regulatory authority over insurance to the states in the McCarran-Ferguson Act of 1945,[35] a number of initiatives starting with the HMO Act imposed layers of federal involvement that have become a substantial force in shaping health insurance. As a result, the regulation of the industry is today a complex federal-state interaction.

Private Accreditation for Managed Care:
The National Committee for Quality Assurance
The separate regulatory schemes administered under federal and state law left gaps in the oversight of managed care arrangements, particularly with regard to quality assurance. With the growing prominence of HMOs and lack of uniform national monitoring, the National Committee for Quality Assurance (NCQA) was created in 1990 as a private accrediting organization to supervise quality.[36] It operates according to a model that is similar to that of the Joint Commission on Accreditation of Health Care Organizations (JCAHO), which accredits hospitals and other facilities. (JCAHO is discussed in more detail in chapter 3 on the regulation of health care institutions.) It seeks to impose quality oversight through collaboration of members of the industry, which can forestall more direct government supervision.

NCQA's first challenge was to determine a way to measure managed care quality. Hospitals maintain facilities and procedures that are easy to identify and evaluate. How do you decide if an HMO, PPO, or other managed care organization is doing its job? Part of NCQA's task was fairly straightforward. Several aspects of HMO operations that are essential to quality service are easy to measure, such as responsiveness to patient inquiries, ease of enrollment, and size of the provider network. There are also features of HMO provider behavior that clearly reflect the quality of patient service and are readily identified, such as the hours that physician offices are open, the responsiveness to telephone calls, and the accuracy and comprehensiveness of medical records. However, while these elements of patient service may be necessary to overall quality, they do not indicate whether acceptable clinical care is actually being rendered.

During the 1990s, NCQA directed much of its effort toward developing and refining a set of data measurements that would reliably reflect the quality of HMO patient care. The Health Employer Data Information Set (HEDIS) is one such set. It examines selected elements of clinical care that are essential to a minimal level of quality, and it was formally included in the accreditation process in 1999. The initial HEDIS data points focused on primary care and, in particular, on the provision of preventive services. They included the frequency with which recommended immunizations are administered to children and with which mammograms and other common screening tests are administered to adults. These data points include clinical elements that are easiest to measure, and their range is limited. However, NCQA continually refines HEDIS to add new elements that reflect a broader range of medical services.

The extent of NCQA's activities has grown steadily since its creation. In 1991, it accredited its first HMO. By 1998, almost 90 percent of all managed care plans collected some HEDIS data elements, and 75 percent of all HMO enrollees participated in plans that were subject to NCQA accreditation review. In 2001, NCQA accredited its first PPO. An accreditation and certification procedure for disease management programs was developed in 2001, and in 2003 NCQA joined JCAHO in a partnership to develop an accreditation process for human research subjects protection programs. There are also accreditation or certification programs for managed behavioral health organizations, medical research facilities, physician organizations, and medical credentials verification organizations.[37]

As the business of health care has become more complex, many new kinds of organizations have found roles in the system. NCQA is the most prominent recent example. It has positioned itself as a private alternative to government regulation for operational aspects of managed care and of a range of allied businesses. Questions remain about the ability of a private association composed of members of the industry being regulated to truly enforce rigorous standards on its own constituents. Nevertheless, NCQA's efforts to develop HEDIS and similar measures of quality make it, at the very least, one of the most innovative bodies in American health care regulation.

The Regulation of Private Insurance

After half a century of evolving regulation, the provisions that apply to traditional private health insurance today are extremely varied and complex. They are based primarily on state oversight, but with extensive federal and private roles. The federal-state balance is particularly intricate and, in some regards, uncertain. However, it is central to the overall regulatory process. It can be viewed as having progressed in a number of discrete stages.

The Federal-State Balance, Step 1: The McCarran-Ferguson Act and the Role of the States

The Constitution grants to the states primary authority to regulate business activities, unless interstate commerce is involved. While insurance can affect commerce across state lines, Congress eliminated any doubt concerning the lines of jurisdiction over it in 1945 when it passed the McCarran-Ferguson Act.[38] That law explicitly placed responsibility for regulating the business of insurance at the state level.

Health insurers, therefore, answer to regulators in fifty states and the District of Columbia, although with some coordination by the National Association of Insurance Commissioners (NAIC), which is described later.

States vary widely in the rigor with which they oversee insurance. Areas of regulatory concern include premium rates, policy language, financial reserves, accounting practices, marketing activities, and unfair claims practices, with each state determining which it will regulate and with what level of intensity. Variations between states are particularly significant in the implementation of new insurance arrangements, such as managed care, which must answer to slightly different, and sometimes inconsistent, regulatory requirements in each jurisdiction.

Effects such as this make the system of state-level insurance regulation controversial. Regulatory variation across jurisdictions may stifle innovation, since multiple regulatory approvals may be needed before a new concept can be implemented. In addition, states with laxer regulatory schemes may let unstable insurers wreak financial havoc that can leave beneficiaries in other states with unpaid claims. On the other hand, regulation closer to the local level may facilitate experimentation that would not be possible under a single federal regulator, which might have difficulty adjusting its focus to address local needs.

The Federal-State Balance, Step 2: The Federal Employee Health Benefits Program (FEHBP)

As a major employer, in fact as the largest single employer in the country, the federal government followed the trend of offering health insurance as an employee benefit beginning in 1960.[39] Because of the size of the federal workforce, 9 million as of 2001, the benefit program that was created presented a tremendous market opportunity for private insurance companies. The program was structured to include as many of them as possible.

FEHBP provides each employee with a set financial contribution that can be applied toward the purchase of any coverage plan within the system.[40] Employees purchasing more expensive plans make up the difference with their own supplemental contributions, and those who select less extensive coverage with lower premiums keep the savings. Any health insurance plan is eligible for inclusion as an option for federal employees, if it meets various coverage criteria. For example, all FEHBP-qualified plans must include prescription drug coverage. As of 2001, the program included seventeen national indemnity insurance plans and a large number of HMOs. However, the number of participating HMOs has declined in recent years from almost 400 in the mid-1990s to 165 in 2002.[41] The FEHBP is administered by the U. S. Office of Personnel Management (OPM), which sets the criteria for participation.[42] It is a small agency with a limited scope of authority; however, management of the FEHBP gives it substantial influence over the nation's private health insurance market, because the criteria that it administers for coverage are often mimicked in the private sector.

The FEHBP is often cited as a possible model for a broader national health insurance system.[43] Supporters see it as a way to bring universal coverage through a private market mechanism. While there would be significant logistical problems in expanding the FEHBP on the scale envisioned by its advocates, this approach continues to attract considerable discussion. Although the FEHBP is a regulatory program governing only the insurers that participate, therefore, its position as the largest employer-sponsored health benefit program in the country causes it to cast a large shadow.

The Federal-State Balance, Step 3: ERISA and the Special Status of Employer-Funded Coverage

Much of the power over health insurance that Congress gave to state regulators through the McCarran-Ferguson Act it later took away, although through blunder rather than design. Among the burdens that state-level regulation created was an inconsistent pattern of regulatory requirements on large employers that self-fund their health insurance coverage. Many national firms have the resources to pay the health care expenses of their workers themselves, without the need for an insurance company to collect premiums and process claims. By effectively eliminating the insurer as middleman, they seek to offer coverage more efficiently and cheaply. However, under state-based insurance regulation, companies that self-insure and have employees in different states would have to comply with the insurance rules of each. In the early 1970s, several companies that offered such self-insured plans sought congressional relief from the burden of state regulation.

Assistance for self-insured health plans came in 1974 in the form of ERISA.[44] Although that law dealt mostly with pension plans, it included a provision exempting self-insured employee health coverage from the state regulation that would otherwise apply under the McCarran-Ferguson Act. The objective was to impose uniform national regulatory standards in place of the varying state rules. However, ERISA implemented only half of this goal. It preempted state regulation of self-insured health benefit plans but failed to create a meaningful alternative national oversight scheme.

Under ERISA, DOL administers a set of reporting requirements for self-insured health plans but with no provision for most of the regulatory areas that the states commonly address, such as premium rates, policy language, and reserve requirements.[45] Self-insured plans must file organizational documents with DOL and annually submit financial results. However, they have considerable latitude to restrict coverage, to ignore state mandates on coverage of specific services, to set aside insufficient reserves for unexpected claim expenses, and to design limited benefit structures.

In 1974, when ERISA was enacted, there were relatively few self-insured health coverage arrangements, so the law's effect on the overall market for health insurance was relatively limited. However, with a relentless rise in health care costs and insurance premiums over the next three decades, self-insured plans proliferated. With their rise, ERISA came to preempt a significant portion of private health insurance from state authority. A dual regulatory system has resulted in which some plans are subject to thorough state oversight, but many others are beholden to almost no oversight at all.

ERISA has created a number of other conflicts between federal and state authority that have been the subject of considerable litigation. The most visible of these involves the reach of state tort law when beneficiaries believe they have been harmed by a self-insured plan's coverage denial.[46] ERISA severely limits the ability of patients to sue the administrator of an employer-sponsored health plan, even when it injects itself into some kinds of medical decision-making.[47] This has added significant uncertainty to the lines of authority in the oversight of private health care finance.

The Federal-State Balance, Step 4: COBRA, HIPAA, and the Growing Web of Incremental Reforms

In enacting ERISA, Congress brought confusion to the line between federal and state jurisdiction in health insurance oversight. In two subsequent laws, it brought the federal government unambiguously into the role of health insurance regulator. These laws responded to gaps in the availability of coverage that have grown into yawning chasms since ERISA's enactment. The linking of health insurance and employment, initiated during World War II and reinforced through ERISA and the tax subsidy for premiums, leaves out a range of people, including not just those who are unemployed but also those who are self-employed and those who are fully employed at firms that do not offer coverage. Moreover, the dependent spouses and children of these workers usually lack coverage along with them.

In two stages, Congress added new federal layers of health insurance regulation to reduce this gap in access to coverage. In 1986, rules governing employer-sponsored health plans were added to a year-end federal spending bill, the Comprehensive Omnibus Budget Reconciliation Act (COBRA).[48] Although this law encompassed many more matters than health coverage, the insurance rules are commonly referred to as the COBRA law. They provide important protections, although within limits, for those who lose coverage through termination of employment along with their dependents. The rules are enforced by DOL. Among COBRA's key provisions is a rule that lets employees who lose health coverage because of a layoff or other involuntary separation from employment continue to participate in their employer's plan for up to eighteen months. This assures displaced workers of uninterrupted access to benefits, although it does not guarantee affordability. They must pay the entire cost of the premium, both the share they had been paying and the share their employer had contributed, plus a small fee. Spouses who lose coverage because of divorce from or death of a covered employee may continue to purchase coverage for up to thirty-six months from the employer's group plan.

COBRA's protections are overseen by DOL. While the COBRA law does not directly regulate the business of insurance, which remains the responsibility of the states, it does add another kind of federal regulation governing the way insurance is provided. COBRA has saved many workers and their family members from falling into the ranks of the uninsured. However, in the fashion of so many other health care regulatory programs, it does so in an incremental manner as part of a complex web of uncoordinated rules.

Continuation of employment-based health insurance has value only so long as the underlying coverage is available. If an employer does not offer health benefits to begin with, then continuation is not an option. For many small companies, health insurance is unobtainable because their workforce includes members with serious and expensive to treat medical conditions. Without a large pool of employees across which to spread the risk, premiums for these firms tend to be prohibitively high. In some cases, insurers may drop coverage for them entirely.

Congress's next focus of attention in the incremental reform of health insurance was the unavailability of coverage for employees with preexisting medical conditions, and for their employers. Having failed to enact the comprehensive health care reform envisioned in the plan proposed by President Bill Clinton in 1993, health reform advocates decided to pursue this and a few other issues as a more modest goal. The Health Insurance Portability and Accountability Act of 1996 (HIPAA)[49] restricted the ability of health insurers to use preexisting consideration in initiating or continuing coverage. (In separate provisions, HIPAA also contains standards for maintaining the privacy of medical records, which are discussed in chapter 7.)

Under HIPAA, insurers may not deny workers insurance because of a preexisting medical condition if they have a sufficient number of years of prior continuous coverage. Similarly, insurers may not deny or refuse to renew coverage for entire employer groups because of the preexisting condition of one of the members, although they may set higher premiums that take account of the greater expected expense. As a companion program to COBRA, the administration of these rules was also assigned to DOL. Congress has also charged DOL with enforcing a few federal enactments that set minimum standards for private health insurance policies with regard to coverage of specific services. They include the Mental Health Parity Act of 1996 concerning lifetime and annual limits on mental health services,[50] the Newborns' and Mothers' Health Protection Act of 1996 concerning hospital stays after childbirth,[51] and the women's Health and Cancer Rights Act of 1998 concerning reconstructive surgery after mastectomies.[52]

Like COBRA, HIPAA has provided important protection for many smaller companies and their workers. However, in the same manner as COBRA, it is an incremental reform with a highly circumscribed target population. Gaps in access to insurance remain for many workers, in particular, those whose employers do not offer health benefits.

The History and Structure of Direct Government Funding: Medicare, Medicaid, and Related Programs

Policy debates over whether the United States should follow the European model of government-funded health insurance continued unabated through the period of private insurance growth during the second half of the twentieth century as they do up to this day. President Harry Truman proposed a national health insurance plan in 1946 but had to settle for a more modest legislative package, primarily including the Hill-Burton hospital funding program, which is described in more detail later in this chapter and in chapter 3. Several other comprehensive plans have been proposed over the years, but none has yet been enacted. However, national health insurance has been adopted for two significant vulnerable populations—the elderly and the poor.

The First Tentative Step to Federal Health Care Funding: The Hill-Burton Act

The one major piece of health care legislation to emerge from the Truman years was the Hospital Survey and Construction Act of 1946, commonly known as the Hill-Burton Act.[53] It did much to improve access to health care, although not on a comprehensive scale.[54] It is significant as the first national health care financing initiative to focus on private providers. The law provided federal funds for hospital construction in underserved regions, both for building new hospitals and for expanding existing ones. The primary beneficiaries were institutions in rural areas, many of which had few if any hospitals at the time. Over the next thirty years, the Hill-Burton Act engendered a massive spurt of hospital construction across the country that succeeded in bringing health care within the geographic reach of millions.

The enduring legacy of Hill-Burton stems as much from its regulatory aspects as from the direct effects of its funding provisions. The law imposed a set of new requirements on hospitals that received funds.[55] Today, it is almost taken for granted that hospitals adhere to the policies that the law implemented, but in 1946 they were considered as innovations. First, the law prohibited discrimination in the provision of hospital services on the basis of race, religion, or national origin. Eighteen years before the federal Civil Rights Act was enacted, Hill-Burton broke new ground in the federal enforcement of equal rights.[56] Beyond nondiscrimination, hospitals were required to offer minimum amounts of uncompensated care to those unable to pay. They were also mandated to maintain emergency rooms open to all.

The rules imposed by the Hill-Burton Act proved to be long-lived. In the 1970s, Congress interpreted the law's regulatory requirements to apply indefinitely to any hospital that had ever accepted any funding.[57] Given the program's expansive generosity, this included the vast majority of hospitals across the country. Since most of those rules implemented policies that are also embodied in other laws, not to mention commonly accepted notions of ethics, this did not create a new hardship. However, in the 1970s, Congress went one step further in declaring that Hill-Burton-funded hospitals could be subject to subsequent regulations as well.[58] In particular, they could be required to participate in the Medicare and Medicaid programs.

Hill-Burton's open access rules for hospitals were only one aspect of the law's enduring regulatory legacy. Perhaps even more significant was the initiation of a policy of government oversight of the distribution of hospitals and health care resources. In implementing the funding provisions of the law, Congress directed that states begin the first experiments with centralized health planning to decide how the funds would be allocated. The experiment bore fruit thirty years later when Congress enacted a national program of government health planning, which formed the basis for certificate-of-need programs to control hospital expansion. (Health planning is discussed in more detail in chapter 3.) The law also set a precedent for active federal involvement in funding health care on a national scale, which helped to lay the eventual groundwork for political acceptance of Medicare and Medicaid. As with many major health care regulatory and funding structures, therefore, the influence of the Hill-Burton Act has endured decades after its initial mission was fulfilled. President Truman may not have carried the post–New Deal goal of national health insurance to fruition, but he achieved much more in shaping American health care than he likely realized.

The Momentum toward Government Health Insurance Coverage in the Early 1960s

After President Truman's efforts in the late 1940s failed to achieve a national plan, serious political concern with the issue did not return until the late 1950s.[59] Attention surfaced in 1960, when Congress passed the Kerr-Mills Act, a limited program of federal support for health care expenses of the indigent elderly.[60] Political momentum for a more comprehensive program started to build again in the early 1960s under President John Kennedy. He sought to reinvigorate the efforts of President Truman, but political opposition to national health insurance remained fierce. Rather than risking defeat for a comprehensive plan that would cover all citizens, he turned to a more limited approach with a focus on those segments of the population most vulnerable to the financial burden of health care costs and least likely to have access to employer-sponsored coverage, the elderly and the poor.

Even with this more restricted agenda, however, proposals for a national health insurance program were thwarted by continuing opposition in Congress.[61] In particular, the American Medical Association (AMA) fought to restrict any new federal initiative to an entirely voluntary program limited to the lower income elderly.[62]

However, the prospects for a new national health insurance program changed dramatically in 1964, with President Lyndon Johnson's landslide victory and the Democrats in control of Congress. A series of compromises was negotiated in early 1965, and by July, a package had been developed and enacted into law.

The Basic Compromise Structure of Medicare and Medicaid

The Medicare and Medicaid programs that emerged represented a set of initiatives with three distinct parts.[63] Medicare Part A covers hospital expenses for everyone over the age of sixty-five. It was expanded in 1972 to include as beneficiaries those who are totally disabled and, as discussed later, those who require kidney dialysis for end-stage renal disease. Medicare Part B covers physician and outpatient services for the same populations, but participation is voluntary and there is an annual premium. While 95 percent of eligible Americans choose to participate and to pay the premium, coverage is not automatic. Under both Part A and Part B, substantial deductibles and copayments apply. The overall structure was modeled on the insurance policies commonly offered at the time by Blue Cross and Blue Shield plans.[64]

As with typical private health insurance plans of 1965, Medicare coverage was not complete. In addition to copayments and deductibles, beneficiaries were on their own in paying for prescription drugs, other than those administered in a hospital or in a physician's office, and for long-term nursing care, other than 100 days immediately following a hospitalization. To fill these gaps, beneficiaries could purchase their own private supplemental insurance policies, commonly called "Medigap" insurance. These policies vary in their generosity, with some covering virtually all health care expenses left unaddressed by Medicare and some primarily absolving patients of responsibility for copayments and deductibles. However, none of the policies cover long-term nursing care. The premiums and benefits available under Medigap policies must comply with federal guidelines and with state insurance regulation. Many retired workers receive equivalent coverage that supplements Medicare under company and union retirement plans.

The final piece of the package is Medicaid, which covers various designated categories of beneficiaries with very low incomes, generally low enough to qualify for welfare. In contrast to Medicare, which is purely federal, Medicaid is operated jointly by the federal government and the states. Overall program parameters are set at the federal level, while implementation and some details of coverage and eligibility are determined by each state. Funding is shared according to a formula, with the federal share covering between half and 70 percent of state program costs. Coverage is not automatic, and beneficiaries must apply to participate. In most states, Medicaid is administered by the department of welfare, although some house it in the department of health and some in a department of aging. The combination of state implementation and federal oversight has engendered considerable tension over the years between state and federal administrators.

Medicaid is technically offered at the discretion of each state, but the generous nature of available federal matching funds has induced all to participate, the last being Arizona in 1991.[65] Not all of those whose incomes fall below the poverty line are automatically eligible to receive benefits. For the most part, they must fall into one of four categories.[66] The first category consists of pregnant women, who may be covered with incomes above the poverty level at each state's discretion, to encourage prenatal care that may produce better health throughout life for the child. As a result of this benefit, Medicaid covers more than one-third of all births in the United States each year.[67] The second category is children, who again may be covered in families with incomes slightly above the poverty level. The third category consists of the poor elderly, who also qualify for Medicare and hence are referred to as "dual eligibles." Medicare provides their basic coverage, but Medicaid contributes premiums, deductibles, copayments, and additional services that Medicare does not provide. Many of these beneficiaries reside in nursing homes, making Medicaid the largest funder of nursing home services in the country. The fourth category is disabled children and adults who qualify for payments under the federal Supplemental Security Income (SSI) program.

States vary considerably in the scope of services that they cover under Medicaid, although a complex set of federal rules limits some of their discretion.[68] Overall, the benefits are more generous than those available under Medicare. In addition to basic physician and hospital services, all states must cover screening programs for children to test for various physical and mental conditions under the Early and Periodic Screening, Diagnosis and Treatment (EPSDT) program.[69] Unlike Medicare, Medicaid programs in all states cover long-term nursing home care. A source of much controversy has been a federal requirement for coverage of some family planning services.[70] Examples of services that some states choose not to cover include podiatry, dental care, and eyeglasses.

The scope of services covered under Medicare and Medicaid has grown over the years, as Congress has repeatedly mandated that they cover new services, including home health care, hospice care, and some screening tests. As new procedures, tests, and devices become available, the federal government reviews them to determine whether they are effective enough to merit reimbursement. This program growth has largely been incremental, overlaying new benefits on the original Medicare and Medicaid structure.

An Early Medicare Coverage Expansion: End-Stage Renal Disease

The first substantial expansion of Medicare's scope came in 1972 with the addition of coverage for kidney dialysis to treat end-stage renal disease (ESRD).[71] The most significant aspect of this benefit from a policy perspective is not the nature of the technology to which it applies but rather the range of beneficiaries whom it assists.[72] Americans of any age, not just those who are elderly, are eligible.

Dialysis cleanses toxins from the blood of patients whose kidneys no longer function. Without it, these patients would die. The technology was perfected for clinical use in the late 1960s, but like many medical miracles, it is extremely expensive. Because of the cost, only a few medical centers around the country were initially able to offer dialysis treatment. Their combined capacity was much smaller than the national need.

The combination of a lifesaving treatment and constraints on its supply created a substantial ethical dilemma. How does a medical center that offers dialysis decide who will live and who will die? Most facilities established committees to allocate this precious, scarce resource among patients, but it is difficult to make such decisions dispassionately. Critics of the system charged that personal biases could not be kept from intruding. This early experience with medical rationing echoes today in debates over insurance coverage for the ever-growing array of expensive miracle technologies. However, few subsequent rationing challenges have been as stark in balancing insurmountable costs against unambiguous fatal outcomes.

The ESRD program resolved the dilemma by guaranteeing dialysis coverage for all who need it.[73] Medicare, with its recently created administrative structure for handling large-scale health insurance coverage, was a natural bureaucratic home for the benefit. In 1978, Congress created a set of ESRD Network Organizations to serve as liaisons between Medicare and providers of ESRD services.[74] Today, there are eighteen Network Organizations that operate on a private basis under contract with the Centers for Medicare & Medicaid Services (CMS) to oversee quality, collect administrative data, and provide technical assistance.[75] All of them belong to the Forum of ESRD Networks, a nonprofit organization that coordinates their activities. In 2003, a total of 311,142 patients received dialysis under the ESRD Program.

Recent Medicare Coverage Expansion:
Managed Care and Prescription Drugs

Starting in the late 1990s, Congress enacted more substantial structural changes to Medicare. Today, it contains two new parts. Part C combines coverage for inpatient and outpatient services for those beneficiaries who choose to receive benefits through private managed care plans. These plans receive a payment from Medicare for each participant they enroll, and they also may collect a premium. The benefits they offer tend to be more generous in scope than those available under Parts A and B, for example, by fully covering outpatient prescription drugs, but reimbursement is subject to the typical constraints of managed care, including review and prior authorization of diagnostic tests and procedures. Part C was called Medicare+Choice under the Balanced Budget Act (BBA) of 1997 but was renamed Medicare Advantage by the Medicare Prescription Drug, Improvement, and Modernization Act (MMA) of 2003.[76]

Part D was enacted as part of the MMA. It represents the first major expansion of Medicare's benefit structure since the program's creation in 1965 by adding reimbursement for outpatient prescription drugs. The coverage is limited in a number of respects, and participation is voluntary and subject to a premium, but it brings substantial new federal funding to an additional aspect of health care.[77] Prior to the enactment of Part D, prescription drugs were covered by Medicaid programs in all states and by pharmaceutical assistance plans for the poor that a few states administer, while Medicare had covered prescription pharmaceuticals only when administered to hospital inpatients or by a physician in an office setting. Under Part D, federal reimbursement is available for prescription drugs obtained on an outpatient basis.

The Part D benefit involves a complex administrative process. It is primarily administered by private companies known as pharmacy benefit managers (PBMs) and by HMOs, which purchase drugs from pharmaceutical manufacturers and arrange for beneficiaries to receive them from retail pharmacies and through mail-order mechanisms. PBMs and HMOs that play this role are designated as prescription drug plans (PDPs). For the most part, the government's role is in oversight rather than direct administration. The MMA explicitly bars it from negotiating prices directly with manufacturers or from actually administering the benefit, except in regions without a participating PDP. However, the oversight role requires numerous detailed decisions concerning which kinds of drugs must be covered, what regions will be served by the PDPs, how coverage will be coordinated with Medicaid, and many other issues that are central to the program's operation. The prescription drug benefit, therefore, creates an intricate relationship between the federal government and a range of private parties, including PBMs, HMOs, pharmaceutical manufacturers, and retail pharmacies. It relies on one of the most complex regulatory schemes in all of American health care.

The set of complex interactions that the MMA implements is particularly intricate in its effect on the relationship between federal oversight and state administration of Medicaid.[78] As described, for health care needs other than prescription drugs, state agencies arrange for the provision of benefits to Medicaid beneficiaries within federal guidelines, and the federal government reimburses a portion of the overall expense according to a legislatively mandated formula. This arrangement applies to beneficiaries who arc dually eligible for both Medicare and Medicaid for those expenses that are covered under Medicaid but not by Medicare. However, the process for funding prescription drugs follows a different pattern.

Dually eligible beneficiaries receive drug coverage under Medicare, rather than under Medicaid as they had prior to passage of the MMA. Unlike other beneficiaries who must affirmatively enroll, they are automatically registered for the drug benefit, since it is a standard component of all state Medicaid programs. However, they pay no premiums to participate, are not subject to deductibles on coverage, and are responsible for only limited copayments. Those who do not select a private plan to administer their drug coverage are randomly assigned to one that operates in their region. The cost of their coverage is assumed by Medicare, but it is then charged back against their state of residence. In other words, the states are required to reimburse the Medicare program for outpatient drug costs incurred by their elderly Medicare beneficiaries.

This recoupment mechanism is commonly referred to as the "clawback." Many states complain that it actually raises their Medicaid costs, since it forces them to pay for prescription drugs without the authority to impose cost-control restrictions, as they had been able to do prior to the MMA. Advocates of the MMA counter that it will streamline coverage to have all Medicare beneficiaries, whether or not they are also eligible for Medicaid, in the same program. Whatever the ultimate effect, the clawback mechanism adds a layer of complexity and an opportunity for potential conflict to the interaction between the state and federal levels of government in the administration of health care finance.

Pervasive Policy Disputes in Structuring Medicare and Medicaid

The compromise structure of Medicare and Medicaid, with different parts and levels of federal, state, and private involvement, addressed a number of sensitive policy issues that challenged Congress when the programs were created. For the most part, they remain contentious today. The underlying philosophical basis for the programs is the most fundamental of them. Liberals have tended to favor a social insurance mechanism for government health care in which general government revenues directly finance a system that covers everyone equally. Conservatives have tended to favor a voluntary insurance system in which government funding supplements premiums paid to private plans by beneficiaries who choose to participate. The complex structure of Medicare and Medicaid includes some aspects of each approach, with hospitalization and indigent care covered fully through direct government reimbursement, and outpatient services for the elderly, prescription drugs, and managed care participation covered for those beneficiaries who select coverage.

Debates rage today about whether Medicare should continue to cover everyone equally or should target its benefits to those in the greatest financial need. Means testing was rejected in 1965 but remains a controversial proposal today. Under the MMA, premiums for Part B are graduated according to income, implementing a partial means basis for receiving benefits. Even without means testing, liberals and conservatives continue to debate whether the same benefit structure should universally apply. Liberals tend to favor the existing arrangement of unified benefits administered by a federal agency, which is consistent with a social insurance model. Some conservatives support changing Medicare into a program that assists beneficiaries in purchasing private insurance policies that can vary in scope.

A second sensitive policy area is the role of the states. Whereas Medicare is administered at the federal level, Medicaid follows a joint approach in which states take the lead in implementation and vary widely in some aspects of administration. At one extreme, the state of Oregon in the 1990s instituted a system of explicit rationing of expensive treatments, which is discussed later in this chapter. Other states use managed care companies to varying degrees to make coverage determinations. Each of these experiments requires a federal waiver of basic Medicaid rules, which have met conflicting responses under different presidential administrations.

Advocates of substantial latitude for states point to the opportunities that these experiments offer to try novel solutions to perennial challenges. Variations in Medicaid administration also enable states to tailor their programs to local needs and values. Advocates of a more standardized program point to the unfairness that variation in the generosity of Medicaid programs creates for poor residents of stingier states, and to the administrative complexity of operating separate programs in each state.

Finally, even within a nationally unified government structure, policy makers continue to debate the appropriate role of the private sector. The compromises of 1965 and those that followed left important functions to private companies. They administer coverage under all parts of Medicare and bear responsibility for a wide range of coverage decisions. Private contractors are selected separately for each state, with those that process benefits under Part A known as "intermediaries" and under Part B as "carriers." Intermediaries and carriers have substantial decision-making latitude in their areas of responsibility. Over the years, private managed care companies have also played a growing role under both Medicare and Medicaid. As discussed, under the Part C Medicare Advantage program, beneficiaries can choose to receive coverage directly from a private managed care plan. Under Medicare Part D, prescription reimbursement is administered primarily by private PDPs. Even under Medicaid, most states now administer benefits through private managed companies, a trend that began in the 1980s.

The results of private administration of benefits are highly controversial. Some contend that the discipline of the market makes private contractors more efficient than government agencies at program administration.[79] Opponents counter that private firms bear costs for expenses such as marketing and executive compensation that actually make them less efficient than the government. The compromises between these views that have been achieved over the years have contributed to the complexity of Medicare and Medicaid administration.

Getting the Programs Off the Ground

Signed into law by President Johnson on July 30, 1965, Medicare was scheduled to be implemented on July 1, 1966. Medicaid was rolled out locally by each of the fifty states, but Medicare required nationwide implementation.[80] Without an administrative structure of their own, Medicare was initially housed in the Social Security Administration (SSA), and Medicaid's federal component in the Social and Rehabilitative Service Administration (SRSA). Both of these were part of the Department of Health, Education, and Welfare (HEW) (now the Department of Health and Human Services [DHHS]).[81]

Since eligibility for hospital coverage under Medicare Part A was automatic, all of the 26 million citizens over the age of sixty-five at the time were deemed covered without any special action on their part. However, coverage for physician services under Part B required that beneficiaries enroll and pay an annual deductible, at that time three dollars. This necessitated a campaign to locate beneficiaries and inform them of their new entitlement. Those most likely to be unaware of the program lived in rural and often inaccessible areas. Therefore, step one of Medicare implementation was a massive publicity and outreach effort to locate millions of elderly citizens in the far corners of the country.

Step two was to enroll providers. SSA used state agencies to certify that hospitals met basic participation standards, including compliance with the newly enacted federal Civil Rights Act.[82] Physicians across the country were notified about their rights under the new program and the rights of their patients. However, this initial effort produced relatively modest results when compared with the program's present size. Only about 35 percent of hospitals and 10 percent of physicians chose to participate.[83]

Step three, which was accomplished concurrently with provider certification, was to implement contracts with insurance companies to serve as carriers and intermediaries to implement the claims payment and coverage determination process. Companies were selected in each state, and most were Blue Cross or Blue Shield plans. This became a lucrative line of business for many of them.

Given the magnitude of the task, SSA needed help from other branches of government, and the overall effort represented a collaboration of work by a number of agencies. Among the others called on to assist in the effort were the Public Health Service, the Welfare Administration, the Internal Revenue Service, the Civil Service Commission, the General Services Administration, the Postal Service, and the Forest Service.[84] Rarely has a domestic policy initiative commanded such broad attention from across the government bureaucracy or reflected as high a level of motivation by the personnel involved.

Beyond the operational logistics of implementing Medicare and Medicaid, SSA faced the task of developing a body of operating policies in areas ranging from provider certification to contract administration by intermediaries and carriers.[85] To provide additional expertise, Congress authorized creation of the Health Insurance Benefits Advisory Council (HIBAC), made up of high-level private officials with varying kinds of relevant expertise. Their input helped to guide policy development.

This new body was housed within SSA, which hired its staff and arranged for it to consult with various constituent groups.

In 1979, responsibility for administering Medicare and the federal portion of Medicaid was transferred to a new agency within DHHS, the Health Care Finance Administration (HCFA). The programs had reached a size that required a dedicated bureaucratic home. HCFA is today known as the Centers for Medicare & Medicaid Services (CMS).

The Programs' Growth

Growth in the size of Medicare and Medicaid since their inception has been dramatic. They are widely popular and now form a pillar of the American health care system and an integral part of the health care regulatory landscape.[86] Medicare alone represents more than one-quarter of all health care spending in America. In 2004, the Medicare budget reached $295 billion, making it the third most expensive federal program after Social Security and defense.[87] It represented more than one-quarter of all health care spending in America. Enrollment that year had grown to more than 42 million from the original 26 million, including 35.4 million who are elderly and 6.3 million who are disabled or receiving kidney dialysis under the ESRD program. This represents one in every seven Americans. The total Medicaid budget in 2003 reached $276 billion, an increase of about one-third from the budget in 2000, and enrollment reached more than 50 million.[88]

In addition to the 50 million people that Medicaid covers, it serves as a safety net for millions more who live on the edge of poverty and are constantly at risk of losing employment-based health insurance coverage. Medicaid is also vitally important to many inner-city and rural hospitals. Were it not for this program, many more indigent patients would appear in emergency rooms with no means of payment. By providing a source of reimbursement for services rendered to them, Medicaid forms a safety net for hospitals as well.

The Evolution of Medicare and Medicare Cost Control

In retrospect it may seem obvious, but at the time of Medicare and Medicaid's implementation, many policy makers were surprised by the rapid rate of spending growth that followed. With a huge new pot of government money available for reimbursement and no external impediments to rendering and billing the government for them, utilization of medical services expanded dramatically. Under the early Medicare program, physician reimbursement was based on a percentage of the prevailing charge for each service rendered. Hospital payments were based on the actual cost of treating beneficiaries. There was no meaningful review of services for necessity as a condition of reimbursement. Inspired by the need to control costs, a series of regulatory innovations in both programs eventually led to a revolution in their financing mechanisms.

Peer Review

The government's first attempt to manage the care rendered under Medicare and Medicaid was fairly modest. It took the form of peer review of the utilization patterns of participating physicians. A demonstration program initiated in 1970 established a network of voluntary physician associations known as Experimental Medical Care Review Organizations (EMCROs) to try out the concept.[89] In 1972, Congress made the system permanent with the establishment of professional standards review organizations (PSROs). They were nonprofit physician-led organizations that reviewed hospital admissions and lengths of stay for Medicare and Medicaid patients for each practitioner within a geographic region.[90] PSROs also examined practice patterns for hospitals and conducted medical care evaluation studies (MCEs) to investigate quality of care.

The sanctions available to PSROs to apply against outlier physicians, however, were fairly mild. Moral pressure was the most commonly used. The strongest remedy was to exclude a wayward physician from continued participation in Medicare and Medicaid, but the implementation of this penalty could require lengthy legal proceedings and so was rarely applied. As a result, PSROs were widely perceived as well-intentioned but largely ineffectual.

In 1982, the PSRO program was downgraded into a voluntary network of autonomous peer review organizations that operated under contract with HCFA to review patterns of utilization on a more sporadic basis.[91] They were also permitted to contract with private insurers and other companies to perform similar services. The groups were renamed professional review organizations (PROs), and their numbers were reduced. While they play a lesser role under Medicare and Medicaid than the predecessor PSROs, some have found stable market niches with a combination of public and private customers. In 1993, Congress formally changed their focus from controlling costs to improving quality, and in 2001, they were again renamed, this time as quality improvement organizations (QIOs).[92]

Prospective Payment

Peer review did little to stem the unrelenting rise in Medicare costs during the 1970s and into the 1980s. Many policy analysts placed the blame on Medicare's underlying incentive structure, which rewarded providers who generated fees for rendering as many services as possible. It became increasingly evident that an approach was needed to limit demand for health care services, since limits on supply through peer review or otherwise seemed hopeless.

The approach that was implemented in the 1980s adopted the strategic approach of managed care. (Prospective payment under Medicare is also discussed in chapter 3 concerning the regulation of health care institutions.) The private insurance market had begun to experiment with managed care cost control techniques in the early 1970s with establishment of the first HMOs. As discussed, the underlying premise of the HMO cost control model is that fixed payments that are set in advance will eliminate the incentive for providers to overtreat.

Payments for treating patients can be set prospectively based on different criteria. HMOs pay primary care physicians through capitation, a set amount per patient, in return for rendering all necessary care. Some European systems pay hospitals based on an annual global budget covering all anticipated costs. Some private insurers reimburse hospitals a predetermined amount for each day of admission, regardless of the services actually provided.

The method that Congress selected as the first prospective payment system (PPS) under Medicare applied to hospital coverage under Part A.[93] Under this arrangement, hospitals were reimbursed based on each patient's diagnosis at discharge. This method, first developed by the New Jersey Medicaid program in the late 1970s, based reimbursement on a list of 465 diagnostic groupings, known as "diagnosis-related groups" (DRGs), which could characterize every Medicare hospitalization. (DRGs are also discussed in terms of their regulatory effects in chapter 3.) The list has since been expanded to include 540 groupings. DRGs are organized by physiological system into twenty-three categories. In addition to the patient's principal diagnosis, they take into account major secondary diagnoses, whether a surgical procedure was performed, and in some cases significant patient demographic characteristics such as age, gender, and discharge status.

To receive payment, the treating hospital assigns a single DRG to each patient at discharge, and each DRG generates a predetermined reimbursement amount. The amount remains constant regardless of the number of days of treatment or the actual services provided, but with a few exceptions. Supplements are permitted for particularly complex "outlier" cases. Teaching hospitals are eligible for additional supplements to cover the indirect cost of training residents and fellows, and for supplements outside of the DRG system to cover education-related direct costs. Hospitals in inner cities and in rural areas that treat a "disproportionate share" of indigent patients may also receive an extra payment.[94] However, as with the underlying DRG payment, these supplements do not vary directly according to the quantity of services actually rendered.

The first step in implementing Medicare prospective payment was enactment of the Tax Equity and Fiscal Responsibility Act (TEFRA) in 1982.[95] That law set per case limits on cost-based reimbursement and directed the Medicare program to develop an implementation plan for a full prospective payment system for hospitals. The DRG system that was devised in response was implemented starting on

October 1, 1983, and phased in over the next four years. Initially it applied only to reimbursement for hospital operating expenses. The system was expanded in 1991 to include capital expenses and in the late 1990s to include outpatient care. Many states now use it in their Medicaid programs.

DRG-based reimbursement is credited with substantially reducing the growth of Medicare hospital spending.[96] However, concurrent with the success of DRGs at controlling hospital costs was a dramatic upturn in the rate of growth in spending for physician and other outpatient services under Medicare Part B.[97] These services remained under a fee-for-service reimbursement model, and hospitals become adept at moving services to the most remunerative setting.

Congress did not authorize a prospective payment system for physician services when the DRG system was established, but it did approve a revised reimbursement approach that was implemented several years later based on an unconventional type of fee schedule. The new approach measured the amount of effort and resources involved in rendering each service and determined a corresponding payment without regard to prevailing rates. This was intended to rationalize the reimbursement structure according to the value actually provided to patients.

The new physician fee schedule was called the Resource-Based Relative Value Scale (RBRVS). It set payments for each service according to three factors—the technical and personnel resources used, the physician training required, and the associated malpractice insurance costs.[98] RBRVS was implemented by HCFA in 1992, with the intent to reimburse for the actual costs of providing each medical service, leaving no room for physicians to use market conditions to inflate fees. An immediate and anticipated effect of RBRVS was to reduce the fees paid for more technical and procedure-oriented services, such as surgery, and to increase fees paid for services with more of a cognitive focus, such as primary care. This result was consistent with an underlying premise of managed care to encourage the provision of services at the least specialized level possible.

RBRVS remains in place today, and its implementation has been highly controversial.[99] A common criticism is that physicians whose fees have declined have compensated by increasing the volume of services that they render. Congress addressed this possibility by directing Medicare to adjust payment rates each year based on utilization trends in each specialty. These adjustments provide a theoretical solution, but lobbying by organizations representing different specialties to override them has tended to limit their effectiveness.

Since its initial implementation, the application of prospective payment to Medicare reimbursement has grown beyond acute-care hospital services. In 1997, as part of the BBA, Congress directed the agency to implement prospective payment arrangements for long-term care and for hospital outpatient care. The long-term care system went into effect in 2000 based on resource utilizations groups (RUGs), which measure the resources needed to care for different categories of patients.[100]

The ambulatory care system was applied starting in 2000 based on ambulatory payment classification groups (APCs), which measure the costs of rendering groupings of related services.

The implementation of each of these prospective payment systems is extremely complex. To determine the payment for each grouping, the financial components of every health care service for which reimbursement may be made must be analyzed, including those rendered in acute inpatient, outpatient, and long-term care settings. Technical corrections are regularly needed. Nevertheless, this approach to reimbursement appears to have succeeded in controlling costs to an extent that alternative methods have not.

Beyond reducing costs, however, prospective payment raises larger issues. Determining payment amounts according to the components of each health care service requires clinical as well as financial expertise. It necessitates decisions on the most appropriate way to deliver services and on the most accurate calculation of costs. Prospective payment scales create their own incentives and disincentives for the use of different specialists, services, and treatments.[101] In creating and administering these scales, Medicare cannot avoid influencing the clinical, as well as financial, aspects of health care. Consequently, under prospective payment the financing of care is inextricably intertwined with the regulation of care.

When Congress created Medicare, it included specific assurances in the legislation that in paying for care, the government would not direct the provision of care.[102] However, paying for a service inevitably creates opportunities for influence, at least indirectly. Since CMS controls such a large proportion of the nation's total health care expenditures, the repercussions of these decisions extend well beyond the care received by beneficiaries of government programs. As a result, Medicare has grown to become much more than a passive facilitator of health care access.

Resolving Payment Issues

In a program of Medicare's size, operational judgments continuously arise. CMS faces numerous decisions on questions ranging from what it will cover to how it will make payments. With coverage extending to more than 40 million people, there is much at stake in the outcomes, and disputes are inevitable. Several bureaucratic mechanisms administer the decision-making process.

Deciding What Will Be Covered

Medicine advances almost every day with new products and procedures. Some perform miracles that are clearly worth their cost, but many are largely ineffective. The Medicare program has to decide which will be eligible for coverage. Decisions on smaller items are made by private intermediaries and carriers operating under contract with CMS for the regions that they administer, but expensive new technologies require uniform national policies.[103] There was a time when the judgment of treating clinicians alone could be relied upon for such determinations, but the growing cost of medical technology has necessitated a more formal assessment process.

In 1998, DHHS established the Medicare Coverage Advisory Committee (MCAC) to provide CMS with outside expertise for coverage determinations of expensive new technologies.[104] The committee includes seventy-eight medical experts and fourteen representatives of industry and consumer interests, who consider medical advances within their areas of knowledge.[105] When a new medical technology is presented for consideration, a smaller committee composed of thirteen to fifteen MCAC members with relevant expertise reviews the medical literature, technology assessments, and other information on effectiveness and appropriateness. Consumer and industry representatives are included as nonvoting members in the group. Based on this review, the committee recommends whether CMS should provide reimbursement and under what conditions. CMS is not bound to follow the committee's advice, but it generally does. Coverage decisions that apply program-wide are known as national coverage determinations (NCDs). They can be initiated by the agency itself or by members of the public, including patients and manufacturers.

Because of the size of Medicare, CMS coverage determinations can have tremendous implications for the availability of new medical treatments and for companies wishing to sell them. The decisions gain even greater weight from their influence on private insurance plans, many of which follow Medicare's lead. Convincing CMS to cover a new product or procedure, therefore, can constitute one of the most important challenges in bringing it to market. The agency's role in deciding on coverage further reinforces its pervasive influence in the overall health care industry.

Administering Prospective Payment

Since Medicare's prospective payment system is extremely complex, its implementation requires numerous determinations that have clinical, financial, and administrative components. Classifying all diagnoses into DRGs is just the start. The DRGs must be ranked according to relative costs to treat, a reference value must be set, the size of supplemental payments must be calculated, and new developments in medical practice must be incorporated when they arise. The RBRVS system for determining physician reimbursement raises similar challenges. These are daunting for an administrative process designed for making only actuarial and accounting decisions.

To assist in the task of administering prospective payment, Congress created two independent advisory bodies as part of the 1983 law that implemented DRG-based reimbursement. The Prospective Payment Assessment Commission (ProPAC) advised HCFA on setting hospital payments and on identifying medically appropriate patterns of resource use. In developing its recommendations, the commission was authorized to conduct and fund research on medical practices. The

Physician Payment Review Commission (PPRC) advised HCFA on physician reimbursement issues.

The BBA merged the two advisory bodies into the Medicare Payment Advisory Commission (MedPAC). This group is charged with advising Congress directly on issues that broadly affect the Medicare program.[106] It also evaluates payments to private managed care plans that participate in Medicare Part C and to physicians under Part B. More generally, it analyzes access to care, quality of care, and other issues affecting the provision of services under Medicare.

MedPAC includes seventeen commission members representing expertise in health care financing and delivery. They are appointed for three-year terms by the U.S. controller general, who leads the Government Accountability Office (GAO), thereby maintaining independence from CMS, the agency whose actions they evaluate. The primary vehicle for disseminating MedPAC recommendations is a pair of reports issued in March and June of each year, which focus on areas of special concern to the commissioners. It issues additional reports on subjects requested by Congress. MedPAC has no direct regulatory authority. It can only advise. However, its recommendations carry considerable weight, and its reports can be extremely influential.

Provider-Specific Disputes

In the complex maze that funnels Medicare reimbursement to those who provide care, what happens when a provider feels that its payment is incorrect? With reimbursement set by CMS, reviewed by MedPAC, and administered by private carriers and intermediaries, there is no obvious place to turn. In enacting prospective payment, Congress sought to limit appeals in the interest of streamlining administration. It directed disputes over individual payments to a single review body and severely restricted broader legal recourse. The Provider Reimbursement Review Board (PRRB) hears appeals of complaints by hospitals and physicians of individual reimbursement decisions made by Medicare carriers and intermediaries and by CMS.[107]

In placing restrictions on review of CMS reimbursement decisions, Congress also limited the direct role of lawyers in the ongoing implementation of prospective payment. However, health care providers were not left entirely without recourse. Political lobbying has replaced legal proceedings in resolving many disputes over Medicare reimbursement policy. The extreme complexity of prospective payment has created opportunities for lobbyists to exert considerable influence over members of Congress and regulators in the range of decisions that they make in setting payment formulas and determining reimbursement amounts. As a result, Medicare prospective payment now consumes a significant amount of congressional attention. Providers may function in a private market, but the market is shaped in large part by politics and regulations emanating from all levels of government.

Experiments with Managed Care

Beyond prospective payment, the apparent overall success of managed care at controlling health care costs in the 1970s and 1980s inspired government policy makers to investigate ways to adopt the HMO model to Medicare and Medicaid more directly. As discussed, this has resulted in a specific role for HMOs under Medicare Part C. As with prospective payment for hospitals, the path was blazed at the state level through Medicaid.

In 1981, Congress gave states the flexibility to experiment with alternative arrangements for delivering health care services under Medicaid, including the use of private HMOs, by requesting a waiver from HCFA.[108] Instead of receiving benefits directly from the state, participants in the program were required to enroll in HMOs, which provided coverage for them under contract. The HMOs could then use all of their cost control armaments, including peer review, prior authorization, and restricted provider networks, to reduce spending in the system. Medicaid programs using managed care were still required to meet basic coverage parameters, but with HCFA's consent, they could take advantage of considerable leeway to structure the administration of benefits.

Over the next decade a growing number of states chose to take advantage of this flexibility so that today, Medicaid coverage administered through private HMOs has become the norm and is used to at least some extent in all states.[109] Many private HMOs now offer plans that are geared specifically to Medicaid patients, and HMOs that focus exclusively on Medicaid have emerged. Many of the Medicaid managed care arrangements are quite complex, with separate companies covering narrow areas of service, such as mental health and prescription drugs, that are "carved out" from the rest of health care.[110] Much of CMS's regulatory activity regarding Medicaid now focuses on reviewing state waiver applications, and much of the work of state Medicaid agencies focuses on preparing them.

HCFA implemented a trial of managed care in the administration of Medicare in the 1980s, which eventually led to the creation of Part C. In 1985, it first offered capitation payments to HMOs to cover Medicare recipients.[111] Under this arrangement, beneficiaries paid premiums to an HMO in lieu of the premium for Part B that they would otherwise pay to HCFA. The premiums were supplemented by additional capitation payments made by HCFA to the HMOs. These plans replaced the copayments and deductibles that otherwise applied under Part B with lower amounts, and some plans included reimbursement for outpatient prescription drugs, which was not available at all under traditional Medicare at that time.

In return, access to care was managed and controlled as it was under private HMO plans.

As discussed, in 1997 Congress restructured these HMO arrangements as part of the BBA into a separate Medicare Part C with the name Medicare+Choice.[112] It permitted a wider range of managed care organizations, including preferred provider organizations and health plans organized by providers, to join HMOs in offering coverage, and it set new formulas for determining the capitation payments paid by HCFA. In 2003, Congress increased funding for the arrangements under the MMA.

The use of managed care under Medicare has proved considerably more controversial than its use under Medicaid. Proposals to expand its availability have reignited debates from the program's creation concerning the appropriate role for the private sector.[113] Proponents of relying on private managed care plans believe that competition among private insurers can bring the efficiency and innovation of the market to a bureaucratic governmental program. Opponents fear that adverse selection will siphon healthy patients from traditional Medicare to HMOs, a trend that could ultimately make the existing program of generous coverage unsustainable. Such controversies over the appropriate role for the private sector have raged since Medicare's inception and will likely continue to do so for the foreseeable future.

The Oregon Experiment

The vast majority of state waivers for Medicaid experiments seek to use private HMOs to administer some or all benefits according to a fairly common pattern. However, one experiment stands out as a revolution in financing health care. In the early 1990s, the state of Oregon asked HCFA for permission to explicitly ration health care for its Medicaid beneficiaries.[114] While rationing has been debated in America as a way to control rising costs and has been used for some time under the National Health Service in England, it had been considered too laden with ethical and emotional overtones to implement in the United States. Oregon set out to change that.

The premise of the Oregon approach was to rationalize health care spending. Some clinical interventions, such as childhood immunizations and antibiotics for strep throat, cost very little in relation to the health benefits that they achieve. Others, such as some kinds of surgery for advanced forms of cancer, are extremely expensive and produce only marginal health gains. The goal of the plan was to reduce spending on the least cost-effective treatments so that the more cost-effective ones could be made more widely available.

To implement the approach, Oregon planned to rank all procedures that Medicaid could cover according to the ratio of cost and benefits. Those falling below a predetermined threshold would be ineligible for reimbursement. The money saved through this rationing process would be used to expand the pool of Medicaid-eligible recipients to include those just above the poverty level. This would bring basic health care, including preventive care, to many pregnant women and poor children who, as healthier adults, would hopefully require fewer health care services in the future.

Oregon's proposal was extremely controversial. While it could produce net health benefits on an overall population basis, it denied to the state's poorest residents treatments for life-threatening conditions that could be obtained by those who were wealthier and privately insured. The state negotiated for several years with HCFA to obtain approval. Some changes were made, most notably to the process for ranking medical procedures. Ultimately, HCFA did approve the plan, and today Oregon administers the only explicit health care rationing program in the United States. No other state has yet followed Oregon's lead, but the plan stands as a bold experiment in the regulation of health care finance.

A Shock to the System: The Balanced Budget Act of 1997

The BBA, which modified the structure of Medicare managed care, produced its most drastic impact on the program by imposing substantial reductions in many elements of reimbursement.[115] The most draconian were in payments to hospitals for most DRGs. In addition, large reductions were made to the supplemental payments that teaching hospitals receive to compensate for the cost of training medical residents and fellows and in the payments to inner-city and rural hospitals for treating a disproportionate share of indigent patients. The effects on hospitals across the country were profound, particularly on those that were part of urban academic medical centers.

The BBA also reduced payments for many elements of outpatient care. It mandated adjustments to aggregate RBRVS payments for various physician specialties and imposed payment caps on reimbursement for the services of physical therapists, occupational therapists, and other allied health professionals. It also directed HCFA to implement prospective payment schemes for ambulatory care and for long-term care, which were previously discussed.

The BBA succeeded in dramatically reducing the rate of growth in Medicare spending.[116] However, critics contended that it was too successful. Some hospitals were pushed to the brink of bankruptcy, and many physicians found that their practices had become unprofitable. Subsequent corrections to the act restored some of the funding cuts but only to a limited extent. The harsher financial environment for many health care providers that the act produced has become an ongoing economic reality. The BBA's impact serves to demonstrate the pervasive reliance on government funding programs that has evolved throughout American health care.

Coming to the Aid of Children:
State Children's Health Insurance Programs

While the BBA focused primarily on cutting costs in government health insurance programs, it expanded coverage in one important area. Congress included a compromise provision to extend health benefits to a segment of the population that was particularly vulnerable and in need of health care. That was the children of families with too few financial resources to obtain private health insurance but too many to qualify for Medicaid. A public investment in basic health care for uninsured children promised a high rate of return in prevention of health care needs later on.

The new coverage program was called the Children's Health Insurance Program (CHIP). In the style of other health care policy compromises such as Medicaid, its administration combined federal oversight and funding with administration as a separate program by each participating state. Consequently, it is more commonly referred as the State Children's Health Insurance Program (SCHIP). While its start was somewhat rocky, SCHIP has made an important contribution to reducing the rate of uninsurance in its target population, and in the country overall.

States receive federal funding for SCHIP under a matching formula that is more generous than Medicaid's, so they have a substantial incentive to participate.[117] Federal rules permit coverage for children in families with incomes up to 200 percent of the federal poverty level. There are also requirements for minimum levels of coverage, limits on the premiums that may be charged, and restrictions on the use of deductibles and copayments, including a prohibition on cost sharing for preventive services and immunizations. Beyond these basic rules, states have considerable flexibility in structuring their SCHIP programs. They can add the new coverage as part of existing Medicaid programs or other state-financed health coverage arrangements, or they can establish entirely new programs. As of 2004, states were about equally split in administering SCHIP plans through Medicaid, through separate plans, and through a combination. States also have a choice between providing SCHIP coverage directly or by subsidizing the purchase of private insurance. However, unlike Medicaid, SCHIP is not an entitlement for those who meet eligibility criteria. States receive a fixed federal contribution and can limit the number of beneficiaries that they cover based on it.

SCHIP provided coverage for more than 3.7 million children by 2003.[118] It is an incremental step toward filling gaps in health insurance coverage, but it marks one of the most substantial expansions of eligibility for public coverage since the passage of Medicare and Medicaid in 1965. However, SCHIP's incremental approach leaves the remaining gaps in access to coverage even more glaring. Some families are now in the awkward position of having health insurance for the children who are within SCHIP's target population, but not for the parents. Nevertheless, much of the growth of American health care regulation has been by such incremental steps, which tend to be more politically feasible than more major policy initiatives.

Current Agency Structure

Centers for Medicare & Medicaid Services (CMS)

The agency that administers Medicare and the federal portions of Medicaid and of SCHIP is disproportionately small in comparison to its mission. CMS finances health care for more than 80 million beneficiaries, almost one in three Americans, and processes more than 900 million claims annually.[119] Yet it had a permanent staff of only 4,219 full-time equivalent employees in 1999.[120] This is almost 500 employees fewer than the agency had in 1980.[121] The total CMS budget is more than $480 billion, of which about $2.7 billion is spent on management. This means that CMS operates its programs with an administrative overhead ratio of about 2 percent. The typical private insurer spends about 11 percent of claims payments on administration, or almost six times as much.[122]

CMS's overhead ratio has declined steadily since Medicare and Medicaid were created.[123] Initially, administration of Part B for physician services consumed 11 percent of claims payments, and Part A for hospitals about 3 percent. The ratios fell in large measure due to the replacement of the complex and cumbersome cost-based reimbursement system with prospective payment.

CMS realizes some of its comparative efficiency by maintaining a lower expense structure than private insurers. It engages in limited advertising, compensates its executives with lower salaries, and has no shareholders to whom it pays dividends. However, other factors are also at work. Much of the work of administering Medicare is accomplished by private carriers and intermediaries that perform most of the actual claims processing. Part of the program's administration is also performed by private HMOs that cover some Medicare beneficiaries under the Medicare Advantage program.[124] More than 65,000 state and local government employees also assist in implementing Medicaid and SCHIP. Overall, therefore, CMS outsources a substantial portion of its responsibilities.

Opponents of major Medicare reform point to the program's low overhead as evidence that it is extremely efficient as presently structured and that the federal government is, indeed, capable of effectively administering a national health insurance program. Proponents of reform believe that added administrative costs in the private sector reflect more aggressive efforts to control medical costs. Whatever the larger policy implications, it is clear that the administration of Medicare is extremely lean.

CMS began operations as the Health Care Finance Administration (HCFA), a component of DHHS, in June 1979 with the transfer of responsibility for Medicare and Medicaid from the SSA and SRSA. It remained in the space that its employees had occupied as part of SSA, which was in Baltimore rather than in Washington, D.C. The Medicaid functions that had been housed in the SRSA headquarters in Washington were moved to Baltimore to join them, and the bulk of CMS's employees remain there today. CMS is one of two major federal health care agencies with primary offices outside of Washington, D.C., and its immediate vicinity, the other being CDC, which maintains its headquarters in Atlanta.

HCFA has been described as a perennially "beleaguered" agency.[125] As an organization composed largely of actuaries and claims administrators, its role lacks glamour. Beneficiaries complain that claims are often wrongly denied, providers complain that payments are regularly missed, and Congress periodically investigates administrative inefficiency. In an attempt to burnish its image, the agency changed its name on 1 July 2001, the thirty-fifth anniversary of the implementation of its component programs, to the Centers for Medicare & Medicaid Services.

Many of CMS's central operations and more than a quarter of its management expense are devoted to finding and prosecuting fraud and abuse in the programs that it administers.[126] The amount that CMS collects in recoveries and the number of physicians and hospitals prosecuted are actually quite small in comparison to the size of the programs.[127] However, the deterrent effect of enforcement can be substantial, as the specter of government fraud investigations is a major factor in much health care business planning. (A more detailed discussion of Medicare fraud and abuse enforcement is contained in chapter 7 on the regulation of health care business relationships.)

CMS's influence on American health care is felt not only in the number of beneficiaries whose care it finances and of providers whose reimbursement it processes but also in the effects of its financial decisions on the actual provision of care. As discussed, the prospective payment systems for hospitals, physicians, and other providers require a multitude of detailed judgments on how services are to be categorized and valued. These judgments are reflected in the relative willingness of providers to offer different services. Decisions on coverage of new technologies and medications determine in large part whether they will be available to the American public, since private insurers usually follow CMS's lead in this regard. By administering the funding of graduate medical education at hospitals as part of Medicare Part A, CMS also plays a major role in shaping the training that America's future physicians receive and the relative attractiveness of different medical specialties.

Department of Labor (DOL)

DOL is responsible for the federal oversight of health insurance. This includes the ERISA law that governs self-insured employer plans and the COBRA and HIPAA laws that protect continuation of coverage. Within the department, the responsible agency is the Employee Benefits Security Administration (EBSA), which was known prior to 2003 as the Pension and Welfare Benefits Administration (PWBA).[128] In addition to these major laws, EBSA also administers the Mental Health Parity Act of 1996, the Newborns' and Mothers' Health Protection Act of 1996, and the Women's Health and Cancer Rights Act of 1998.

ERISA is a complex law that addresses pensions as well as health benefits. While EBSA has primary responsibility for regulating health coverage plans, the Internal Revenue Service (IRS) and the Pension Benefit Guarantee Corporation (PBGC) play roles in enforcing other aspects of the law. It is a reflection of the growing importance of oversight of health insurance at the federal level that EBSA was upgraded at the time of its name change in 2003 to a subcabinet position, and its chief was designated as an assistant secretary.[129]

State Insurance Departments

Every state has an agency that regulates insurance. These are usually of medium size compared with other regulatory bodies. Their focus is on financial aspects of insurance company operations, particularly on the amount of financial reserves that insurers must maintain to cover the cost of paying claims. The scope of authority of state insurance departments varies widely.[130] Some review premiums before they may be implemented, and some evaluate the actual language of insurance policies before it may be used. Other states require that premiums and policy language be filed with the insurance department for possible later review, and some merely require notification with no departmental review authority.

Variation among states in insurance regulation is perhaps most pronounced in its political dimension. Some states elect their insurance commissioners, while others rely on gubernatorial appointments. The insurance commissioner of California, for example, is elected, and as a result, insurance regulatory issues often receive considerable media attention during election campaigns. Since they are not appointed by the governor and may belong to the opposing party, elected insurance commissioners often advocate positions contrary to those of their state's chief executive. By way of contrast, Pennsylvania's commissioner is appointed by the governor and tends to pursue policies that are consistent with the governor's policy agenda.

Since the financial aspects of insurance are regulated primarily at the state level, companies that operate nationally may face fifty different sets of conflicting laws and regulations. To achieve some measure of consistency, the commissioners of all state insurance departments belong to a private nonprofit organization known as the National Association of Insurance Commissioners (NAIC).[131] This group develops uniform laws that are recommended for adoption across all states, and in some instances recommends specific regulatory policies. Committees of the NAIC permit state regulators to collaboratively address areas of common concern, such as regulatory policy toward managed care. Although the NAIC has no regulatory or enforcement authority itself and no power to adjudicate actual disputes, its recommendations are often given substantial weight by regulators and legislators, so it can be extremely influential in setting national policy on insurance regulation.

Perennial Policy Conflicts

In health care, as in all industries, to understand the underlying dynamics, you have to follow the money. The flow of financial resources determines what is produced and to whom it is allocated. The financial resources that underpin American health care flow through a collection of different mechanisms, some public and some private. The system is often characterized as a free-market model, yet the government insures more people than do all private insurance companies combined. However, the line between the public and private spheres can be difficult to draw. Within the major government programs, private contractors perform many of the most essential functions. On the other hand, private insurance is heavily regulated and is itself the product of a series of government policy initiatives, including tax preferences and special regulatory status under ERISA. Overall, in health care, the money flows along a complex and convoluted path in which a wide array of entities is involved.

The trail of regulatory oversight that shapes American health care finance is as essential to the dynamics of health care provision as any other factor, including the direct regulation of clinical practice. The financers of health care, once largely passive conduits of money, now actively direct the services that they fund. In one sense, both government and private payers merely act as pass-through mechanisms, with the government programs taking tax dollars and private insurers taking premiums and funneling them to providers. However, the payment structure through which the funds flow exerts tremendous influence on the behavior of those receiving them.[132] Managed care, prospective payment, utilization review, and a host of other mechanisms have turned health care payers into active partners in the provision of clinical care.

Who gave the financers of health care the right to manage the care that they fund? Medicare, Medicaid, and private payers are staffed largely by actuaries and other financial experts, not by clinicians. Are patients well served when another partner shapes their care? Clinicians, after all, are not considered qualified to determine the structure of health care finance.

Although patients and caregivers may complain, in directing compensation to providers, payers must decide what kinds of care legitimately warrant reimbursement. To neglect this role would be to burden the ultimate sources of funding, taxpayers and premium payers, with unjustifiable expenses. In the days before health care placed excessive demands on government budgets and employer benefit programs, there was no compelling need to police reimbursement. Under the financial constraints that have grown over the past two decades, no financing mechanism can survive without carefully considering what it is paying for.

However, to acknowledge that financing inevitably blends into oversight is not to say that any particular scheme is efficient or fair. HMOs are criticized for their intrusiveness into clinical decision making. CMS prospective payment policies may encourage providers to emphasize some services over others that are needed but less generously reimbursed. The challenge is to balance the imperative to control costs with the demands of health care quality and equity.

Of greater concern, despite the bewildering array of public and private programs that address pieces of the financing of health care, each year almost one in six Americans has no coverage at all. The total as of 2003 was almost 45 million.[133] Lack of insurance presents a growing crisis for the American health care system that is found in no other industrialized country. The huge government investment in subsidizing health coverage is approaching $800 million annually when Medicare, Medicaid, SCHIP, FEHBP, Veterans' Administration, military and Indian health care, and the tax subsidy are combined.[134] It operates in combination with the extensive regulatory apparatus that oversees the provision of private insurance. However, a gaping hole in coverage perennially remains. Despite a series of policy initiatives over the past several decades, it only seems to keep getting deeper.

5

Regulation of Drugs and
Health Care Products

The history of progress in food and drug regulation over the past
century is largely the history of the development of science, not the
enactment of statutory provisions.
—P. B. Hutt, *Journal of the Association of Food and Drug Officials*

The quality of the health care that Americans receive depends as much on the tools that clinicians have available as on the clinicians themselves. Without its array of diagnostic and therapeutic products, modern medicine would be quite different. The borders of science are constantly expanding with new drugs, devices, and machines that push the limits of therapeutic possibilities. They redefine medical practice as they proliferate.

While the products that shape modern medicine determine the quality of much of our health care, they are also major drivers of its costs. Over the past several decades, their use has grown dramatically. Drugs, for example, represented 6.6 percent of total American health care spending in 1992, when patients received 1.9 billion prescriptions. In 2002, they represented more than 10 percent, and 3.3 billion prescriptions were written. Total spending on prescription drugs rose from about $45 billion in 1990 to more than $140 billion in 2001.[1]

The central challenge for regulation in this area has historically been to determine whether the products are safe and effective. Americans have come to expect that widely used medical products have received some form of government scrutiny and that passing this scrutiny implies suitability for use. However, it was not always this way. Until the beginning of the twentieth century, drugs and devices received little or no regulatory review, either before or after they entered the market. Even drugs that were known to be ineffective and dangerous escaped government oversight. A series of revelations and scandals over the next sixty years changed that situation, so that today the regulation of drugs and devices, despite some gaps, is as rigorous as it is for any aspect of health care.

In recent years, a new regulatory force has entered the picture. As health care costs have grown, driven in part by advances in technology, payers of care have begun to play a more active role in policing its use. Large health maintenance organizations (HMOs) and the major federal payment programs, Medicare and Medicaid, are becoming particularly vigilant. Even after a drug or device has been approved as safe and effective, its manufacturer must often convince those who will pay the bill that it is worth its cost. As a result, an added layer of regulatory pressure is emerging to address the economics of medical products.

With the stakes in terms of health and cost so high, the regulatory structure that oversees drugs and devices today is extensive. Different but related processes oversee the safety and efficacy of products before and after they reach the market, the intellectual property protections for those who develop new technologies, and the access that patients have to them. The resulting system shapes not only the market for drugs and devices but, as technology continues to command a central place in medical practice, the entire character of American health care.

History and Structure of Food, Drug, and Device Regulation

Regulation of food and drugs dates back as far as recorded history. The laws of Hammurabi in the eighteenth century B.C. addressed the cultivation of corn and its use in commerce.[2] The problem of food adulteration was recognized in the literature of Theophrastus, a pupil of Plato and Aristotle, who investigated its artificial preservation.[3] Other early writings on food adulteration include those of Pliny the Elder concerning additives, preservatives, artificial oils, and wine, and those of Galen, a Greek physician who practiced in Rome during the second century, on food hazards.[4] In 1202, King John of England enacted the first English food law, the Assize of Bread, which prohibited adulteration of bread with other ingredients and also regulated its weight.[5]

The earliest food and drug laws in America date to the colonial period. Since internal food trade within the colonies was rare at this time, most laws were concerned with exports. In a prelude to controversies over American federalism that arose decades later, laws varied greatly from state to state, and firms complained that they had to manufacture according to different procedures in each.[6] The variation in rules between states became more problematic as interstate trade gradually increased.

Congress enacted the first broadly based ban on food and drug adulteration, the Import Drugs Act of 1848, during the Mexican-American War.[7] Two years before passage of the law, Dr. M. J. Bailey, a New York customs inspector, had testified before Congress that the majority of drugs imported into the United States were dangerously adulterated, deteriorated, ineffective, or worthless, and he argued that America, lacking the regulation that was then widespread in Europe, had become "the world's dumping ground for counterfeit, contaminated, diluted, and decomposed drug materials."[8] In support of his claims, he cited shipments of the painkiller opium that had been reduced to one-third of the original potency or were "infested with live worms."[9] Dr. Bailey's concerns were echoed by Ohio congressman and physician Dr. T. O. Edwards, who reported that disease and death among soldiers in the Mexican-American War were partly due to fraud in medical supplies.[10] Rather than attempting to fix domestic problems with drug adulteration, however, Congress set limits on foreign drugs. The Import Drugs Act provided for inspections of drugs at ports and for the destruction, detention, or exportation of drugs that did not meet the standards of the U.S. Pharmacopeia, a compendium of all recognized medications.[11] Because of its limited applications, however, the law was largely ineffective.[12]

The First Steps toward a Comprehensive Law

The movement toward today's regulatory scheme for food and drugs began with the appointment in 1862 of Dr. Charles Weatherill by President Abraham Lincoln to found the Bureau of Chemistry in the U.S. Department of Agriculture (USDA). This new body was directed to investigate the safety of foods, drugs, and animal feed on a national level.[13] The bureau's first investigations were into adulterated agricultural commodities beginning in 1867.[14] In 1880, Peter Collier, the department's chief chemist, issued the first call for a national food and drug law. His proposal was defeated in Congress, but more than 100 subsequent bills were introduced over the next twenty-five years until success was finally achieved in the wake of a major scandal.

The first step toward enactment of a comprehensive food and drug law was fairly modest. By 1900, the use of vaccinations to combat a number of diseases had become widespread. The head of the U.S. Hygienic Laboratory (later to become part of the National Institutes of Health [NIH]), which conducted research on vaccination methods, expressed concerns about continued unregulated growth in the production of vaccines.[15] His fears of public health consequences proved to be warranted. In October 1901, errors were made in the manufacture of diphtheria vaccine in a St. Louis laboratory that resulted in the deaths of thirteen children.[16] Hundreds of reports of similar incidents soon became public. In 1902, Congress passed the first national law to regulate a pharmaceutical product, the Biologics Control Act, which established licensing procedures for the manufacture and distribution of vaccines and permitted government officials to inspect laboratories and factories.[17] It was widely praised by both public health officials and vaccine manufacturers, and its initial success brought heightened public support for proposals to implement more comprehensive regulation.[18]

The next step, enactment of a federal law covering all foods and drugs, resulted from another scandal. The public was prepared for bad news about the safety of foods and drugs by a series of exposés published in 1905 and 1906 in the popular magazine *Collier's Weekly* on harm caused by two popular cold remedies.[19] The articles were widely read and kept in the public's eye by the American Medical Association (AMA), which distributed reprints. The major scandal that directly led Congress to act was revealed by the work of Upton Sinclair, whose book *The Jungle,* published in 1904, exposed dangerous and unsanitary conditions in the meatpacking industry.[20] In response to the resulting public outcry, President Theodore Roosevelt ordered government inspections of several facilities, which confirmed the findings.[21] This validation of threats to public health, along with pressure from the AMA and from the Bureau of Chemistry's chief chemist at the time, Harvey W. Wiley, persuaded Congress to enact the Pure Food and Drug Act in 1906.[22] A companion law, the Meat Inspection Act, was passed the same day.[23]

The Pure Food and Drug Act contained an overall prohibition against "adulteration and misbranding of foods and drugs in interstate commerce."[24] For foods, it required that ingredients be listed on packages. For drugs, it mandated the listing of especially dangerous ingredients such as alcohol, heroin, and cocaine, but it did not actually ban any of them from use. The law also prohibited labels for foods and drugs that were false or misleading and required that drugs be manufactured in accordance with standards set by the U.S. Pharmacopocia.[25] The law was administered by the Bureau of Chemistry.

Early enforcement of the law, however, faced several obstacles. The first was a decision by the Supreme Court in 1911 in the case of *United States v. Johnson,*[26] which ruled that it applied only to statements about the composition of a drug, not to false therapeutic claims.[27] Congress responded by passing the Shirley Amendment in 1912, which prohibited false therapeutic claims that were intended to defraud the consumer, but the law still turned out to be a weak enforcement tool, since intent is often difficult to prove. The effectiveness of the 1906 law was also hindered by Congress's failure to authorize funds for enforcement. Moreover, many manufacturers were able to use brochures and advertisements to promote false claims, since they were not considered labeling under the act.

Incremental steps in food and drug legislation continued over the next two decades. In 1914, Congress passed the Harrison Narcotics Tax Act, which required prescriptions before patients could obtain products containing more than minimal amounts of narcotic substances.[28] That law also mandated that physicians and pharmacists maintain records of prescriptions issued and dispensed. In 1927, the bureaucratic organization of the Bureau of Chemistry moved closer to that of the present Food and Drug Administration (FDA), when it was reorganized into two units. One of them, the Food, Drug and Insecticide Administration, handled all regulatory functions. In 1930, the name of this unit was changed to the Food and Drug Administration, and the unit was authorized by Congress to set standards for packaging of most canned foods.[29]

Comprehensive Regulation Arrives with the 1938 Food, Drug, and Cosmetic Act

The movement to overhaul and strengthen the FDA's statutory authority began in earnest in 1933 with the administration of President Franklin Roosevelt. The agency developed a legislative proposal that year to strengthen its authority, but Congress declined to act on it. As with past food and drug legislation, it took a public scandal to move the political process forward.

The scandal occurred in 1937 and involved a product known as elixir of sulfanilamide, an antibiotic preparation for administration to children.[30] To make the drug palatable for younger patients, it was prepared in liquid form through use of a solvent, diethylene glycol, which can be lethal. Prior to marketing, however, the preparation had been tested only for fragrance and taste, not for toxicity. By December 1937, 107 deaths in fifteen states, mostly of children, had been attributed to the drug. It was estimated that if the entire supply had been used, the number of deaths would have reached 4,000.[31] Since the existing regulatory structure did not require premarket testing of drugs, the FDA had no authority to step in before the drug reached consumers.

The public outcry prodded Congress to act. In 1938, it passed the Food, Drug, and Cosmetic Act, which revamped the oversight of foods and drugs and established the basic regulatory structure that governs pharmaceuticals today.[32] Among the law's provisions were procedures for review of the safety of new drugs before they came to market, extension of the FDA's scope of authority to include cosmetics and therapeutic devices, elimination of the requirement that the government prove fraud to prosecute false claims, new authority for the FDA to inspect factories and to obtain court injunctions against the distribution of unsafe or adulterated products, and expansion of FDA standard-setting authority for quality and packaging of food. A separate law, the Wheeler-Lea Act, authorized the Federal Trade Commission (FTC) to regulate advertising of products subject to FDA oversight other than prescription drugs.[33] With these laws, the regulation of food, drugs, and cosmetics took a quantum leap.

The central element of the 1938 law is the authority that it grants the FDA to evaluate new drugs for safety before they reach the market. Agency regulations implement the procedures under which this is accomplished.[34] To convince the FDA that a drug should be approved, manufacturers must conduct tests on human subjects, known as clinical trials. The agency supervises the tests and reviews the data generated at the end of the process to determine whether the product is safe enough for sale. Safety alone was originally considered in reviewing drugs, but, as discussed later, amendments to the law passed in 1962 added efficacy as a criterion. Since new drugs are tested in human subjects, the FDA also regulates the safety of the trials themselves through a network of institutional review boards (IRBs) at each institution that sponsors testing. (The role of IRBs in the regulation of research is discussed in more detail in chapter 8.)

Under the 1938 act and related laws and regulations, the path that a drug follows from discovery to marketing is a long one.[35] When a manufacturer finds a compound that holds therapeutic promise, its first action is to apply for a patent with the federal Patent and Trademark Office (PTO). Without this protection, the discovery could fall into the public domain, eliminating its profit potential. Once legal protection for the discovery has been obtained, the next step is to begin experiments in animals. Although it is a standard part of the process, this step was not legally mandated until 1962. If therapeutic potential and safety are confirmed, the drug is ready for testing in humans. To do so, the manufacturer must receive the first in a series of FDA approvals, an investigational new drug (IND) exemption, which permits the drug's administration to human research subjects. A similar procedure applies to new medical devices.

With an IND exemption, a drug or device formally enters the process of clinical trials. Three phases of trials must be completed before a drug can be approved for sale, and a fourth continues after marketing.[36] Phase I tests for safety in a small group of healthy volunteers. Generally, fewer than 100 subjects are studied, and often many fewer than that. Investigators seek to determine whether larger trials can safely be conducted to gauge the compound's actual effects and, if they can be, to establish a safe dosage range, preferred route of administration, and possible toxicities. About one-third of all drugs are abandoned by the end of phase I because of safety concerns.

Phase II also uses small samples of subjects, but these are patients who actually suffer from the target condition. This phase looks for the first indications that the drug acts as intended, while still monitoring for adverse effects. If the drug seems to have a clinical benefit, the optimum dosage range and route of administration are further refined. Only about one-third of candidate drugs survive to the end of this phase of testing.

Phase III is the most comprehensive in the process. The drug is given to a large sample of subjects, sometimes numbering in the thousands, and is administered as it would be in actual clinical practice in physicians' offices and hospitals. Testing in this phase can take several years. It assesses safety in a much larger study sample and gauges actual clinical effectiveness and dosage range. Only about one-quarter of drugs that entered the original winnowing process emerge when this phase of testing is complete.

For those drugs that appear safe, and as of 1962 effective as well, the manufacturer must then file a new drug application (NDA) with the FDA.[37] In reviewing the application, the agency considers all the data from all the clinical trials in light of the drug's intended use. In most cases, an advisory committee composed of experts in the therapeutic area involved first reviews the data and offers a recommendation to the agency. Although advisory committee recommendations are not binding, it is unusual for the agency to reject them. Approval, when granted, is very specific. The drug may be marketed only for delineated conditions or symptoms, which are known as indications for use. In some cases, it may be promoted only for specified patient populations, according to age, gender, or other factors. The labeling must list these limitations as well as known side effects and factors that would present a heightened risk of adverse reactions or that would limit effectiveness, which are known as contraindications.

FDA rules also restrict many of the details of drug promotion and advertising.[38] A drug's scientific and brand names must be approved, both must appear in all marketing materials, and the size of the typeface used to list them must meet specifications. All printed promotions must list indications, contraindications, and side effects. The more recent phenomenon of advertising drugs directly to patients is subject to further restrictions, which are discussed later in this chapter. A twist in the regulatory framework permits physicians to prescribe an approved drug for any use, even one not covered by the FDA's approval, although the manufacturer may encourage them to do so only under strict limits. Promotion of a drug by its manufacturer for a new indication or in a new patient population generally requires a new FDA approval in the form of a supplemental NDA.

The penalties for manufacturers that violate the conditions of drug approvals can be severe.[39] Heavy fines can be assessed, as well as injunctions against further sales of the product and even confiscations of existing inventories. In extreme cases, corporate officers can face criminal penalties. No marketing activity is as heavily regulated in America as that of prescription drugs.

Even after a new drug has reached the market, surveillance of it continues, although in a looser form.[40] A fourth phase of clinical trials requires that manufacturers collect data on adverse reactions of which they become aware. Patterns of commonly occurring or severe side effects must be reported to the FDA. In response, the agency can require that new warnings be included in the drug's labeling or, when serious risks are uncovered, that a drug be pulled from the market. Continuing surveillance of a new drug's effects is an important supplement to the process of premarket review. Adverse drug effects may not appear until years after a product has reached the market, when it has been used by a much larger number of patients and over a longer period of time than can be studied in premarket clinical trials.

The process of postmarket surveillance is controversial.[41] Agency critics claim that this phase of oversight is too lax and that many drugs remain on the market longer than they should.[42] Although it is referred to as the fourth phase of clinical trials, postmarket assessment does not require actual testing and instead depends largely on voluntary reporting. Systematic study of drugs after approval is most commonly conducted to evaluate side effects in populations that were not included in earlier testing, such as children, and to gather data for approval to market a product for a new use. Postmarketing safety studies are legally required only in two instances—for significant new drugs that were given "fast-track" approval and those requiring review of pediatric hazards. The FDA approves some drugs on the condition that continued testing explore suspected late-appearing side effects, but follow-through in enforcing such conditions has been inconsistent.[43] The agency lacks clear authority to directly require clinical testing for safety after a drug has been approved.

Filling Regulatory Gaps: Amendments after 1938

Over the decades after 1938, gaps in the new scheme for overseeing drug safety gradually became apparent. The first involved drugs that are at the safest end of the spectrum of risk. Products that emerge from the FDA regulatory process and reach the market differ greatly in the level of hazard that they pose. Some are safe enough for consumers to use without medical guidance, but many can be safely used only under clinical supervision. The 1938 act made no distinction.

In 1951, Congress passed the Durham-Humphrey Amendment, which established procedures through which the FDA could determine which drugs were safe enough to be sold directly to patients "over the counter" (OTC) and which should continue to require a prescription.[44] The law established three criteria to guide the agency in deciding whether a drug could be sold for use without medical oversight. The criteria were whether it is habit forming, whether its potential toxicity is excessive, and whether its initial approval was limited to use only under the guidance of a physician. The law also prohibited refills without the authorization of the prescribing practitioner. Though the amendment addressed a fairly technical issue, it effectively removed a considerable amount of regulatory uncertainty.[45]

Over the course of the 1950s, additional amendments clarified and strengthened other provisions of the 1938 law. In 1953, the Factory Inspection Amendment required the FDA to provide manufacturers with written reports of the results of inspections. In 1954, the Miller Pesticide Amendment established procedures for setting limits for pesticide residues on raw agricultural products. The FDA's bureaucratic home also changed during this time. In 1940, it had been transferred from the Department of Agriculture to the Federal Security Agency. In 1953, it moved to the Department of Health, Education, and Welfare (DHEW), now the Department of Health and Human Services (DHHS), where it remains today.

A Special Concern with Food Safety Challenges Regulators

One set of amendments to the 1938 act passed in the late 1950s created a new regulatory paradigm that challenged regulators for years to come. Advances in toxicology had begun to reveal a connection between some substances found in the environment and the development of cancer. Of particular concern were substances commonly found in foods. Ingestion of small amounts of potential carcinogens in the food supply may be inevitable, but additives to foods pose a risk that can be more easily isolated and curtailed. In 1958, Congress enacted the Food Additives Amendment, commonly known as the Delaney Clause after the congressman who proposed it.[46] The law banned the use of any carcinogenic substance as a food additive, regardless of dose. In 1960, the Color Additive Amendment extended the prohibition to food colorings.[47] These provisions were unusual in their absolutist approach. Any amount of a carcinogen, no matter how small, was banned, regardless of its strength and with no discretion for regulators.

Over the decades after passage of the Delaney Clause, advances in toxicology made it possible to detect increasingly minute traces of carcinogens. It gradually became evident that almost no food could be guaranteed to have none. In 1969, the FDA found itself compelled to ban the widely used artificial sweetener saccharin because of evidence that it could be carcinogenic in high doses, even though those doses were much larger than any that consumers would be likely to ingest.[48] Critics of the absolutist approach argued that the law went too far. In 1977, Congress passed the Saccharin Study and Labeling Act, which overturned the ban as long as a warning label was included in the product's packaging.[49] Congress repealed the warning requirement in 1996 and the same year passed the Food Quality Protection Act, which eliminated the application of the Delaney Clause to pesticides.[50]

Absolutist regulatory schemes reduce the chance that interest groups can dilute a public safety initiative. With no regulatory discretion, an agency has no choice but to act as prescribed by Congress. Discretion can be useful, however, when competing considerations become apparent. Scientific progress raises subtleties and nuances that can make regulatory policies that initially appeared straightforward seem to be more complex over time.

Policing Drug Efficacy: The 1962 Kefauver-Harris Amendments

After a series of refinements in the 1950s, the 1938 act faced its first major overhaul in 1962. The Kefauver-Harris Amendments had their origin in 1959 in a series of hearings conducted by Tennessee senator Estes Kefauver, which covered a wide range of topics, including allegations of price-fixing, deceptive promotion practices, and ineffective FDA enforcement.[51] Subsequent to the hearings, Senator Kefauver proposed legislation to address a range of perceived abuses in the pharmaceutical industry, including requirements that drugs be proved efficacious as well as safe before receiving approval and limits on the extent of patent protection. His proposal initially generated little support, until a public scandal once again arose to catalyze the legislative process.

The scandal came in 1962 and involved the drug thalidomide, a sleeping pill often prescribed to pregnant women. By 1962, it had been approved abroad and was awaiting FDA approval in the United States. However, reports began to appear that year linking it to serious birth defects in more than 5,000 babies worldwide.[52] The FDA official in charge of reviewing thalidomide's NDA, Dr. Frances Kelsey, became suspicious when she discovered that the drug had not been tested in animals. Since the FDA was required at that time to hand down a decision within sixty days of submission of an NDA, Dr. Kelsey repeatedly asked the manufacturer for more data, which bought more time for review. It was during these delays that data accumulated from several countries indicating significant safety concerns.[53] Once these reports reached the press, the NDA was withdrawn.

In response to the publicity, Congress reconsidered Senator Kefauver's concerns. The Senate Judiciary Committee amended a pending food and drug reform bill to include new provisions that strengthened FDA's authority in several regards, and Congress enacted the bill as the Kefauver-Harris Amendment. Among the most significant provisions, the law abolished the sixty-day time limit for FDA new drug reviews, permitted the FDA to order a drug off the market if there was evidence of an imminent danger to the public or of false labeling, prohibited drug testing on humans before animal testing had been conducted, and required that all advertising carry labeling on possible side effects. Other key features required that drug companies register their manufacturing facilities with the FDA and be inspected at least once every two years, that records be maintained and made available for inspection, that reports of adverse drug effects be promptly transmitted to the FDA, and that informed consent be obtained before a patient could participate in a clinical trial. The most substantial change of all altered the foundation of FDA oversight. The law mandated that effectiveness as well as safety of new drugs be demonstrated in order to gain FDA approval.[54]

The requirement that manufacturers establish drug efficacy as part of the approval process placed a significant new burden on the FDA. Not only did it have a new criterion to evaluate in subsequent NDAs, but it was also required to review all drugs that it had previously approved between 1938 and 1962, when only proof of safety was required.[55] To accomplish the retroactive assessments, the agency initiated a massive drug efficacy study implementation (DESI) review that was not completed until the 1970s.

The Kefauver-Harris Amendment of 1962 represented the most comprehensive expansion of the basic 1938 regulatory scheme up to that time. The addition of efficacy as a required element of NDAs transformed not only the regulatory process but also the way drugs are developed, tested, and marketed. As a result, the environment in which the pharmaceutical industry operates and the way it does business became considerably more complex.

Regulatory Refinements to the 1962 Law

Although the basic structure of the 1962 amendments remains in place today, Congress has enacted several important but less sweeping refinements to FDA jurisdiction. In 1970, it created the Environmental Protection Agency (EPA), which assumed the FDA's responsibility for regulating pesticides. (For a discussion of the EPA's role in regulating pollution, see chapter 6 on public health.) In 1971, the Bureau of Radiological Health, which regulates radiation exposure from electronic products, was transferred from the Public Health Service in HEW to the FDA. In 1972, Congress transferred to the FDA from NIH regulatory authority over vaccines, blood products, and other biologics, which gave the agency responsibility for issuing licenses to manufacturers and suppliers, including blood banks, and for requiring that products be tested for potency and safety before being released for sale.[56] In 1973, Congress transferred authority to regulate the safety of various consumer products such as toys, fabrics, and potential poisons from the FDA, where it had resided since 1927, to the newly created Consumer Product Safety Commission (CPSC).[57]

The most significant expansion of FDA authority after the 1962 amendments was contained in the Medical Device Amendments of 1976.[58] That law mandated that devices, including diagnostic products, be registered with the agency and required that some receive premarket approval.[59] The result was the creation of a process for testing and approval of devices that is parallel to that for drugs.[60] In the same law, however, Congress also reduced FDA authority over vitamins, minerals, and food supplements by including the Vitamin Amendments, which exempted these products from the agency's review. Disputes over the appropriate scope of FDA jurisdiction with regard to these products arose again in the 1990s concerning the regulation of herbal supplements, which is discussed later in this chapter.

Regulation of pharmaceuticals has continued to engender considerable political attention with increasing intensity in recent years. Ironically, debates have returned to many of the themes raised by Senator Kefauver in his 1959 hearings about drug pricing, marketing, and FDA effectiveness. The most recent addition to the political mix is the issue of financing drug use through insurance. The pace of legislation in this and other areas has accelerated in recent decades as pharmaceutical products have come to play an expanding role in the delivery of health care.

The FDA's First Entry into Economic Regulation:
The Hatch-Waxman Act of 1984

Manufacturers would not invest the huge sums needed to develop new drugs without the protection of patents that provide a period of exclusive marketing rights. The legally sanctioned monopoly that patents confer allows drug companies to recoup their costs and earn a profit on their investment. A patent prohibits anyone other than the patent holder from making or selling a product for twenty years from the date of its filing.[61] It is, in essence, a government regulation that forbids market competition on a temporary basis.

Competition in the market for a drug arrives when the patent expires and companies other than the one that developed the product are legally permitted to manufacture and sell copies, which are known as "generic" versions. Manufacturers of original, or "pioneer," drugs are eager to delay this point as long as possible. A particular concern for them is that in practice the patent monopoly for pharmaceutical products can actually last for far less than the full twenty years. Since patents are obtained as soon as a new molecular entity is discovered, they begin to run before any testing starts. By the time all clinical trials have been completed and FDA approval has been obtained, ten to fifteen years may have elapsed, leaving the firm with a shortened period of patent protection while the drug is actually on the market.

The challenge from generic competition, however, was left uncertain under the 1938 law and 1962 amendments. The law did not clarify whether generic drugs are considered new drugs that must complete all phases of testing and receive another FDA approval prior to marketing, or are close enough to the pioneer product that they can piggyback on its testing and review. If new drug approval procedures are required for generics, it could take an additional ten years or more after patent expiration before they are able to reach the market. However, if they are treated as new versions of approved products, generic companies would reap a windfall at the expense of pioneer companies that paid for the initial drug development and testing.

Between 1962 and 1984, the FDA resolved the issue in favor of manufacturers of pioneer drugs by requiring that generic companies submit original clinical data on safety and efficacy for drugs they wished to copy. As a result, only 35 percent of new drugs approved during this time faced generic competition.[62] In effect, monopoly protection could last long after patent expiration, while the benefits of price competition were lost. The issue came to a head in a 1983 Supreme Court decision in the case of *United States v. Generix Drug Corporation*,[63] in which the Court confirmed that generic drugs are new drugs, subject to the full regulatory review process. The court reasoned that although generic drugs rely on the same active ingredient as the original product, they are usually packaged with coatings and fillers, known as "excipients," that are different. The active ingredient in its new container may be released at a different rate or to a different extent, changing its "bioavailability." The entire pill, therefore, not just the active molecule, constitutes the actual product.

With the Supreme Court's decision, the prospect of market-based price competition for drugs began to seem illusory. To facilitate a viable generic industry, Congress responded the following year by enacting the Drug Price Competition and Patent Term Restoration Act of 1984, commonly known as the Hatch-Waxman Act.[64] Its goal was to strike a balance between the interests of generic and pioneer drug firms in order to facilitate a vibrant role for both.[65] Given the importance of fostering as widespread a mechanism for generic competition as possible, in 1988 Congress passed the Generic Animal Drug and Patent Term Restoration Act, which struck a similar balance for veterinary drugs.[66]

The most significant benefit that the Hatch-Waxman Act gave to generic manufacturers was a streamlined review process that eliminated the dilemma posed by the *Generix* decision. Applications to the FDA for approval of generic versions of brand-name drugs could now dispense with the first two phases of clinical testing and rely instead on the data already filed with the application for the original product. Phase III clinical studies were still required but focused just on bioavailability of the generic copy rather than overall efficacy of the active ingredient. Moreover, these tests were permitted to begin while the patent on the original drug was still in effect, so with proper planning, the generic drug could be approved to enter the market as soon as the patent expired. The most significant benefit that the law gave to brand manufacturers was an extension of patent terms up to an additional five years to account for time lost in the FDA approval process.

Other elements of the trade-off between benefits for brand and generic drug companies were more complex and more controversial. As the decision in the *Generix* case noted, pharmaceutical products contain more than just the active ingredient. Each of the excipients, including fillers, coatings, colorings, and other inert components, is usually subject to a patent of its own. If filed after the patent for the active molecule, their protection extends to a later date. Even after waiting for the original patent to expire, therefore, a generic manufacturer may still risk an infringement lawsuit if it copies one of these other ingredients.

To assist generic companies in navigating the minefield of patents waiting to be infringed, the act required that brand manufacturers list all patents related to their approved drugs with the FDA. The agency, in turn, makes the lists available to the public in a document known as the Orange Book. Before marketing a copy of a medication, a generic manufacturer must certify that it is infringing none of the patents listed, either because they will have expired prior to marketing or because the patented ingredient will not be used.

Brand manufacturers, however, may disagree that a generic product avoids all infringement. The Hatch-Waxman Act gave them an advantage in pursing such claims. Upon filing a lawsuit alleging infringement of a patent listed in the Orange Book, a brand manufacturer receives an automatic extension of its exclusive right to market the drug up to an additional thirty months or until the litigation is resolved if that is sooner. To balance the equation, if a generic manufacturer challenges a patent and wins, it receives 180 days of marketing exclusivity for its product, during which no other generic version of the same drug may compete. These provisions have encouraged the filing of many lawsuits by companies seeking to use these provisions to gain a marketing advantage.

Overall, the Hatch-Waxman Act has dramatically reshaped the market for generic drugs. In 1984, the year of its passage, generics represented 18.6 percent of the total American pharmaceutical market. In 1997, the share was 44.3 percent.[67] The act is also credited with enhancing competition in the brand-name industry, by encouraging companies to fill their pipelines with new drugs that do not face impeding generic threats.[68] Today, generic drugs are an integral part of many health care cost control strategies.

The implications of the Hatch-Waxman Act go beyond the effects on drug costs. The law also begins to alter the scope of FDA responsibility, as the agency is injected into intellectual property disputes. The filing of patents is the traditional province of the PTO. This agency decides whether a new invention meets the criteria for patent protection by being original, nonobvious, and potentially useful, although its judgments are subject to court review if a patent challenge is filed.[69] The FDA's traditional role is to decide whether a new drug, regardless of its patent protection, is safe and effective. These are separate tasks requiring distinct kinds of expertise. Under the Hatch-Waxman Act, however, the FDA also serves as a keeper of drug patent records in the Orange Book. The agency does not police the validity of the patents that the Orange Book contains, but its role in administering this registry gives it responsibility for overseeing the bureaucratic mechanism around which many pharmaceutical intellectual property disputes revolve. The Hatch-Waxman Act thereby began to merge the regulatory functions of safety assurance and economic oversight. As the financing of pharmaceutical access occupies an increasing share of the attention of policy makers, the confounding of these missions will likely take on increasing significance in shaping the drug industry.

Further Refinements to the FDA Regulatory Process

In addition to the Hatch-Waxman Act, Congress enacted a series of other laws refining FDA drug regulation through the 1980s and 1990s. Some addressed minor issues, but several affected the regulatory process in significant ways. Increasingly, the thrust continued to be economics rather than traditional safety concerns.

The Orphan Drug Act

As massive as America's pharmaceutical research enterprise has become, its economic structure is not well equipped to address some kinds of health care needs. Of particular concern is research into treatments for rare diseases. These conditions present a difficult target for investment because of the limited potential market, since few patients are affected. Many devastating illnesses that may be prime candidates for pharmacologic research are not widespread, such as Huntington's disease, myoclonus, Lou Gehrig's disease, Tourette's syndrome, and muscular dystrophy.[70] Lacking lucrative marketing possibilities, drugs for these conditions are known as "orphan drugs."

To address the plight of patients with rare conditions, Congress in 1983 enacted a plan to create special incentives to induce manufacturers to develop drugs to treat them. The Orphan Drug Act authorized grants, tax credits, and seven years of additional market exclusivity beyond patent expiration for drugs targeted to treat rare diseases.[71] The act was later amended to specifically define an orphan drug as one designed to treat an ailment that affects 200,000 people or fewer.[72] The law appears to have worked as intended, as the FDA has approved more than 800 orphan drugs to date.[73] These are medications that might not have been developed without legislative assistance.

Refinements to Safety Rules

In 1987, Congress revisited the issue of drug safety in passing the Prescription Drug Marketing Act, which limited the distribution of drugs beyond conventional retail sale.[74] It banned the diversion of prescription drugs from legitimate channels, prohibited the sale of manufacturer samples, and restricted reimportation of American drugs back from foreign countries to which they had been sent. Reimportation can be attractive to consumers because drugs are sold in most foreign countries at much lower prices than they are in the United States. Since most other countries directly regulate the prices that drug manufacturers can charge, reimportation gives Americans the chance to piggyback on foreign price controls. It is a highly controversial practice that, as described later, continues to inspire legislative responses.

In 1990, Congress passed two significant additional refinements to the law governing food and drug safety. The Nutrition Labeling and Education Act required that all food packages include nutrition information, and it standardized the use of labeling terms with health implications, such as "low fat" and "light."[75] The Safe Medical Devices Act required that institutions such as hospitals and nursing homes that use medical devices report problems to the FDA, and it gave the agency new authority to order recalls.[76] Manufacturers of implanted devices were also required to conduct postmarket surveillance and to establish systems to locate patients so they can be warned of hazards if they appear.

The Status of Herbal Supplements:
What Is a Food and What Is a Drug?

As FDA review of drugs grew in rigor over the years, the question continued to arise as to what, exactly, is a "drug." The Food, Drug, and Cosmetic Act defined drugs as "articles intended for use in the diagnosis, cure, mitigation, treatment, or prevention of disease in man or other animals" and "articles (other than food) intended to affect the structure or any function of the body of man or other animals."[77] This leaves room for interpretation concerning several kinds of products, most notably herbal remedies. Manufacturers claim that these products help to cure, treat, or prevent disease, but they are sold as dietary supplements, which implies that they are really foods, that do not face premarket review.

In 1994, Congress decided that herbal remedies sold as dietary supplements are more like foods than like drugs. The Dietary Supplement Health and Education Act (DSHEA) created a special regulatory structure for these products that is somewhat more stringent than that for foods in general but considerably less stringent than that for drugs.[78] The act directed the FDA to promulgate good manufacturing practice regulations and authorized it to review safety and efficacy for supplements that are already on the market. However, the law included no requirement for premarket testing and approval, as there is for drugs.[79] Manufacturers are not obligated to record, investigate, or even report to the FDA information that they receive on adverse events, and existing regulations do not contain a penalty for withholding the information.[80]

Herbal supplement manufacturers are allowed to advertise claims that their products improve health and strengthen the body against illness, but not that they treat a specific disease. If the FDA finds that a product poses an "unreasonable risk of injury or illness," it must notify the manufacturer and then allow for a hearing. If the agency wishes to proceed further, it must first go to court, where it bears the burden of proving that the product is dangerous. In the event of a public health emergency, the FDA is not permitted to take the product off the market but must ask the secretary of DHHS to do so, a process that necessitates an evidentiary hearing.[81] The dietary supplement industry feels that it is fully regulated under this system, but some consumer advocates believe that the full drug oversight process should apply.[82]

Speeding the Review Process:
The Prescription Drug User Fee Act

With a growing number of new drugs being developed and the market opened for more generic copies, demands on the FDA approval process began to increase dramatically by the late 1980s. Manufacturers complained that the result was greater delays that impaired their ability to bring drugs to market. With the clock ticking on patents, regulatory inertia presents a special burden for pharmaceutical companies. In 1992, Congress responded by passing the Prescription Drug User Fee Act (PDUFA), which sought to speed the process at manufacturers' expense.[83] The act set new time limits on the FDA to complete its reviews of NDAs. To provide the resources needed to meet the tighter deadlines, the agency was directed to hire more reviewers for its staff with funds raised from user fees levied on applicants.[84] The trade-off succeeded in speeding new drug reviews; however, it also raised concerns that the reviews were so speedy that they failed to adequately assess all risks.[85]

PDUFA was initially implemented for a five-year period, but its perceived success led Congress in 1997 to reauthorize it as part of the Food and Drug Administration Modernization Act (FDAMA).[86] That law went further than reauthorizing PDUFA by implementing some of the most significant reforms in FDA practices since the 1962 act. FDAMA accelerated the review of medical devices, putting them on a parallel footing with drugs, and it made important changes to the oversight of pharmaceutical marketing. However, it also softened food regulation by replacing a premarket approval with a premarket notification requirement for packaging. Nevertheless, it is the drug marketing provisions that had the greatest effect and that may lead to a fundamental realignment in the relationship between manufacturers, physicians, and patients.

Drugs, Marketing, and a Revolution in Consumer Information

As the provision of health care is increasingly driven by the use and manipulation of information, so is its pharmaceutical component. Traditionally, it was physicians who assessed and filtered data on prescription drugs, leaving their patients to passively respond. In recent years, however, patients have gained increasing access to information that enables them to act as more equal partners in deciding on their treatments. Through the Internet and other sources, new kinds of information are available today that did not previously exist or were difficult for the public to obtain until the last few years. The regulatory structure governing pharmaceuticals has had to react to keep pace.[87]

Off-Label Prescribing: Who Should
Decide the Best Use of Drugs?

In its provisions on marketing, FDAMA helped to revolutionize the way drugs are promoted to patients and physicians. It is an anomaly of the American pharmaceutical regulatory scheme that manufacturers are permitted to market drugs only for those clinical indications and patient populations that the FDA approves, but once a drug is on the market, physicians may prescribe it for any application for any patient. There is no direct regulatory limit on physician prescribing decisions. When a product is prescribed in a way that varies from its FDA-approved labeling, it is considered as being used "off label."

In some cases, doctors use this flexibility to prescribe a drug that has been approved for one condition to treat another one that is closely related. For example, a drug approved to treat one form of cancer may be prescribed to treat another. In other cases, doctors use a drug in a different age-group, perhaps by prescribing one that is approved for use in adults to an adolescent. In some situations, physicians prescribe drugs for conditions that are entirely unrelated to their original application. For example, the FDA originally approved the drug minoxidil for treating high blood pressure, but anecdotal reports suggested its effectiveness in restarting hair growth. Long before the FDA approved its relabeling, many physicians were already prescribing minoxidil to treat baldness.[88]

Before 1997, the FDA prohibited manufacturers from promoting their drugs for off-label uses. The reasoning was that the clinical trials that support a drug's application for approval only assess a specific type of use in a particular kind of patient. Use of a drug to treat a different condition would have no systematic testing of safety or efficacy behind it. If manufacturers wished to market a product for a new use, they were required to submit results of new clinical trials. They complained, however, that research evaluating off-label claims is frequently published in reputable scientific journals, even if the findings were not part of FDA-supervised studies, and they sought the right to at least direct physicians to such information.

FDAMA offered a compromise. For the first time, manufacturers were permitted to disseminate peer-reviewed scholarly journal articles that evaluate off-label uses of their products, if the company commits that it will file, within a reasonable time, an application with the FDA for permission to promote that use. Companies were also permitted to provide information on economic factors related to use of their products to institutional purchasers such as managed care organizations. In 1999, these restrictions were loosened further under a federal court ruling in a challenge to the act. In the case of *Washington Legal Foundation v. Shalala*,[89] the U.S. District Court for the District of Columbia found that the constitutional protection of free speech permits drug manufacturers wider latitude to promote off-label uses. The court held that they may disseminate research articles that were published in a peer reviewed journal or a medical textbook as long as the promotions disclose that an off-label use has not been approved by the FDA and are not false or misleading. Any economic analyses must disclose the sponsor's interest in the product.

FDAMA and the subsequent court decision bring new freedom to manufacturers in drug marketing. They loosened the FDA's restrictions on advertising and enabled more information to flow to prescribers and their patients. Whether the information is used wisely remains to be seen. Of even greater significance, however, by permitting greater latitude in the dissemination of information, the changes in marketing practices may begin to alter the relationships between patients, providers, and manufacturers.

Direct-to-Consumer Advertising: Trying to Put Patients in the Driver's Seat

Promotion of off-label drug uses is only part of the ongoing transformation of pharmaceutical marketing. A change that is more widely visible to the public is the recently sanctioned ability of manufacturers to advertise prescription products directly to consumers, a practice commonly known as "direct-to-consumer" (DTC) advertising. Traditionally, drug companies aimed their marketing exclusively at physicians, who made purchasing judgments for their patients. However, it has become increasingly evident that patients who request specific products can actively influence physician decisions.

There are no laws that explicitly prevent manufacturers from advertising their products directly to consumers. However, the FDA has the authority to punish companies for false or misleading advertising, and it can use this legal power to impose sanctions for DTC promotions that it deems overly aggressive. DTC advertisements first appeared on a limited basis in the early 1980s. In response to concerns about their accuracy and clarity, the agency requested that the industry refrain from the practice to permit time for a review.[90] This voluntary moratorium was lifted in 1985, and by the early 1990s, DTC advertisements had become widespread. Most of the ads were in the print media, but television campaigns began in the mid-1990s, raising the practice's profile. With television's wide reach, the potential for consumer confusion and the possibility of harm from misleading advertisements was substantially increased.

Two FDA directives, one issued in 1999 and one in 2001, set the rules under which DTC advertisements on television would be considered acceptable.[91] They take the form of guidance rather than actual regulations, because of the agency's limited authority to explicitly regulate advertising before it is released. However, the directives offer important advice to companies that can help them to avoid the possibility of an FDA investigation and prosecution down the road. The first directive advised companies to reference in their advertisements four sources where consumers can obtain more information on the drug being promoted, including a toll-free telephone number, a Web site, and a print advertisement, as well as encouragement to consult with a health care professional.[92] The second permitted companies to use the wording contained in FDA-approved labeling to summarize a drug's uses and risks in print advertisements, as long as the full labeling is reprinted in another accessible printed form with a discussion of risks.[93] These requirements make DTC advertisements, whether on television or in print, long and complex, but they ensure that large amounts of relevant information on advertised drugs are available in a readily accessible form to patients.

Access to Clinical Trials: Giving Patients
a Head Start in Obtaining New Drugs

Beyond the broad-based marketing of FDA-approved drugs, there have been calls for public information to achieve another kind of patient access to medications on a targeted basis. The most cutting-edge drugs are those still in clinical testing and for which approval has not yet been obtained. While safety and efficacy data are not yet complete, many of these drugs show therapeutic promise well before the FDA has had its final say. Patients who participate in the testing may have access to advanced medications years before the drugs actually reach the market. The clinical research enterprise in America is huge, and at any given time, hundreds of drugs are being tested at sites across the country. Most physicians, even experts in their fields, have difficulty keeping track of what might be available to a patient as a participant in a research study. If patients could be more effectively matched with clinical trials, both they and the researchers conducting the trials stand to benefit.

To resolve the impediments to communication of clinical trial opportunities, FDAMA directed the NIH to establish a public registry of trials, both those that are federally funded and those that are privately financed, that includes drugs for serious or life-threatening conditions.[94] The goal was to open the world of clinical trials to those who can benefit most directly. The registry has been implemented, although the listing of private trials has proceeded at a slower pace than originally anticipated. The effort represents a promising start at expanding patient access to a new realm of medical information.

Other provisions in FDAMA seek to increase the speed with which new breakthrough medications reach patients. In addition to authorizing creation of a publicly available database of clinical trials, the act directed the FDA to maintain a program to put important new life-saving medications on "fast-track" status to speed their regulatory approval.[95] A separate program on compassionate use permits patients with life-threatening conditions to receive medications and devices that are still being tested in clinical trials, even when they are not participating as subjects in the trials.[96]

FDAMA and the Needs of Children

FDAMA's reach included several other gaps in the regulatory process. First among them was the testing of drugs in children. Manufacturers study most pharmaceutical products in adult subjects, because they usually represent the most likely target patient population. Many products, however, are also appropriate for pediatric use. Determining which drugs are safe and effective in children and setting dosing recommendations for them is not an easy task. The physiology of children is different from that of adults in many ways other than just size and weight.[97] A drug that works in an adult may be useless or even dangerous in a child.

The pediatric market for most drugs is much smaller than the adult market, so there has historically been little incentive for manufacturers to explicitly enter it. They have left it to physicians to prescribe drugs to children based largely on guesswork as to safety, effectiveness, and dosage. FDAMA contained provisions designed to change that. It gave manufacturers that test a drug in children according to FDA-approved procedures an additional six months of marketing exclusivity beyond the expiration of the patent.[98] Technically, this period is not an actual patent extension but rather a period during which the agency may not approve any application for a generic copy. The economic effect for manufacturers, however, is the same, and it can be worth millions of dollars in sales. The response from companies was extremely positive. During the first year after FDAMA's implementation, the FDA received more than 150 requests for approval of proposed pediatric studies.[99]

FDAMA's pediatric exclusivity provision is a voluntary mechanism. In 1999, the FDA issued a related regulation, known as the Pediatric Rule, which permits the agency to affirmatively require pediatric testing of new drugs and of biologic products.[100] Tests can be mandated when they have not been conducted voluntarily either under the FDAMA exclusivity provision or otherwise and the drug may provide a benefit to a substantial number of children or could present a significant risk.[101] The Pediatric Rule is credited with inducing more pediatric drug studies than FDAMA, although the two regulatory programs continue to leave gaps, especially with respect to older drugs for which patent protection has expired and with it the incentive of a marketing exclusivity extension.[102]

The Next Regulatory Frontier: Financing of Drugs

The greatest medical miracles are of little value if no one can afford to pay for them. The use of prescription drugs has risen steadily over the past decade, and the cost of drugs has mushroomed along with it.[103] For those with health insurance that covers drugs, cost is of little concern, but for those without this coverage, essential treatments may be financially out of reach. About one-third of Americans who are covered by private health insurance do not have a prescription benefit.[104]

The Medicare Prescription Drug Benefit
In 2003, Congress added a benefit for outpatient prescription drugs to Medicare through the Medicare Prescription Drug, Improvement, and Modernization Act (MMA).[105] Drugs administered to hospital inpatients and in physicians' offices had previously been covered but not those obtained directly by patients from pharmacists. The MMA's coverage includes various limitations, including substantial copayments and deductibles, but it will make drugs more accessible for millions of elderly patients. (The law is discussed in more detail in chapter 4 on the regulation of health care finance.) It does not directly address the regulation of safety and efficacy, but the FDA's mission is likely to be affected nonetheless in important ways. In particu-

lar, wider use of medications will raise the public profile of the screening process through which drugs reach the market.

The Regulation of Reimportation:
Consumers Try to Beat the Pricing System

The United States is the only industrialized country that does not directly regulate drug prices.[106] As a result, prices in the United States for brand-name drugs tend to be considerably higher than anywhere else. With lower costs abroad, some Americans have found it financially advantageous to make purchases outside of the country and to bring their drugs back in. In doing so, they "reimport" their medications, often at a substantial savings. The easiest route for reimportation back to America is through Canada, which is a car or bus ride away for many who live in northern states. The draw of lower prices has brought increasing numbers of Americans to Canadian pharmacies, some through actual travel and some through Web sites.

Reimportation challenges the market-based pricing of drugs in the United States. In essence, it brings foreign price controls into the American market. If practiced on a wide enough scale, it could make the American pricing structure meaningless. Manufacturers have expressed concern about the long-term effects on their profits. They have also challenged the practice of reimportation based on safety concerns. Once drugs leave the country, they are no longer subject to FDA oversight of their transportation and storage. When the drugs return, the agency is unable to provide assurances that they were not mishandled. While individual purchases made in person at foreign pharmacies may pose a minimal hazard, larger scale purchases over the Internet may involve unknown sellers that operate outside of the reach of American regulation.

The Prescription Drug Marketing Act of 1988 severely restricted the ability of Americans to reimport prescription drugs, although it is rarely enforced against individual purchasers of medications intended for personal use.[107] In 2000, Congress passed the Medicine Equity and Drug Safety Act to permit reimportation on a wider scale.[108] It directed the FDA to develop regulations to permit wholesalers to reimport drugs from foreign countries for resale in the United States, if safety can be assured. The agency declined to issue rules under the act, however, based on a determination that it cannot assure safety at an adequate level. The MMA added a further directive to the FDA to promulgate regulations permitting reimportation, but again under the condition that it find that safety can be safeguarded, which it has been reluctant to do.[109] Nevertheless, calls to legalize a reimportation process that is not contingent on an FDA safety determination remain widespread. Advocates see little risk from drugs sold in Canada and other Western countries. They perceive the issue as one of economics, not of safety.

By making the FDA the arbiter of reimportation hazards, Congress has added to the agency's budding economic mission. A regulatory decision that facilitates foreign purchases of prescription drugs could have profound effects on American prices. The issue may often be framed in terms of regulating safety, but it also strikes at the heart of the system of market-based pricing and America's status as the lone holdout in a world of countries that control drug prices.

Agency Structure

Food and Drug Administration

The FDA, a component of DHHS, today exerts regulatory influence over almost one-quarter of the nation's economy. It has a staff of 9,100 employees and a budget of $1.7 billion, of which $40 million comes from user fees charged under PDUFA. It employs a range of professionals, including chemists, physicians, and pharmacists. The agency inspects 16,000 facilities each year and oversees 95,000 different businesses.[110] It also answers more than 70,000 consumer questions, 40,000 requests for data under the Freedom of Information Act, and 180 citizens' petitions each year.[111]

The FDA performs its work through six centers that address broad areas of regulatory responsibility. They are listed in table 5.1. In addition to its headquarters in Rockville, Maryland, outside of Washington, DC, the FDA has field offices across the country. The agency is headed by a commissioner who is appointed by the president subject to Senate confirmation.

The key FDA office for the regulation of drugs is the Center for Drug Evaluation and Research (CDER), which is the largest of the agency's centers. It employs a staff of more than 1,500 in five offices and six divisions. CDER oversees all aspects of drug development and production, including manufacturing, testing and research, and advertising. It contains an office that oversees generic drugs and a division that regulates over-the-counter products. In terms of the FDA's other areas of responsibility, food safety, foodborne illness, nutrition, and labeling fall under the supervision of the Center for Food Safety and Applied Nutrition; the safety of medical devices belongs to the Center for Devices and Radiological Health;

Table 5.1
FDA Centers

Center for Food Safety and Applied Nutrition
Center for Drug Evaluation and Research
Center for Veterinary Medicine
Center for Devices and Radiological Health
Center for Biologics Evaluation and Research
National Center for Toxicological Research

Source: http://www.fda.gov/opacom/7org.html
(7 August 2006).

the safety of the blood supply, vaccines, and transplant tissues is the responsibility of Center for Biologics Evaluation and Research; and animal therapeutics and various other veterinary public health concerns are regulated by the Center for Veterinary Medicine.[112]

State Oversight of Prescribing

The actual prescribing of drugs by physicians is regulated by the states. They grant licenses for clinical practice that include the authority to write prescriptions. States also grant other kinds of health care professionals the power to prescribe, including dentists in all states, nurse practitioners and physician assistants in some, and psychologists in two states, New Mexico and Louisiana.[113] The pharmacists who actually fill prescriptions are also licensed by each state.[114] The authority to write or fill a prescription is limited to the state that has issued the license, although practitioners may be licensed in more than one. An exception is practice within the military. A license from any state is legally sufficient to prescribe or to fill prescriptions for patients in any military facility.

Related Regulation of Foods and Other Products

A number of other agencies oversee aspects of the safety of foods and of consumer products. Advertising of health care products other than prescription drugs and devices is the province of the Federal Trade Commission (FTC).[115] The labeling and quality of alcoholic beverages are regulated by the Bureau of Alcohol, Tobacco, and Firearms, which is a component of the Department of Treasury.[116] The actual sale of alcohol is regulated by each state. The safety of household products other than those that fall under FDA jurisdiction is regulated by the CPSC.[117] Meat and poultry safety is overseen by the Food Safety and Inspection Service in USDA.[118]

EPA regulates the safety and effectiveness of pesticides, a responsibility that had resided in the FDA prior to EPA's founding in 1970. (EPA's role in regulating pollution is described in more detail in chapter 6 on public health.) This agency also sets tolerance levels for pesticide residues in foods. The FDA and USDA are together responsible for monitoring the food supply for residues that exceed permissible thresholds. The EPA also sets national standards for drinking water, while the FDA oversees the safety of bottled water.

Regulation of Controlled Substances

The most significant aspect of pharmaceutical regulation that falls outside of the FDA's jurisdiction is the control of narcotics. This is the responsibility of the Drug Enforcement Administration (DEA), a component of the Department of Justice

(DOJ). DEA is larger than FDA, with 10,000 employees and a total annual budget of more than $2 billion. It enforces criminal laws regarding the possession and manufacture of controlled substances, including those that are outlawed for any purpose, such as heroin, and those that may be used in medical settings, such as methadone. In order to prescribe controlled substances, physicians must register with DEA, which can monitor their use of these drugs.

DEA has had a tortuous bureaucratic history. It grew out of the Bureau of Internal Revenue within the Department of Treasury.[119] This was the first agency to administer the Harrison Narcotics Tax Act of 1914, which mandated prescriptions for narcotics and increased the record-keeping requirements for physicians who prescribed them and for pharmacists who dispensed them. The unit within the bureau that enforced the act was renamed the Bureau of Prohibition in 1927, when alcohol was outlawed nationwide. The enforcement function for drugs was split from that office and placed in a new Bureau of Narcotics in 1930. In 1968, the agency merged with the FDA's Bureau of Drug Abuse Control to form the Bureau of Narcotics and Dangerous Drugs, which was placed in the DOJ. In 1973, it was reconstituted as the DEA with the incorporation of four other drug enforcement agencies, including the drug investigation unit of the U.S. Customs Service in the Department of Treasury, the Narcotics Advance Research Management Team in the Executive Office of the President, and the Office of National Narcotics Intelligence and the Office of Drug Abuse Law Enforcement in DOJ.

The DEA's evolution reflects the different attitudes of policy makers toward the hazards of narcotics and toward those of other kinds of drugs. Many nonnarcotic prescription drugs can be as dangerous as narcotics if taken improperly. Some are even obtained illicitly for recreational use despite widely known serious health risks. Narcotics, however, are perceived as presenting a separate and special concern, as their regulation and the enforcement structure surrounding them reflects.

Overriding Policy Debates: Does FDA Regulation Strike the Right Balance?

As with many aspects of health care regulation, the oversight of medical products reflects a process of balancing.[120] Too great a concern with safety can stifle innovation, but too lax a concern can lead to public health tragedies. How many new drugs are worth the possibility of another elixir of sulfanilamide or thalidomide? The regulatory scheme must weigh the risk of harm from the medicines that we use against the lost benefits of therapeutic breakthroughs that are delayed.

Prescription drugs are regulated to an extent not applied to any other kind of product. They may not reach the market until they have undergone years of costly government-supervised testing from which only a small fraction survive. After arriving on the market, their distribution and use are carefully monitored and documented, and the government can withdraw approval that it has previously granted. Every aspect of marketing is controlled and scrutinized down to the choice of product name and the size of the typeface used when it appears in print. Even beyond the FDA, numerous other agencies at both the state and federal levels add more layers of oversight.

Despite this huge regulatory burden, America's pharmaceutical industry remains fundamentally robust and strong. It is perennially among the most profitable.[121] Perhaps the rigorous government oversight actually reinforces the industry's strength. Many useless and dangerous drugs reached the market prior to enactment of the Food, Drug, and Cosmetic Act of 1938. Public confidence in the drugs that are available would be tenuous without the assurance of an exacting regulatory process. If the public fears that each new product could be the next thalidomide, the use of medications by patients and the willingness of health care professionals to prescribe them could diminish significantly.

In manufacturing products on which customers rely for their life and health, the pharmaceutical industry must command the public's trust to a greater extent than most. Only a disinterested third-party expert can provide the oversight on which such trust can rest. Polls indicate that the public trusts the FDA more than any other federal agency.[122] The administration of food and drug regulation is complex and perhaps uneven, requiring numerous reforms and refinements over time. However, without the assurance of vigilant outside oversight, the market for drugs in America would be very different, and likely much smaller, than it is today.

The regulation of drugs is also vulnerable to arbitrary distinctions that can undermine its credibility. Policy makers must categorize products in ways that often reflect politics as much as science. As the system now stands, chemicals that are classified as drugs may be sold but only after the completion of a long series of clinical trials and an approval process in which risks are weighed against clinical benefits. If they are classified as dietary supplements, even if they are promoted as having health effects similar to those of drugs, they may be sold without premarket testing and with only minimal postmarketing oversight. A few chemicals that act like drugs have been determined by Congress to fall into a special class that presents such serious hazards that they are treated as controlled substances, with less regulatory discretion over permitted uses. Although they may at times seem arbitrary, however, regulatory distinctions in a field as complex as pharmaceuticals are inevitable. Politics and science will always influence the process.

Over the coming years, substantial new challenges will force legislators and regulators to make increasingly difficult distinctions. New products based on new technologies, most notably the emerging science of genetics, will proliferate.[123] The process of drug development in terms of both the underlying science and the economics of research and development will evolve in response. Policy makers will have to weigh the promotion of innovation against the reduction of hazards in new ways, and the mix of policy and science will involve growing complexity. If history is a guide, our tolerance for risk will initially be high, but at the first sign of scandal, the legislative and regulatory reaction will be strong. Achieving the best regulatory balance will be a crucial task so that clinicians remain equipped with the safest and most effective medical technologies that science can provide.

6

Regulation of Public Health

Public health prevents epidemics and the spread of disease, protects against environmental hazards, prevents injuries, promotes and encourages healthy behaviors, responds to disasters and assists communities in recovery, and assures the quality and accessibility of health services.
—U. S. Department of Health and Human Services,
"Public Health in America"

In its earliest form, health care regulation in America addressed widespread threats to the public at large. While each decade has brought a cascade of new health care challenges, protection of the population from such threats, especially those of epidemic diseases, has never fully faded as an underlying concern.[1] In the scramble to shape a system that delivers the best health care to each individual, it is easy to forget our perennial vulnerability to illnesses that attack on a large scale and our early successes in defeating some of them. At times, though, there are unpleasant reminders.

The movement to control public health threats stems largely from advances in the ability to understand them. Scientists achieved many breakthroughs in knowledge about germs and infection during the late nineteenth century. These established the basis for sanitation, quarantine, and immunization in controlling disease outbreaks. Further knowledge demonstrated how food safety and nutrition could also help to prevent or cope with epidemics on a large scale. During the middle and late twentieth century, scientists achieved breakthroughs in knowledge about the causes of many chronic conditions. They were able to discern relationships between environmental factors such as tobacco, asbestos, and poor nutrition and diseases such as cancer, lung disease, heart disease, and a range of other slow-developing illnesses. Environmental protection and occupational exposure limits flowed as policy consequences.

While the history of public health regulation concerns policy reactions to advancing knowledge of disease causation, it also reflects, as does much of American health care regulation, a dynamic and often unstable balance of federal, state, and local authority. Science does not necessarily trump politics. The story of public health regulation in America is one of a government role that repeatedly bursts into the country's consciousness, often with dramatic political conflicts and consequences, despite the tendency of many to take it for granted or to remain blissfully ignorant of the activities involved. Time and again, advances in scientific understanding demand attention of one sort or another. (An overview of the historical changes in public health and its regulation over the past two centuries is contained in appendix B.)

History of Public Health Regulation

The First Steps in Public Health: States Take Center Stage to Fight Infectious Diseases

In 1892, William H. Park of the New York City Department of Health discovered that nearly half the diphtheria patients at one city hospital had been misdiagnosed.[2] Putting them next to real diphtheria patients in hospital wards actually created the risk of acquiring the disease. This finding made the importance of accurate diagnostic testing clear. A few years later, Charles V. Chapin, the health commissioner of Providence, Rhode Island, opined that all dirt is not equally dangerous.[3] We could best prevent contagious diseases by cleaning filth that is most likely to carry germs, rather than by fumigating everything.

The history of the nineteenth century leading up to these advances was filled with similar discoveries that corrected medical misconceptions. Public policy followed closely behind with regulatory programs to apply the emerging science to practice.[4] At the start of the nineteenth century, the goal of these programs seemed unimaginable—to protect the public's health on a wide scale. By the end of the century, public health regulation was putting the goal within reach.

Early government public health efforts were sporadic and local.[5] For example, the city of New York was granted authority by the state legislature in 1798 to pass health regulations in response to a yellow fever epidemic that killed 1,600 people. In 1805, a city inspector of health was appointed along with an advisory board of health. The inspector collected vital statistics and oversaw sanitation. Between 1810 and 1838, health inspectors were part of the police department. In 1866, the Metropolitan Board of Health was created out of the advisory board of health. It was replaced in 1870 by the New York City Health Department, which forms the nucleus of the agency that exists today.[6]

Germs like to travel with their hosts, and the greatest infectious disease threats to nineteenth-century America were in the port cities.[7] The first state health agency was established in New Orleans in 1855, although it achieved only limited success.[8] Massachusetts created the first permanent state health board in 1869. The earliest federal role can be traced to the decision to centralize the administration of marine hospitals under a supervising surgeon general of the Marine Hospital Service in 1870. Over the years, that office grew tremendously in scope and is today known as the Surgeon General's.

The federal-state balance in public health regulation shifted decisively toward the states just a few years later. In response to outbreaks of cholera and yellow fever in 1878, Congress gave the Marine Hospital Service the authority to quarantine ships, but subject to local overrides.[9] A yellow fever outbreak in New Orleans in 1879 led Congress to take the further step of establishing the National Board of Health. In 1883, however, the surgeon general, jealous of the new board's authority, convinced Congress to dissolve it. States also argued at the time that public health was not an appropriate federal concern. In the ensuing federal regulatory void, state and local governments took the lead and kept it from then on. By 1928, there were 204 county and local health departments in seventeen states. Today there are over 3,000 of them.[10]

Great scientific progress was made in the 1880s and 1890s with the discoveries of bacteria that caused several major diseases, including typhoid, cholera, tuberculosis, malaria, leprosy, and plague. The germ theory of disease was proposed and achieved increasing acceptance. State health departments grew rapidly in response, and in many instances borrowed officers from the Marine Hospital Service for guidance. With this model of states in the lead and federal officials in supporting roles, the structure of federal-state partnerships for public health protection began to take hold.

Early and Mid–Twentieth Century:
The Federal Government Finds Its Role

In addition to supporting state efforts with money and manpower, the federal government began to focus on public health aspects of areas in which it had traditionally exercised authority but with other primary goals, such as protecting national borders and interstate commerce. In 1891, the Department of Immigration sought the Marine Hospital Service's help in screening immigrants at the processing station on Ellis Island in New York. In 1912, Congress formally changed the service's name and defined a new scope of responsibility. The agency became the Public Health Service (PHS), as it is still known today, and was given authority to investigate the spread of diseases, including the role of sanitation and sewage, "and the pollution either directly or indirectly of the navigable streams and lakes of the United States."[11]

The newly renamed Public Health Service quickly found a range of public health challenges to address on a national scale. World War I focused attention on venereal disease, which led to the establishment in 1918 of the Division of Venereal Disease to promote sex education. Capabilities in epidemiology and biostatistics were expanded through the 1920s to better track national disease outbreaks. In 1929,

Congress added the Narcotics Division, which was later renamed the Division of Mental Hygiene.[12]

In its original role of directly providing hospital care, the Marine Hospital Service had required personnel. In peacetime, without direct access to military staff, this created the need for a dedicated corps of health care professionals. That need was filled in 1889 by the creation of the U.S. Public Health Service Commissioned Corps. The corps originally included only physicians, who were designated as medical officers. They were appointed by the president with the advice and consent of the Senate after passing several examinations.[13]

By 1900, the corps included about 100 commissioned officers. Their screening reflects contemporary attitudes toward professional competence. All survived an ordeal of rigorous tests not only of their medical skills but of general knowledge as well. One successful applicant, Dr. Victor Heiser, described his experience in 1898 in which a group of forty-two applicants were winnowed down.[14] Thirty were disqualified for physical reasons. Ten survived to be quizzed on a range of general skills, from reading aloud in French to knowledge of the Rosetta stone. They were then observed on medical skills, including diagnosing patients and identifying bacteria and parasites under a microscope. Three survived to be offered commissions.

Focus on Food

The need for a wider federal public health role gradually became evident as scientists began to clarify ways in which disease-causing organisms travel from state to state. Agricultural products, especially food, provide the best ride. Several states, including New York, Massachusetts, and Georgia, began inspecting agricultural products as early as 1819. In the 1870s, a few states began to inspect dairy products. A regulatory gap remained, however, in controlling items that moved in interstate commerce.

Revelations in the late nineteenth century and early twentieth century of unsanitary conditions in meatpacking plants, of poisonous preservatives and dyes in foods, and of worthless or dangerous patent medicines led to calls for a more active federal role in these areas. By 1880, senior officials of the U.S. Department of Agriculture (USDA) called for a system of national food and drug regulation. Although these calls were not fulfilled until the enactment of the first comprehensive federal food and drug law in 1906 (see chapter 5 on the regulation of drugs), the first tentative steps were taken in the 1890s. In 1890 and 1891, laws were enacted in a few states mandating meat and poultry inspections. In 1898, a federal official, Dr. Harvey Wiley of the USDA, helped to coordinate state activities by heading the Committee on Food Standards of the Association of Official Agricultural Chemists that set standards intended for incorporation into state food safety laws.

The movement toward federal involvement in food safety received a strong impetus in 1904 from the publication of Upton Sinclair's novel *The Jungle,* an exposé of unsafe and unsanitary conditions in the meatpacking industry.[15] The abuses that Sinclair described shock readers even today. The result was passage in 1906 of the Pure Food and Drug Act and the Meat Inspection Act, which together greatly expanded the USDA's regulatory and inspection roles. Among the most significant effects of these laws was implementation of the Hazard Analysis and Critical Control Point program, which included regulations addressing animal feed, use of uncontaminated water in food processing, effective use of food preservatives, improved sanitation of food-processing equipment and facilities, and surveillance of food handling and preparation. (Aspects of these laws concerning the regulation of drugs are discussed in chapter 5.) While their own role was growing, federal officials also continued to support food safety efforts at the state level. In 1924, the PHS helped Alabama develop a milk sanitation program, which developed voluntary sanitation standards for interstate shipment of grade A milk.[16] These standards have since been incorporated into mandatory milk safety standards in every state.

Scientific advances in the early decades of the twentieth century revealed that food safety is not merely a question of what not to eat. Staying healthy also depends on eating enough of the right things. During that period, scientists found that substandard nutrition can cause a range of diseases. In 1917, the USDA issued its first dietary recommendations based on five food groups, followed by a recommendation for including iodine in salt in 1924. Federal legislation in the 1920s assisted states in employing nutritionists, and in the 1930s food relief and school feeding programs were established. President Franklin Roosevelt convened the National Nutrition Conference for Defense in 1941, which recommended that wheat flour be enriched with vitamins and iron.[17]

These programs reduced food-related diseases dramatically. One of the greatest achievements in this regard concerned pellagra, a potentially lethal condition once considered infectious but that, in the 1930s, was found to result from a deficiency in niacin.[18] Once this nutrient was used to fortify flour, the incidence of pellagra dropped to zero by the late 1940s, after an estimated 3 million cases and 100,000 deaths between 1906 and 1940.

The USDA's food safety and nutrition programs continue to the present day, although they have never risen to prominence in the public's awareness, and the department is rarely thought of as a major public health agency. Other areas of health policy are considered more glamorous, while food safety and nutrition are often regarded as concerns that primarily affect less developed countries. Nevertheless, the preventive role of guarding against foodborne pathogens and ensuring adequate nutrition has saved millions from illness or death and represents an unsung triumph of early public health regulation. Its very success is what causes it to be taken for granted.

World War II and Worldwide Diseases

World War II produced yet another set of challenges for public health and a new impetus for an expanded federal role. The PHS's personnel and mission expanded significantly, as a new set of health issues, this time on a global scale, caused it to double in size. A 1942 malaria campaign that the service pioneered in the southern United States was exported to tropical areas around the world through the Malaria Control in War Areas program, the first worldwide public health initiative. The PHS also supported the war effort by developing standards for nurses and hiring 65,000 of them. In 1944, the fast-growing agency was reorganized to include the Office of Surgeon General and three bureaus—one for medical services, one for state services, and one for the new and expanding National Institutes of Health (NIH), which funded medical research throughout the country.[19] (See chapter 8 for a discussion of NIH's role in funding and regulating research.)

Another important development during World War II was the broadening of the National Health Service Commissioned Corps to include nonphysicians, such as nurses, medical scientists, dieticians, and physical therapists. Its size jumped from 625 officers to 2,600. After the war, however, the corps' popularity began to wane, as its cost and the quality of its facilities and care were increasingly questioned. By 1966, only eight of twenty-one hospitals remained open, and in 1971, a plan was developed for its dissolution. It was ultimately rescued from oblivion in 1972 with reorganization and a new name, the National Health Service Corps, which included noncommissioned staff.[20]

A more far-reaching development for the evolution of American public health regulation came in 1946, when the malaria control program expanded its mission and was renamed the Communicable Disease Center, or CDC for short. The program, formed to combat a disease endemic to warm climates, was based in Atlanta, where it employed 4,300 people. President Roosevelt sought to expand its mission into a national public health role based largely on his confidence in its leader, Dr. Joseph Mountin. Having no interest in trading the swamps of Georgia for the swamps of the Potomac, Dr. Mountin insisted on remaining where he was. The president agreed, Emory University donated land for offices, and the CDC has stayed in Atlanta ever since, representing the largest federal health agency based outside of the Washington, D.C., area.[21]

Over the years, several other agencies were added to the expanding PHS. Among these, the Indian Health Service (IHS) provides health care on and near reservations for Native Americans through a network of hospitals and clinics. The Health Resources and Services Administration (HRSA) monitors the nation's health care workforce and tracks the supply of physicians, nurses, and other health care professionals. It also administers funding for state programs in maternal and child health, human resource development, and primary care access. Overall, the PHS's reach now extends throughout the American health care system, in contrast to its more limited original role of providing support for state public health activities, or that of its predecessor, the Marine Hospital Service, of caring for sick sailors.[22]

Middle and Late Twentieth Century: Chronic Disease Control Rises on the Agenda

As public health policy responded to advances in knowledge about the causes of infectious diseases during the late 1880s, improved understanding of many chronic diseases led to a set of new policy challenges in the mid–twentieth century. In contrast to infectious diseases that manifest themselves rapidly, chronic diseases appear over time. They include conditions such as cancer, neurological disorders, and diabetes that can lead to progressive deterioration of physiological functions, including failure of organs and, in many cases, to death. Scientists had suspected for many decades that some kinds of environmental exposures could lead to such lethal degenerative conditions. In particular, they increasingly thought that various forms of cancer could result from exposure to an array of toxic substances, such as tobacco smoke. Led by new data and theories of chronic disease causation, public health policy began to take on a new meaning as the twentieth century progressed.

The year 1964 was a turning point. While it may have come as no surprise to epidemiologists and toxicologists who had been following the research, the surgeon general publicly reported that year a causal link between cigarette smoking and lung cancer.[23] The tobacco industry disputed the conclusions for many years, but the implications for public policy were clear. The government's public health establishment had taken a position on a question of chronic disease causation, and the apparatus that evolved to address the infectious disease threat would be deployed to meet this new kind of public health challenge.

At the CDC, the Epidemiology Branch, which had tracked infectious disease outbreaks, was expanded to include research into chronic diseases.[24] Other new programs were added to the agency's mission to address family planning, leukemia, and birth defects. The broadening of focus from infectious disease control was formally recognized in 1970 with a new name for the agency, the Centers for Disease Control. New areas of attention included indoor air quality, tobacco, asbestos, lead-based paint, and vinyl chloride exposure.[25] In 1983, the agency established the Violence Epidemiology Branch, in 1986 the Office of Smoking and Health, and in 1988 the Center for Chronic Disease Prevention and Health Promotion. In 1987, the National Center for Health Statistics, which collects and maintains vital statistics on a national basis, was moved under CDC's umbrella from the central office of the Department of Health and Human Services (DHHS). By 1992, the expanded mission was clear enough that the agency's name was changed again, this time to the Centers for Disease Control and Prevention. With its identity having become firmly established, however, the familiar CDC acronym was retained.[26]

During the same period, food safety and nutrition programs shifted their emphasis toward controlling the long-term risks of heart disease, cancer, and other illnesses related to high fat consumption and obesity.[27] Food labeling took on new importance in warning consumers of fat, salt, and caloric content. Public information campaigns by several agencies, including the USDA, the National Cancer Institute, and the CDC, began to focus on reducing saturated fat intake and maintaining a healthy weight. Nutritional deficiencies having been largely conquered in the United States, the focus of food safety centered on the role of dietary excesses.

Environmental Concern

Another milestone in the transition of public health policy toward chronic disease causation was the creation of the Environmental Protection Agency (EPA) in 1970. EPA administered several sweeping pieces of legislation that sought to limit public exposures to environmental hazards that pose long-term health risks. These included the National Environmental Protection Act, which required "environmental impact assessments" of all new government projects to balance predicted benefits against possible harm to the environment;[28] the Clean Water Act, which directed the government to set discharge standards for emissions into streams and other waterways;[29] and the Clean Air Act, under which discharge standards were set for emissions into the air from smokestacks, automobiles, and other sources.[30] In 1976, Congress passed the Resource Conservation and Recovery Act requiring EPA-issued permits for the operation of waste disposal facilities.[31]

EPA gained prominence in 1980 in the wake of a toxic waste scandal at Love Canal near Buffalo, New York. Press reports contained allegations of adverse health effects on local residents from an abandoned waste disposal site located near a residential area, and the public became sensitized to its vulnerability to improperly discarded hazardous waste.[32] In response, Congress passed the Comprehensive Environmental Response, Compensation and Liability Act (CERCLA), commonly known as "Superfund."[33] That law fostered a huge national effort to identify and clean toxic waste sites throughout the country, many of which had been festering without remediation for decades. EPA's budget and mission grew rapidly, and the expansive liability provisions of the law, which sought to pin blame on responsible private parties, greatly increased its legal activities as well.

The Superfund law also created a new agency under CDC's jurisdiction to assess health hazards at toxic waste sites. The Agency for Toxic Substances and Disease Registry (ATSDR) studies ways to prevent further exposures and illness from hazardous substances and monitors exposures and related diseases.[34] It serves as the research arm for EPA investigation and enforcement efforts.

In addition to the federal EPA, most states have established their own environmental protection structures.[35] In some instances, these duplicate federal regulations, and in others they fill gaps in regulatory coverage. Many states also have their own Superfund programs, and most have special regulations for tracking and managing medical waste, which are important to the operation of hospitals, physicians' offices, and other kinds of health care facilities. Unlike public health efforts to combat infectious diseases, however, most environmental protection continues to be led at the federal level.

Workplace Health

Chronic disease prevention through toxic exposure limitations was also expanded with the establishment in 1970, the same year as EPA's creation, of the Occupational Safety and Health Administration (OSHA).[36] Those who work on a daily basis with hazardous substances experience much higher exposure levels than the general public, with consequently greater health risks. Epidemiological studies published in the 1960s and 1970s strongly linked a few commonly encountered industrial chemicals, including benzene, lead, and polyvinyl chloride, with various forms of cancer.[37] OSHA set its own exposure standards, distinct from EPA's, for those who work with such substances, as well as safety standards for preventing accidents and infections. This standard setting is supported by research conducted by the National Institute of Occupational Safety and Health (NIOSH), a component of CDC.

Mental Health

Until the latter half of the twentieth century, the health care system's response to mental illness was primarily to separate patients from society rather than to treat them.[38] Few effective therapies were available. Psychotherapy, which gained prominence in the first half of the century, could help patients with milder conditions, but there were no reliable tools for dealing with severe mental diseases that prevented patients from functioning in society. Those suffering from schizophrenia and other severe mental afflictions could only be placed in long-term care hospitals that offered little hope of recovery. The same was true of patients with addictions to drugs or alcohol, for which confinement without therapy was usually the only available remedy.

This situation began to change in the early 1950s with development of the first medications to treat symptoms of schizophrenia, depression, and severe anxiety.[39] Antipsychotic drugs spared schizophrenic patients from some of the most severe manifestations of their illness and permitted some to function in society. Drugs for depression alleviated the effects of this condition for many, as did tranquilizers for severe anxiety. Treatments such as methadone were also developed for some forms of drug addiction, although their effectiveness remains controversial. All these medications can produce severe side effects, and none offers a complete cure, so the new psychoactive medicines were far from panaceas. However, they represented a giant step forward from the meager therapeutic armamentarium that preceded them.

Over the next several decades, the variety and effectiveness of psychoactive medications steadily increased. At the same time, other therapeutic techniques, including behavioral treatments, also advanced. By the end of the twentieth century, many kinds of mental illness, including addictions, had become treatable, if not curable, conditions.[40]

In response to the availability of treatments, the paradigm for mental health services shifted from one that favored institutionalization in most cases to one that encouraged community residence whenever possible.[41] Without actual cures, though, patients who were returned to society continued to need support services that they could access on an outpatient basis. To provide this resource, Congress in the 1960s authorized the establishment of a network in each state of community mental health centers to administer psychoactive medications, provide counseling, and offer other support services.[42] The Mental Retardation Facilities and Community Mental Health Centers Construction Act of 1964 provided the initial funding to construct these facilities.[43] However, over the succeeding decades, operational funding varied considerably with political changes at the federal level.[44]

In 1992, Congress created a new agency to coordinate the oversight and funding of mental health and substance abuse services at the federal level, the Substance Abuse and Mental Health Services Administration (SAMHSA).[45] It functions as a component of DHHS. Much of its work involves the administration of block grants to states that support community-based treatment programs. SAMHSA operates through four component offices.[46] The Center for Mental Health Services (CMHS) supports community programs for patients with serious mental illness and services for their families. The Center for Substance Abuse Prevention (CSAP) funds educational programs to prevent alcohol and drug abuse. The Center for Substance Abuse Treatment (CSAT) supports community-based addiction treatment centers. The Office of Applied Studies (OAS) collects and analyzes data on substance abuse practices.

Mental illness remains a difficult chronic disease challenge for the health care system. The array of pharmacological and behavioral treatments continues to grow, but for the most part therapies offer relief from symptoms rather than cures. Many of those with severe mental illnesses have been returned from institutions to communities where they are capable of functioning to only a marginal degree. Large numbers of these patients who have been "deinstitutionalized" are unable to find and maintain permanent residences, and they live on streets and in shelters in a state of homelessness. They continue to need public services, but the responsibility has shifted to a large extent from health care programs to the welfare and criminal justice systems. In light of this, some critics question the overall benefit of moving their care from custodial settings to outpatient treatment. Nevertheless, newly available therapies have enabled many with severe mental illnesses and addictions to lead productive lives that otherwise would not have been possible. For large numbers of them, the network of publicly funded community resources provides support that is essential to this result.

Beyond the severely ill who are candidates for institutionalization, mental impairments of one form or another are estimated to affect almost 54 million Americans, or almost 20 percent of the population.[47] While in many cases the conditions involved are quite mild, almost half of those who have them are limited in their ability to perform essential functions, commonly referred to as "activities of daily living." The overall system of services that the government provides has been described by a presidential commission as a fragmented array of forty-two different programs that operate with little or no coordination.[48] Mental health has historically received less attention and funding than other aspects of public health, and despite recent advances in scientific understanding of its causes and nature and improvements in its treatment, this pattern still prevails.

Public Health Today: Coming Full Circle

The recent regulatory preoccupation with chronic diseases can be seen, somewhat ironically, as a consequence of the triumph of American public health over the past 100 years. Had the country not made so much progress in the late nineteenth and early twentieth centuries in controlling infectious hazards, it would not have the luxury of turning its attention to more complex, slower-developing ailments. With antibiotics, sanitation, inoculations, disease reporting, and other tools, the American public health infrastructure can look back with pride at a threat largely contained. As an example of this success, the incidence of typhoid fever, which peaked at 45 per 100,000 in the 1920s, was at zero in 1960.[49]

The sense of triumph, however, may be starting to fade, since the threat of infectious diseases has been making a comeback. Some of the diseases that constitute this threat are new, and some straddle the line between acute and chronic. Acquired immune deficiency syndrome (AIDS), first identified in 1981, poses a major infectious disease burden consuming huge amounts of public resources. In a further irony, as we have begun to develop effective treatments, it has taken on the characteristics of a chronic condition requiring longer-term approaches to control. Ebola, West Nile virus, and other new infectious diseases with shorter clinical courses have appeared with growing regularity as international travel has increased. Formerly controlled infections, most prominently tuberculosis, are returning with greater virulence in antibiotic-resistant forms. It appears that the need to control infections has not gone away; it just went into hiding for a while. Many of the lessons learned and public policies implemented more than a hundred years ago may need to be revisited.

As if new natural threats of disease were not enough, we now also face dangers from infectious diseases that are spread, and even manufactured, intentionally. The use of diseases as weapons has joined the list of public health challenges, as bioterrorism has become a reality and biological warfare a serious threat. The infrastructure that the United States developed to respond to nature's devastation is now called on for protection from human actions. In response, the system of federal, state, and local coordination of regulation and research, of monitoring, and of reporting will significantly evolve yet again with the creation in 2002 of the federal Department of Homeland Security (DHS), whose structure is discussed later in this chapter. As public health becomes a matter of national defense, a new set of public crises is about to push American health care regulation into different and uncharted territory.

The Structure and Function of Public Health Agencies

In keeping with the history of federal-state tension in the United States, primary responsibility for maintaining America's public health infrastructure remains divided between the federal government and the states.[50] The actual implementation of many programs is at the state and local levels, but essential elements, including funding, coordination, data reporting, and standard setting in key areas, are provided by federal agencies. The interplay between levels of government forms a constant source of conflict that will likely intensify as public health challenges become more complex.

The Federal Level

Public Health Research, Surveillance, and Coordination:
The Centers for Disease Control and Prevention (CDC)
CDC increasingly forms the hub around which public health regulation in America revolves. Its mission is to "promote health and quality of life by preventing and controlling disease, injury and disability."[51] Organizationally, it is part of the PHS, which in turn is a component of DHHS. CDC's Atlanta headquarters is the farthest from Washington, D.C., of any federal health agency, lending it at least the perception of greater independence.

Although not large by federal standards, CDC has grown considerably over the years. It now includes twelve centers, institutes, and offices and employs 8,500 people in 170 occupations.[52] Its basic organization is summarized in table 6.1. It is among the most interdisciplinary agencies in American government. Of its staff, 5,600 work in the Atlanta headquarters and the rest in facilities spread throughout the country

Table 6.1
CDC Centers, Institutes, and Offices

Component	Mission
Office of the Director	Overall direction for the agency
National Center on Birth Defects and Developmental Disabilities	National leadership for preventing birth defects and developmental disabilities
National Center for Chronic Disease Prevention and Health Promotion	Prevent premature death and disability from chronic diseases and promote healthy behaviors
National Center for Environmental Health	Prevent disease and death resulting from interactions with the environment
National Center for Health Statistics	Provide statistical information to guide policies
National Center for HIV, STD, and TB Prevention	Prevent and control HIV infection, sexually transmitted diseases, and tuberculosis
National Center for Infectious Diseases	Prevent illness, disability, and death from infectious diseases in the United States and worldwide
National Center for Injury Prevention and Control	Prevent death and disability from nonoccupational injuries
National Immunization Program	Prevent disease, disability, and death from vaccine-preventable diseases
National Institute for Occupational Safety and Health	Ensure workplace safety and health through research and prevention
Epidemiology Program Office	Coordinate public health surveillance, support in scientific communications, and training in surveillance and epidemiology
Public Health Program Practice Office	Strengthen community practice of public health

Source: http://www.cdc.gov/about/cio.htm (25 May 2006).

from Alaska to Puerto Rico. Its activities span a range of research, health monitoring, and support for state public health efforts. The agency boasts among its recent accomplishments helping local health officials identify West Nile disease, a sometimes lethal virus that first appeared in the United States in 1999, publishing *Emerging Infectious Disease Journal* online and in four languages, operating the National Vital Statistics System, and coordinating state efforts in bioterrorism response.

CDC's history has been marked by numerous other significant accomplishments. It helped develop the polio vaccine and influenza shots in the 1950s.[53] Polio, which is most commonly found in children, is a highly contagious disease that is often fatal and can cause permanent paralysis of the legs and other parts of the body in those who survive. It was widespread throughout the world, including the United States, prior to the development of a vaccine.[54] In the wake of large-scale immunization efforts, there were no reported cases of polio in the United States between 1979 and 2005.

In 1951, CDC established the Epidemic Intelligence Service to provide twenty-four-hour-a-day on-call investigations of disease outbreaks. In 1961, it began publishing the weekly *Morbidity and Mortality Weekly Report,* which compiles data supplied by public health officials throughout the country into national snapshots of trends that may not be evident at the state or local levels and which published the first report of AIDS.

Perhaps CDC's greatest triumph was a program begun in the 1960s to eradicate smallpox. Coordinated with public health agencies in several other countries, the program succeeded on a worldwide scale when the last case of this disease was reported in 1977 in Somalia. Since then, CDC has been charged with guarding one of two remaining vials of the virus that were retained for possible future research, the other being kept in what was then the Soviet Union and is today Russia.[55] Unfortunately, smallpox may make a comeback as a weapon of bioterrorism, possibly reversing CDC's, and one of humankind's, greatest accomplishments in the sphere of health. Nevertheless, having seen a disease eradicated as a threat once, we now know that it can be done.

CDC has also helped to solve numerous medical mysteries and is called in regularly by state and local health departments for authoritative medical detective work. As discussed, it was primarily responsible for identifying the organism that causes Legionnaire's disease, a lethal respiratory illness that first attracted medical attention when it struck attendees at an American Legion convention in Philadelphia in 1976. In 1981, CDC and the California Department of Health helped to classify AIDS as a new disease. This condition devastates the immune system and initially drew public attention as an affliction primarily of gay men. The cause of AIDS continued to baffle physicians and scientists for several years after the first patient was diagnosed. While initial cases were concentrated in the gay community, other vulnerable groups were soon identified, including recipients of blood donations and intravenous drug users who shared needles. By relentlessly destroying the immune system of patients, AIDS leaves them vulnerable to a range of serious and deadly infections. Identification of the condition led to discovery of the virus that causes it, human immunodeficiency virus (HIV), which in turn facilitated several steps that helped to control its spread. These included screening tests to identify those who are infected, tests to find the virus in donated blood, and drugs that can significantly slow the disease's progression.[56]

Public Health Manpower: Health Resources and Services Administration (HRSA) and National Health Service Corps

Most public health regulatory agencies, whether their mission is to issue rules, conduct research, or maintain data, operate far from the sphere of the individual patient. While they are crucial to the health of millions of people from a population perspective, their roles do not put them close to clinical care provision on a day-to-day basis. Government involvement in providing medical services to the civilian population grew quite gradually, in part because of opposition from the organized medical profession, which feared competition.[57] Public health hospitals, including those of the Marine

Hospital Service, were founded in the earliest days of the nation but served only targeted populations. In 1932, a local health department in New York State became the first to offer medical services to indigent residents, a role that historically had been played by private nonprofit dispensaries dating back to the late eighteenth century. But for some time, this was not followed elsewhere to a significant extent.

In the 1960s, the situation started to change. A national network of neighborhood community health centers was established to offer some primary care services to indigent patients under the federal Office of Equal Opportunity. In the early 1970s, these centers were transferred to HRSA, and over the next several years their numbers grew substantially.[58] While they have never become a sizable part of American public health efforts when compared with regulatory programs, these clinics and similar ones established by state and local health departments have made clinical care provision part of the government's public health role.

When the community health network was created, a senior PHS physician, Dr. Laurence Platt, proposed a National Health Service Corps to staff it that would incorporate the National Health Service Commissioned Corps, which had been slated for dissolution. His idea was to send health professionals to underserved areas of the country, where they would have an opportunity to serve a social need and to provide patients with better access to care.[59] As an inducement to join, physicians and other health professionals in training were given scholarships and low-interest loans in return for service in the corps.

The proposal for the new corps led to a restructuring that produced two federal agencies with missions to provide health care services directly to needy patients. One was Dr. Platt's National Health Service Corps, which provided health care manpower. The other was HRSA, which maintained the corps and administered several of PHS's existing service delivery programs, including those for maternal and child health and migrant health.

As of 1980, the National Health Service Corps had 2,080 health care providers in the field. It was supporting the education of another 6,000 through its educational loan programs.[60] Today there are 2,700 providers, but the number of loans has fallen to 3,600.[61] The number of community health centers had grown to 872 that year from 157 in 1974. Among other missions, the corps helped to move personnel into community health centers and away from hospitals, which had been part of the PHS's original mission.

As home to the corps and other health manpower agencies, HRSA has as its overall objective providing health care resources for medically underserved populations. It supports a network of 643 community and migrant health centers and 144 primary care programs for the homeless and residents of public housing. It also oversees the nation's organ transplant system, which is operated by the United Network for Organ Sharing (UNOS), a private nonprofit organization (described in more detail in chapter 3); administers Ryan White CARE Act programs for children with AIDS; administers maternal and child health programs to promote prenatal care, nutrition, and other childhood preventive services; and provides funds to the states for human resource development in health care, maternal and child health, and primary care access.[62]

The agency now has 1,366 employees in its Washington, D.C., headquarters and 744 in regional field offices (not including National Health Service Corps members).[63] Its primary operations are divided into five bureaus. They are described in table 6.2.

Food Safety and Nutrition: United States Department of Agriculture (USDA)

The USDA is a large cabinet-level agency with a broad set of components stretching from the National Forest Service to the Rural Business-Cooperative Service. Three constituent agencies promote and regulate food safety and nutrition—the Food Safety and Inspection Service (FSIS), the Food and Nutrition Service (FNS), and the Center for Nutrition Policy and Promotion (CNPP). In addition, the Economic Research Service (ERS) conducts research on food assistance and nutrition.[64]

Table 6.2
HRSA Bureaus

Bureau	Areas of Responsibility
Bureau of Primary Health Care	Community health centers, black lung clinics, migrant health centers, public housing primary care, mental health and substance abuse services, obstetrical and gynecological care
Maternal and Child Health Bureau	Oversight and assistance for funding programs
HIV/AIDS Bureau	Funds for areas disproportionately affected by AIDS, assistance for states in improving services for AIDS patients, assistance in access to AIDS drugs, support for innovative AIDS service delivery models and training of providers, support for nonreimbursed dental programs
Bureau of Health Professions	National Health Service Corps, grants for health professional education, promotes health professionals in underserved communities, research on health workforce issues
Healthcare Systems Bureau	Construction assistance for health facilities, manages Organ Procurement and Transplantation Network, Scientific Registry of Transplant Recipients, and National Marrow Donor Program, state health insurance planning grants, administers National Childhood Vaccine Injury Act of 1986

Source: http://www.hrsa.gov/about/orgchart.htm (25 May 2006).

The FSIS ensures the quality of meat, poultry, and egg products through inspections of all products sold in interstate commerce and through labeling requirements.[65] It also reinspects imported goods. In addition to the inspection of foods, the FSIS sets requirements for slaughtering and processing plants with regard to sanitation and temperature, inspects them for contamination, and conducts epidemiological investigations of foodborne disease outbreaks in cooperation with the CDC. Reflecting the magnitude of the task, FSIS currently employs more than 7,600 workers to serve as inspectors.

As with much other public health regulation, authority for meat and poultry inspections is divided between the federal government and the states. Under the federal Meat Inspection Act and the Poultry Products Inspection Act, plants can apply for either federal or state inspection for products produced for intrastate commerce.[66] To qualify as an alternative to federal oversight, a state's requirements must be at least as stringent as those of the FSIS. Currently, twenty-seven states operate their own inspection programs. Almost 6,500 plants are inspected under the federal program and about 2,100 by the states. FSIS provides half of the operating funds for the state programs, along with training and other assistance.

To complement the inspections, the FSIS operates the Foodborne Disease Active Surveillance Network in conjunction with CDC, the Food and Drug Administration (FDA), and state health departments to track the sources of food-related illnesses. It also conducts consumer education programs regarding foodborne pathogens and safe food-handling techniques. These programs emphasize warnings for populations that are particularly vulnerable, such as the elderly, pregnant women, and young children. The FSIS also maintains two advisory committees on scientific aspects of food hazards—the National Advisory Committee on Meat and Poultry Inspection and the National Advisory Committee on Microbiological Criteria for Foods.

The FNS operates five nutrition programs for needy populations.[67] To implement them, it relies heavily on coordination with state, local, and private organizations. The programs include food stamps for low-income families; child nutrition assistance for day care, after-school, and summer programs; team nutrition to educate schoolchildren; supplemental nutrition for women, infants, and children; and food distribution to low-income families, emergency feeding programs, Indian reservations, and the elderly.

The CNPP was founded in 1994.[68] Its mission is to provide scientific support for nutrition programs, which is particularly important in correcting erroneous advice that can reach the public through the popular press. The center develops and coordinates nutrition policy within USDA, assesses the cost-effectiveness of government-sponsored nutrition programs, assesses the cost of food for American families, investigates techniques for effective nutrition communication, and evaluates the nutrition content of the American food supply, an initiative that in its original form dates back to 1909. It also publishes reports on nutrition and nutrition expenditures by families and issues dietary guidelines, including the Food Guide Pyramid, which graphically represents the components of a well-balanced diet.[69]

Public Health and National Defense: The Department of Homeland Security (DHS)

A new element in the regulatory landscape is the intersection of health care and national defense. Americans have become increasingly aware that biological agents can be used for military purposes. More fundamentally, a wide-scale disease outbreak, whether of man-made or natural origin, could pose a serious threat to large numbers of people and to the country's economic base. Public health officials repeatedly warn that an uncontrolled outbreak of a condition such as severe acute respiratory syndrome (SARS), West Nile virus, or influenza could spread rapidly to a large portion of the population, removing many people from the workforce and placing unsustainable demands on the health care system.

Congress created DHS as a cabinet-level agency in 2002 to coordinate the protection of American citizens within the country's borders. While the impetus for creating the agency was the terrorist attacks of 11 September 2001, its mission also encompasses protection from many kinds of natural disasters. DHS is responsible for overseeing the country's network of first responders who act in response to disasters, including biological attacks and major disease outbreaks.[70] Its component agencies include the Federal Emergency Management Agency (FEMA), which administers disaster relief.

Among DHS's overall tasks is to establish a national response plan for all public hazards.[71] In the event of a serious public health emergency, DHS would play a major role in orchestrating the activities of several health care regulatory agencies, including the CDC, which monitors disease outbreaks; the FDA, which supervises the production and distribution of vaccines; and the PHS, which provides staff for many public hospitals and clinics. As a result, although it does not directly regulate health care, DHS could play an important role in directing the overall health care system should an emergency arise.

Environmental Health: Environmental Protection Agency (EPA)

EPA's conception can be tied to the first celebration of a novel holiday.[72] On 22 April 1970, hundreds of thousands of demonstrators nationwide, including 100,000 in New York's Union Square, celebrated the first Earth Day by rallying support for efforts to reduce pollution and clean the environment. The event revealed a huge and previously unsuspected following for this cause, and it has led to annual observances ever since, although on a smaller scale than the first. Less than eight months after the first Earth Day, the movement achieved a major political accomplishment when a new agency with a mission devoted to protecting the environment opened its doors on 2 December 1970.[73]

The legislative drumbeat leading to EPA's creation had been building for some time. In 1947, Congress passed the federal Insecticide, Fungicide, and Rodenticide Act, giving the FDA authority to regulate these hazardous products.[74] In 1948, the federal Water Pollution Control Act, also known as the Clean Water Act, was enacted, followed in 1955 by the Clean Air Act. In 1965, the Shoreline Erosion Protection Act and the Solid Waste Disposal Act were passed, and in 1967 the Air Quality Act.[75] As a precursor to creating EPA, in 1969 Congress passed the National Environmental Policy Act (NEPA), under which a three-member Environmental Quality Council was established to review and approve environmental impact statements for all federal projects affecting the environment.[76] As a reflection of the growing prominence of national environmental concerns, the council was given representation in the president's cabinet. The focus of environmental policy had shifted from simply conserving natural resources to proactively protecting and improving the country's natural environment.

In forming EPA, Congress incorporated into it several existing agencies and functions. From the Interior Department came the Water Quality Administration, including pesticide regulation. From the Department of Health, Education, and Welfare (now DHHS) came the National Air Pollution Control Administration. From the FDA came pesticide research, the Bureau of Solid Waste Management, the Bureau of Water Hygiene, and parts of the Bureau of Radiological Health. USDA contributed its pesticide regulatory activities under the Agricultural Research Service. The Atomic Energy Commission (now the Nuclear Regulatory Commission) and the Federal Radiation Council retained their separate status but coordinated with the new agency the development and enforcement of radiation criteria and standards. Finally, the newly formed Council on Environmental Quality transferred its ecological research activities to EPA.[77]

EPA now employs 18,000 people in its Washington, D.C., headquarters, ten regional offices, and seventeen laboratories around the country. More than half of the agency's employees are engineers, scientists, and environmental protection professionals. Bureaucratically, it is structured into seventeen offices as described in table 6.3. The administrator is appointed by the president, subject to confirmation by the Senate.[78]

With this extensive infrastructure and set of resources, EPA's work spans a range of environmental protection activities. Its core functions include setting and enforcing emission standards for pollutants under the Clean Air and Clean Water Acts, regulating the content of and warnings for pesticides, licensing waste disposal sites, implementing the cleanup of Superfund sites, and reviewing environmental impact statements for federal projects. It also supports numerous initiatives that disseminate research and information on environmental issues. These include developing detailed data on global warming, helping state and local responders to plan for bioterrorism threats, providing public information on lead poisoning, and operating the National Environmental Supercomputing Center to support global environmental research.[79]

Table 6.3
EPA Offices

Office	Areas of Responsibility
Office of the Administrator	Overall supervision for the agency
Office of Policy, Economics and Innovation	Information on regulatory development and economic analyses
Office of Administration and Resources Management	The agency's human, financial and physical resources
Office of Air and Radiation	Air and radiation protection programs
American Indian Environmental Office	Indian public health and environmental protection with emphasis on tribal capacity to administer programs
Chief Financial Officer	Planning, budgeting, analysis and accountability, as well as financial management
Office of Enforcement and Compliance Assurance	Compliance with environmental laws
Office of Environmental Justice	Environmental protection for communities comprised predominantly of people of color or low income populations
Office of Environmental Information	Center of excellence to advance the use of information as a a strategic resource at the Agency
History Office	The agency's institutional memory
Office of Inspector General	Audits and investigations of agency programs and operations
Office of International Affairs	Agency involvement in international policies and programs that cut across offices and regions
Office of Prevention, Pesticides and Toxic Substances	Toxic substance control and public information on chemical risks
Office of Research and Development	Research and development needs of operating programs
Sciences Policy Council	Cross-media, cross-program and cross-disciplinary science policy issues
Office of Solid Waste and Emergency Response	Land disposal of hazardous wastes, underground storage tanks, solid waste management, and Superfund program
Office of Water	National water programs, technical policies, regulations relating to water quality, and protection of wetlands, marine, and estuarine areas

Source: http://www.epa.gov/epahome/locate1.htm (25 May 2006).

The regulation of pollution often brings with it heavy financial burdens on those who are regulated. Emission limits may require the use of expensive technology, which can also limit production efficiency; cleanup of hazardous waste sites under the Superfund program is always expensive; and other EPA-administered programs, including the licensing of waste disposal facilities, can impose heavy costs as well. Disputes over environmental compliance costs have placed EPA in the center of much political controversy and litigation. Lengthy court battles, often reaching the Supreme Court, have characterized much of the agency's work.[80] In particular, the Superfund program, which assigns liability for cleanup costs to private parties, has engendered its own area of law, with EPA enforcement policies at the center. Much of EPA's policy making, therefore, is shaped as much by the courts as by the traditional administrative rule-making process.

In an attempt to make environmental regulation more efficient and responsive and less prone to litigious interference, an experiment begun in the 1990s moved some of EPA's regulatory work away from formal standard setting into a more market-based approach. The agency was authorized to issue pollution allowances that permit holders to emit predetermined levels of waste into the air or water in return for a fee. The allowances can be bought, sold, and traded between polluting businesses as each determines its own best trade-offs of costs for technology to reduce emissions against costs for obtaining the credits. The aggregate amount of allowances available in a region is subject to an overall cap, which is set slightly below the historical overall emission level. At the end of a compliance period, which can last up to five years, each polluting source must demonstrate that it owns allowances at least equal to its discharges.[81]

An allowance program was initiated for sulfur dioxide nationally in 1990 and for sulfur dioxide and nitrogen oxide in the Los Angeles area in 1994. A cooperative program of northeastern states for nitrogen oxide was begun in 1999. This approach has significantly reduced EPA's administrative costs for emission control and may have avoided litigation that individual enforcement actions would have entailed. The agency is considering expanding this approach into other areas.[82]

Environmental Monitoring: Agency for Toxic
Substances and Disease Registry (ATSDR)
ATSDR is one of a handful of federal agencies with a mission of research and data gathering but with no actual regulatory authority. Its original mandate under the 1980 Superfund law was to assess health hazards at toxic waste sites, investigate ways to prevent further exposure and illness, and expand knowledge about the health effects of hazardous substances. Subsequent laws expanded the list of activities slightly to include tasks such as providing public health assessments of licensed hazardous waste facilities and maintaining toxicology databases. The agency is headquartered in Atlanta alongside CDC, with ten regional field offices. It employs a relatively small staff of 400 professionals, including epidemiologists, physicians, and toxicologists.[83]

The overall mission of the agency is now to provide data and advice on toxic exposures. It maintains the National Exposure Registry of hazardous substances and of people exposed to them. (Identities are protected under the federal Privacy Act.) In response to specific releases of toxic substances, its officials help to determine if members of a community were exposed, educates residents and professionals, and makes recommendations to the EPA, which in turn has the regulatory authority to penalize or close plants or businesses. The agency also provides an ombudsman to investigate community concerns about environmental health hazards and business concerns about environmental regulations. In keeping with the pattern of federal-state relationships in public health, it maintains partnerships with twenty-three states to conduct public health assessments and to provide guidance and technical assistance to local health departments.[84]

Workplace Health: Occupational Safety and Health Administration (OSHA)

OSHA came into being right on the heels of EPA, on 29 December 1970.[85] Unlike EPA, which is an independent agency, OSHA is part of the Department of Labor (DOL). Its primary mission is to mandate standards to protect the safety and health of workers in businesses engaged in interstate commerce. The agency also conducts inspections and assesses fines to enforce compliance with its standards. OSHA also approves, monitors, and funds occupational safety and health plans implemented by the states. In late 1972, the first three such plans were approved in South Carolina, Montana, and Oregon. Today, twenty-four states have plans.[86]

The Occupational Safety and Health Act, which created the agency, is also significant for the underlying obligation that it places on employers.[87] The "general duty clause" requires that workers be provided a safe workplace, over and above the employer's compliance with any specific regulation. This broad language fills any holes that may be left in OSHA's regulatory scheme by creating a legal standard that all businesses must meet. Failure to meet the standard can, in itself, engender liability to injured workers. The act further requires employers to prominently post information on employee rights to a safe and healthy work environment, as well as information on contacting the agency for complaints.

Very soon after its creation, OSHA adopted its first standards on 17 January 1971. This move was sweeping and engendered some controversy. The agency faced the challenge of protecting millions of workers in a short time frame. Without the time or resources to conduct the research needed to fully support this effort, it adopted the existing rules of various industry trade organizations. Many of the rules were overly specific and in some instances seemed trivial. Some were so detailed that compliance was almost impossible. Over time, many of these standards were revised and refined, but the agency got off to a somewhat rocky start.[88]

OSHA operates in tandem with a sister agency that conducts research to support its regulations. The studies sponsored by the National Institute for Occupational Safety and Health (NIOSH) are aimed at developing new occupational standards, which it recommends to OSHA for implementation. To retain its independence from the regulatory arm, NIOSH is part of the CDC rather than DOL.[89]

Bureaucratically, OSHA's structure includes ten offices and directorates, which are listed in table 6.4. Much of OSHA's resources are devoted to inspections. It has 2,370 employees, of whom 1,170 are inspectors. The twenty-four state-run plans have a total of 2,948 employees, including 1,275 inspectors.[90]

Among OSHA's most controversial activities have been its efforts to protect workers from chronic diseases. Through the 1960s and 1970s, research findings accumulated linking several kinds of workplace toxic exposures to various chronic conditions, many of them fatal.[91] Benzene has been linked with leukemia, polyvinyl chloride with pancreatic cancer, lead with severe anemia, solvents with brain damage, and a range of other chemicals with many other ills. No one faces a greater risk of exposure than those whose work involves daily contact.

As with much government policy toward chronic disease prevention, including that of EPA, OSHA must balance known risks against unknown variables. Scientific data can move the argument only so far. At some point, experts disagree. When that point is reached, a government agency charged with protecting public health must make educated assumptions on how to weigh health risks against the costs of exposure reduction. This dilemma becomes particularly acute when, as is often the

Table 6.4
OSHA Offices

Office/Directorate	Areas of Responsibility
Office of Assistant Secretary	Overall agency management, public affairs, equal employment opportunity
Directorate of Administrative Programs	Personnel, program budgeting, and financial management
Directorate of Construction	Construction standards and compliance, engineering services
Directorate of Compliance Programs	Investigations, compliance assistance
Directorate of Federal-State Operations	Consultations, assistance to states, training and education
Directorate of Health Standards Programs	Risk assessment, risk education technology, standards analysis and promulgation
Directorate of Information Technology	Management data systems, statistics
Directorate for Policy	Academic and professional affairs, program evaluation, regulatory analysis
Directorate of Safety Standards Programs	Establishing safety standards
Directorate of Technical Support	Technical support, support for occupational health nursing and occupational medicine, science and technology assessment

Source: http://www.osha.gov/html/oshdir.html (25 May 2006).

case, the costs of risk reduction are high. OSHA must often draw a difficult line between industry concerns over cost and the worries of workers, organized labor, and public interest organizations over health. Not surprisingly, the path of OSHA, like that of EPA, has been largely paved with litigation.

A few milestones on OSHA's road stand out. In a closely watched legal contest, in 1980 the Supreme Court ruled that the agency does not have to balance costs and benefits in issuing toxic exposure standards.[92] Health considerations alone can be determinative. In the mid-1980s, OSHA issued its first standard calling for biological monitoring of individual workers for toxic exposures rather than measurements of ambient toxin levels.[93] The workplace limits for lead represented the first tentative steps toward individualized physiological analysis of harm. Many businesses saw an expensive new burden, while many workers feared for their medical privacy. During the final days of the Clinton administration in 2001, the agency issued its first regulations to limit repetitive stress injuries that can lead to carpal tunnel syndrome and similar orthopedic impairments.[94] Later that year, the Bush administration rescinded the rules to study less intrusive approaches. Few other agencies face as complex and politically charged a set of policy trade-offs.

OSHA also faces a challenge in bringing public health protections to the health care industry itself. Hospitals, physicians' offices, and other health care settings present workers with unique health risks from infections. Direct contact with patients and with bodily fluids, such as blood, presents hazards to physicians, nurses, and even nonmedical personnel. A detailed set of OSHA regulations governs the operation of health care facilities, with emphasis on the handling of body fluids.[95] Some health care settings present further risks from the implements of treatment, including radioactive and toxic substances.

State and Local Health Departments

If the work of public health is trench warfare, then the trenches run through state capitals. There are fifty-five state-level health agencies in the United States, one for each state and one each for the District of Columbia, Guam, Puerto Rico, American Samoa, and the Virgin Islands.[96] Most oversee local agencies at the municipal or county level. They also develop programs, monitor them, regulate and fund them, and license health care facilities and institutions, while local governments deliver many of the actual services. (The regulation of clinical professionals is described in chapter 2 and of institutions in chapter 3.) The exception is the smallest state geographically, Rhode Island, which has no local agencies and spends 40 percent of its public health budget funding private organizations.

The largest portion of funding for public health efforts in most states is derived from federal grants for various health promotion activities.[97] The remainder comes from state tax revenues and from license and related fees. As discussed earlier, CDC provides funds for the prevention of communicable and chronic diseases and injuries and serves as an expert resource when needed. HRSA funds state programs in maternal and child health, human resource development, and primary care access. Funding sources for local public health departments vary considerably, with the largest share typically coming from the state, some of which represents a pass-through of federal funds, and the remainder coming from local tax revenue.[98]

Each state has put its own stamp on its public health bureaucracy, but there are common themes.[99] Each has a health commissioner or secretary of health who is advised by a state health officer, generally a licensed physician. In some states, the two positions are combined. About half of the states place policy-making and funding authority in a separate board of health, whereas the other half incorporate it into the agency. Most state health departments focus solely on public health, but many, including California's Department of Health Services, include related areas such as mental health services, environmental health, disability services, and the state's Medicaid program.[100] Medicaid perennially overshadows public health in its share of state budget funds, so health departments with Medicaid administration responsibility tend to be substantially more visible.[101]

The typical core public health functions of state and local health agencies are data gathering, education, standard setting, and licensure, as summarized in table 6.5.[102] Many also devote considerable resources to directly providing services through pri-

Table 6.5
Core State and Local Public Health Functions

State Departments	Local Departments
Collect and analyze health statistics to determine the health status and general health situation of the public	Maintain vital statistics
	Control communicable diseases
Provide general education to the public on matters of public health importance	Implement environmental sanitation
	Provide maternal and child health services
Maintain state laboratories to conduct certain specialized tests that are required by state public health law	Implement health education programs
	Operate public clinics that provide primary care and preventive services
Establish and police public health standards for the state as a whole	
Grant licenses to health care professionals and institutions throughout the state and monitor and inspect the performance of personnel and institutions as appropriate	
Establish general policy for local government public health units and provide them with financial support	

mary care clinics that address the needs of indigent patients, including many who receive benefits under Medicaid. However, recent changes in the structure of Medicaid programs in most states have lessened this aspect of health department missions.[103] Medicaid is now administered predominantly through managed care plans that assign beneficiaries to primary care providers, reducing their reliance on public clinics. (The history and structure of Medicaid are discussed in chapter 4.) As a result, the prominence of providing primary care services as a public health function is receding in many states in favor of more traditional population-based programs such immunizations, preventive screening, prenatal nutrition, and addiction counseling.

A fairly representative state health department is that of Pennsylvania. Its Bureau of Community Health Systems within the Department of Health operates through six district offices that coordinate and administer support to fifty-seven community health centers.[104] The district offices also maintain data from local health statistics reporting, investigate communicable disease outbreaks, perform epidemiological studies, and implement chronic disease prevention and intervention programs. Overall, there is about one health center in each county in the state; however, they differ considerably in funding level and service provision. There are also nine city and county health departments in the state created by local governments. They operate independently of the Bureau of Community Health Systems but often work collaboratively with the state-run centers.

In New York, overall policy is set at the state level, but actual service provision is the responsibility of the counties.[105] The New York State Association of County Health Officials provides training and technical support for county efforts and administers grants from the state Department of Health. There are fifty-eight county and city health departments that provide services ranging from indoor and outdoor air sampling to free breast examinations, childhood lead screening, Lyme disease education, compilations of health statistics, and water supply inspections.[106]

California's public health bureaucracy has a very different structure.[107] Fifteen agencies with health-related responsibilities are placed under one umbrella in the Health and Human Services Agency. These range from the Department of Aging to the Department of Mental Health to the Department of Social Services and are summarized in table 6.6. Among these components is the Department of Health Services (DHS), which performs most of the core functions of public health provision and regulation. As the key health agency for the country's most populous state, DHS has more than 5,000 employees in its headquarters and its more than sixty field offices. It is divided into fourteen programs and support areas that cover functions such as licensing, health information dissemination, strategic planning, prevention services, and support for primary care. It also administers the state's Medicaid program under the name Medi-Cal, a task that most states assign to their welfare department. With regard to service provision, DHS supports local health care providers,

Table 6.6
California Health and Human Services Agency

Department	Key Functions
Department of Aging	Administers home and community-based services for senior citizens
Department of Alcohol and Drug Programs	Develops, administers, and supports prevention and treatment programs
Department of Child Support Services	Supports services and collection activities for children
Department of Community Services and Development	Develops resources for low-income communities
Department of Developmental Services	Provides services and support for children and adults with developmental disabilities
Emergency Medical Services Authority	Administers a statewide system of coordinated emergency medical care, injury prevention, and disaster medical response
Employment Development Department	Administers job placement and referrals, unemployment insurance, disability insurance, employment and training, labor market information, and payroll taxes
Health and Human Services Data Center	Maintains information technology for health and human services agencies
Department of Mental Health	Provides advocacy, education, and provision of mental health services
Department of Rehabilitation	Provides services and advocacy to promote employment, independent living, and equality for individuals with disabilities
Department of Social Services	Administers state and federal programs for health care, social services, public assistance, job training, and rehabilitation
Managed Risk Medical Insurance Board	Administers three health care insurance programs for needy populations
Statewide Health Planning and Development	Oversees safety of health care facilities, administers loans for facilities, supports training of primary care health professionals, and collects data on facilities
Workforce Investment Board	Provides advice and assistance in planning, coordinating, and monitoring workforce development programs and services
Department of Health Services	Administers oversight of activities related to the provision of health care services

Source: http://www.dhs.ca.gov/home/caboutcdhs/dcfault.htm (25 May 2006).

community organizations, and local health departments with technical expertise and resources.

Perennial Policy Issues

While protection of public health was the original foundation for American health care regulation, many of its core functions have been relegated to the backwaters of health policy. The great communicable disease threats of the nineteenth century that gave the impetus to public health protection have seemed to be largely contained or conquered. Public attention to infectious threats has diminished over the past century from the days when use of mandatory inoculations, quarantine, and sanitation were still untested and controversial policies. The continuing governmental role of monitoring, educating, and licensing has gradually given way in the public's eye to policies affecting more dramatic aspects of health care. Over the past several decades, the news media have been filled with reports on newer issues, from financing for high-technology heroic care, to researching cures for chronic diseases, to safeguarding patients' rights. The exception has been environmental protection, which receives considerable press attention, but even there, the public focus tends to be on natural resources and environmental aesthetics rather than on preventing disease.

The return of infectious public health threats to America's collective consciousness has been relatively sudden and certainly unwelcome. The public became increasingly aware starting in the 1990s of the emergence of drug-resistant bacteria, newly discovered exotic disease-causing organisms, and disease dissemination as a military tactic. Unlike the old public health tools of the nineteenth century, defenses against these threats are not likely to be effective on a local basis. National coordination and international cooperation are necessary parts of the arsenal. Where will this move public health policy? Four themes that have shaped public health debates over the past hundred years are likely to remain prominent.

State-Federal Balance

The conflict between federal and state authority permeates American political history. Alexis de Tocqueville, a French observer of early America, saw it in the 1820s, and debates revolve around it today.[108] The Tenth Amendment to the U.S. Constitution reserves to the states all powers not granted to the federal government.[109] This was intended to permit states leeway in enacting and enforcing laws that respond to varying local needs, a concern that is particularly applicable to health care. There is considerable regional variation in American attitudes and values toward health and the responsibility of government to protect it.

Over the years, state primacy has played an important role in shaping public policy in many areas, except with regard to the fields of explicit constitutional federal authority, such as interstate commerce and national defense. As society has become more complex, however, state primacy has become increasingly difficult to maintain in many areas of government concern. There are fewer and fewer fields of economic and social activity that do not affect interstate commerce, making uniform national policy more important. A tremendous amount of local health regulation can now be seen as having national dimensions.

Early efforts to combat infectious diseases addressed local crises, and federal initiatives were largely superfluous.[110] Epidemics, even when serious, tended to stay in single regions, and state and local control over governmental responses seemed feasible. Health challenges today are rarely so confined or so simple. New foreign viruses, like West Nile, arrive from overseas and spread throughout the country. Toxic chemicals and wastes linked to chronic diseases are transported nationwide. Pollutants spread through rivers, lakes, and air. Germs used as implements of bioterrorism are sent across state lines, and victims can disperse to seek care. Yet clinical care is usually provided locally. Physicians and hospitals are licensed and regulated by the states, and their patient bases tend to be close by. The clinical responses to public health threats, therefore, are not an area of direct federal involvement.

The key challenge in the future will be to coordinate efforts at all levels of government. Each aspect of public health regulation should have its governmental home under America's federalist system. In the early twentieth century, the division of responsibility in health care was easier to make, as the major disease challenges were more localized. Today, much more is known about health and disease, and so it is evident to a greater extent how complicated their regulation and control can be. As time goes by, it likely will be necessary to redefine many regulatory homes for public health functions.

Population Health versus Individual Health

Public health regulation is the area of health policy most concerned with the aggregate health of populations. It is in the very nature of concern for "the public." While aggregate health and individual health are generally compatible goals, at many times they compete. In a world of finite resources, health care funds spent on population-based prevention represent dollars not spent on the care of those who have already become ill. Overall, the United States spends much more on clinical care for the sick than on preventive health measures.[111] Whether or not our balance is appropriate depends on personal values. What is undeniable is that trade-offs must be made.

Where will our resources be focused in the next round of public health challenges? Will public policy try to prevent the greatest amount of sickness from occurring in the face of new infections, drug-resistant diseases, toxic substances, and biological attacks, or will it be directed to providing the best care possible to those in the most medical need? While American health care spending on treatment dwarfs that on prevention, it is usually less financially efficient. Prevention, when it is effective, spreads the greatest good to the greatest number, but to give this approach primacy, it is necessary to make less available to those who are already ill.

As a tool of public health, mass inoculation programs to combat infectious diseases cost much less per life saved than medical treatment for individual victims.

This is not to mention the dramatically reduced toll in human suffering. Perhaps this is why historically the amount of government public health activity involving direct provision of care has been overshadowed by preventive programs.[112] Nevertheless, preventive programs fail to reach many people. Often those not reached are the ones most vulnerable to health threats and least able to obtain care when it is needed, in particular those who are elderly and of low income. Government involvement in direct care provision has increased over the past several decades with the expansion of the National Health Service Corps and the federally supported network of community primary care centers. As the plight of those in need of direct services becomes increasingly central to policy debates, population-based prevention and individual care provision may more visibly compete for government public health resources.

The newest public health threats especially demand a preventive approach. Defense against a biological attack would be useless if treatment were delayed until large numbers of people became ill. Preventing the spread of an artificially propagated infectious agent before the population is debilitated and the health care service delivery system is strained would be essential. Fighting drug-resistant pathogens—microorganisms that have evolved to withstand treatment—can only succeed through prevention. The response to new foreign organisms must depend on the nature of the illnesses they cause, but intercepting them before they cause diseases is clearly a more effective response than waiting to develop new treatments.

Chronic disease threats present special concerns of cost. It is estimated that more than half of all cancers are caused by environmental and lifestyle factors, and many other chronic conditions, including heart disease, diabetes, and asthma, have been shown to have large behavioral and environmental components.[113] Treatments for all these conditions are advancing rapidly but are almost always very expensive. Because of the long-term nature of chronic diseases, the expenditure continues over time. As America's overburdened health care system seeks to control costs, prevention becomes an important financial as well as clinical consideration. Money that is spent treating conditions that could have been prevented is money that is not available to improve the quality of care or to expand access to care.

Acute versus Chronic Diseases

The history of American public health in the late twentieth century traces a shift from the control of infectious and acute conditions to chronic ones. The methods, approaches, and costs of responding to each type of illness are very different. Infectious diseases tend to result from rapid, identifiable exposures, and their clinical courses tend to be quick. In contrast, the behavioral and environmental factors behind many chronic conditions can occur over long periods, and the resulting chronic diseases can develop over decades. Strategies for prevention and treatment must vary significantly.

Moreover, whereas the causes of most acute conditions, especially infectious ones, are often clear, the current state of scientific knowledge leaves the causes of many chronic conditions and the effects of many toxic exposures more clouded. It is not always obvious what kinds of factors should be controlled and which are relatively harmless. Even when dealing with known environmental risks, scientists must address matters of degree. How high or prolonged must an exposure be before it should be considered hazardous? Infectious exposures are more commonly matters of all or nothing. Environmental factors also often reflect large individual variation. Whether due to genetic makeup or prior environmental experiences, some individuals are naturally immune to specific causative agents, while others need only limited encounters with a substance for ill effects to manifest themselves. Public health responses to chronic diseases face many of the scientific uncertainties that infectious disease control faced a hundred years ago.

Chronic disease prevention also tends to involve more significant costs than infection control. EPA and OSHA face this challenge constantly when setting exposure limits or implementing the cleanup of toxic waste sites and workplaces. As medications have moved AIDS from a short-term illness with an inevitably fatal course to a long-term chronic condition, the cost of treatment has risen dramatically. Public health at the beginning of the twenty-first century, therefore, is not only more scientifically complex but also much more expensive.

Public versus Private Sector Role

Government approaches to public health protection in the late nineteenth century often faced conflicts with an alternative approach, that of reliance on the private sector.[114] Organized medicine was an early adversary of some public health initiatives out of concern that they would take autonomy, and business, away from private physicians. To this day, much health policy balances government involvement against private initiatives.

The direct provision of health care in America has traditionally been an area of private sector concern, and since the battles of the late nineteenth century, government public health activity has tended to stay away from it. The federal and state governments do provide some care, but this tends to be the exception. The National Health Service Corps, the Veterans Administration, Indian Health Service hospitals, and military hospitals directly provide health care to targeted segments of the population, but their efforts represent a small fraction of total health care provision in America. Public health protection, with its focus on populations and preventive health, is more naturally conducted as a direct government activity. The mass inoculations and quarantine programs of the late nineteenth century, for example, were essentially police activities conducted in conjunction with law enforcement. The biodefense challenges of the early twenty-first century are part of national defense. It would be difficult for private businesses to carry out these activities on their own.

New public health challenges will make the public-private balance more difficult to strike. Issues such as biodefense, drug-resistant infectious organisms, foreign pathogens, and chronic disease prevention require population-based approaches that intersect with the direct provision of care. Numerous conflicts between the traditional government and private roles lie on the horizon. For instance, in trying to limit overuse of antibiotics that produce drug-resistant strains, should CDC tell private physicians how to practice? In defending against biological warfare threats, are mass immunizations best delivered in public clinics or private physician offices? Are medically underserved regions best helped with National Health Service Corps physicians or incentives for more private practitioners? Is pollution control best accomplished with regulations mandating discharge limits or with tradable pollution credits?

The U.S. health care system has a more extensive and complex mixture of governmental and private roles than almost any other industry. Despite historical conflicts, in many areas of public health the government and private industry work in tandem. New challenges may cause the government and private roles to become even more intertwined. However, rather than engendering friction, emerging imperatives may move public health regulation to rely increasingly on constructive public-private partnerships.

Overall Lessons for Health Policy

With all these issues, delicate balances will have to be struck. Once struck, they must constantly be revisited and adjusted as circumstances change. Public health regulation is anything but obsolete. EPA and OSHA repeatedly find themselves in the middle of highly contentious political battles. Infectious disease control has grabbed national attention as a key to prevention of pandemics and biodefense. The challenges of public health continue to burst onto the scene and, when they do, to touch some of our most sensitive policy concerns.

7

Regulation of Health Care
Business Relationships

Unlike regular consumer goods, health care also has powerful moral
dimensions that compel its use.
—U. Reinhardt, *Health Affairs*

The notion that health care is a business is not new. Providers have always needed
payment in some form for their services, and they continually compete with one
another in the market for patients. However, the complexity of health care's commercial side has grown dramatically in recent decades. Before the twentieth century,
physicians functioned largely as independent practitioners, hospitals were almost
all charitable welfare institutions, effective pharmaceutical products were few, and
large-scale insurance arrangements did not exist. In health care, it was an economically simpler time.

Today, American health care is an industry that consumes almost one-sixth of
the nation's gross domestic product.[1] Business arrangements, such as managed care
and provider networks, often shape the provision of services as much as the training
and skill of clinicians. Only a minority of physicians still practice on their own, few
hospitals function outside of larger health systems, and pharmaceutical products are
revolutionizing the nature of care. The foundation of America's health care system
now rests to a large extent on the economic relationships between its components.

The driving force behind the commercial transformation of American health
care was the development of insurance. Before the appearance of Blue Cross and
Blue Shield plans in the 1930s, most patients paid for physician and hospital services directly out of their own pockets. By the end of the 1950s, private health insurance through employer groups was common. In these early arrangements, however,
insurance plans passively paid bills for services and did not directly interject them-

selves into the management of clinical care. That dynamic began to change after the enactment of Medicare and Medicaid in the mid-1960s. By the 1970s, the seeds of a revolution in private health care finance in the form of managed care had been planted, and by the 1990s, American health care emerged with a new and complex economic structure.

The business side of health care answers to a range of laws and regulations that apply to all business transactions. These include laws governing corporations that prescribe the relationships between stockholders, directors, and management; securities laws that govern the sale of stock; and employment laws that regulate relationships between health care entities and their workers. They also include the Sarbanes-Oxley Act, which imposes standards for accounting practices.[2] This web of federal and state statutes and regulations applies to all health care entities, whether they are physician practices, hospitals, or pharmaceutical companies.

Four main areas of business regulation are unique in their application to health care, and these are the focus of this chapter. These are the prohibitions against fraud and abuse in billing government payers for health care services, the antitrust restrictions on anticompetitive behavior, the rules governing charitable tax-exempt organizations, and the protection of patient privacy. Health care business arrangements are regulated in these areas in ways that are different than those of most other kinds of commercial enterprises.

History of Health Care Business Regulation

Before the late 1970s, most physicians practiced on their own or with one or two colleagues.[3] Group practices were the exception, and physician employment arrangements were unusual. This was the legacy of the profession since its standardization in the late nineteenth and early twentieth centuries with the enactment of licensure laws. There was virtually no direct government oversight of clinical behavior, and most financial arrangements were fairly straightforward. Physicians billed patients for the services that they rendered and were paid either by the patient directly or by the patient's insurance company. They admitted patients to hospitals at which they maintained clinical privileges but with which they had no direct financial relationship. Hospitals provided physicians with a place to admit patients and to perform procedures, and physicians in turn provided the institutions with a source of patients. Each partner in the relationship billed for its own services, the hospital for room, board, and ancillary services, and the physician for treatments rendered.

Most hospitals were structured as nonprofit tax-exempt corporations. With only rare exceptions did they employ their physicians or enter into complex financial arrangements with them. Most functioned as stand-alone entities, and multihospital health systems were largely unheard of.

Patient records at this time were maintained on paper, and copies were made only occasionally. With no electronic storage, not to mention e-mail and faxes with which to transmit clinical information, the chances of unauthorized distribution of sensitive medical data were more limited. Instantaneous worldwide transmission over the Internet was not a concern.

With the financial dealings fairly simple, business regulation of physicians and hospitals was rudimentary. Much of health care, in fact, could be characterized as a cottage industry. Growing economic complexity engendered two legal developments during the 1970s that brought health care commercial arrangements under the purview of regulators quite precipitously.

Control of Business Predators:
The Origins of Health Care Antitrust

Although the first and most significant antitrust law, the Sherman Act, was passed by Congress in 1890, antitrust enforcement did not become a priority of government law enforcement until the first decade of the twentieth century when President Theodore Roosevelt made "trust busting" a major focus of his administration. Policy issues related to antitrust continued to play a major role in political debates after President Roosevelt left office and were a topic of considerable interest in the 1912 presidential election. Congress passed a series of additional antitrust laws over the next several decades. Both the Federal Trade Commission Act, which created the Federal Trade Commission (FTC), and the Clayton Act, which limited mergers and acquisitions, were enacted in 1914 during the administration of President Woodrow Wilson.[4]

The FTC began business in 1915 by incorporating the work of the Bureau of Corporations of the Department of Commerce, which had been established in 1903.[5] The early FTC conducted investigations, published reports, and brought administrative cases against companies that used unfair and anticompetitive business practices. In 1973, Congress expanded the agency's power by granting it authority to seek preliminary and permanent injunctions against mergers that might harm competition. In 1975, the Federal Trade Commission Improvement Act gave the agency the authority to seek civil penalties for violations of trade rules.[6] In 1976, the Hart-Scott-Rodino Act required that companies notify the agency in advance of proposed larger mergers and imposed a waiting period before such mergers could be consummated to facilitate review of economic and legal consequences.[7]

Until 1975, courts considered physicians to be largely immune from the antitrust laws. This attitude gave doctors the latitude to set prices among themselves, to control advertising within the profession, and to impose restrictions on acceptable business dealings. The reasoning of courts in permitting this leeway was that physicians were practitioners of a "learned profession," and as such had a higher ethical calling than mere commercial success. Learned professionals, including lawyers as well as doctors, were presumed to be guided by the ethical guidelines of their professions to put the interests of their customers, whether clients or patients, first. In a 1975 decision in the case of *Goldfarb v. Virginia State Bar,* the Supreme Court changed that presumption.[8] The Court found that a restriction imposed by the Virginia Bar Association on advertising by lawyers constituted an illegal restraint of trade under the antitrust laws. The learned professions doctrine was no longer recognized as a defense. By extension, the reasoning reached medicine as another learned profession. Health care had legally come into its own as a business, treated for purposes of antitrust enforcement like any other.

Application of the antitrust laws brought three federal statutes to bear on the health care industry. The most significant was the Sherman Act, which has two operating provisions.[9] Section 1 addresses collusive conduct by competitors in the same market. They are prohibited from engaging in any "contract, combination or conspiracy" that may restrain trade. Over time, courts have interpreted this language to forbid such activities as price-fixing, group boycotts, tying arrangements between products, and market allocation agreements. Section 2 addresses unilateral conduct that is intended to create or maintain a monopoly. This applies to firms that gain large market shares through willful acts that subvert competition, such as threats, intimidation, or coercion of competitors, suppliers, or customers. It does not apply to straightforward competitive success. The second law is the Clayton Act, section 7 of which forbids mergers and acquisitions that may substantially lessen competition or tend to create a monopoly.[10] The final one is the Federal Trade Commission Act, section 5 of which outlaws unfair or deceptive acts or practices, including anticompetitive actions covered by the Sherman and Clayton Acts.[11]

Oversight of Financial Integrity: Prohibitions on Fraud and Abuse

Two years after the *Goldfarb* decision, the law of business regulation struck health care again, this time on another front. Medicare and Medicaid had injected billions of dollars into the health care system to pay for services provided to the elderly and poor. Under the original structure of these programs, physicians were reimbursed as they were under private insurance, with a fee for each service rendered. However, physicians are in a position to decide for themselves what services they will perform and to advise patients to obtain services from other providers for additional care. There is no financial disincentive to the physician from making referrals and, under comprehensive insurance coverage, little financial obstacle to patients in accepting them. The opportunities for excessive utilization at taxpayer expense are substantial.[12]

Medicare and Medicaid created two kinds of temptation for unscrupulous physicians. The first is to commit outright fraud, that is, to lie in their claims for reimbursement by seeking fees for services that were not rendered or that were performed at a lesser level of intensity than that claimed. The second is to abuse their ability to refer patients to other providers by making recommendations not on the basis of the patient's medical needs but on the basis of financial inducements commonly known as "kickbacks." The same temptations exist when a patient is covered by private insurance, but the size of those programs is not as great.

Fraud and abuse have posed challenges to the administration of Medicare and Medicaid since their inception, more so for Medicare because the fees it pays to providers are higher. In response to reports that these practices were rampant and growing, Congress substantially strengthened the statutory penalties in 1977.[13] The new law changed the classification of the underlying crime from a misdemeanor to a felony. It also defined the crime of abusing referral discretion in return for a kickback more broadly to encompass a much larger collection of behaviors. Under the 1977 amendment, anyone who willfully solicits, receives, offers, or pays "any remuneration (including any kickback, bribe or rebate) directly or indirectly, overtly or covertly, in cash or in kind," to make or to solicit a referral may be imprisoned for up to five years and subject to a fine of up to $25,000.[14] Even with subsequent refinements that are discussed later in this chapter, this law remains a formidable check on referral abuses.

Hospitals as Businesses: Scrutiny of Tax-Exempt Status

Regulation of the business practices of hospitals also expanded at this time. As businesses, hospitals face the same array of corporate rules as any other incorporated entity. However, most hospitals operate as nonprofit charitable enterprises, and as such they face another layer of oversight from the federal Internal Revenue Service (IRS). Charitable institutions receive an array of legal benefits. They pay no, or limited, taxes and are eligible to receive tax-deductible donations, to issue tax-exempt bonds, and to receive research grants from federal funding agencies and private foundations. Before receiving these benefits, an institution must be formally recognized by the IRS as a charity, commonly under section 501(c)(3) of the Internal Revenue Code.[15] In the 1970s and 1980s, the IRS assumed a more active role in enforcing standards for hospitals and other health care organizations on which it had conferred this status. In the dawning era of managed care and complex financial relationships, the IRS no longer automatically accepted the notion that hospitals serve a charitable mission. A series of regulatory rulings required hospitals to provide minimum amounts of free care to indigent patients, to engage in active community outreach, and to order their financial dealings with physicians according to emerging legal standards.

A New Frontier in Health Care Business Regulation: Data Privacy

With the laws of antitrust, fraud, and abuse, and tax exemption brought fully to bear on health care, the complexity of business regulation grew substantially through the 1980s and 1990s. Each area has its own set of rules and its own set of regulatory enforcers, and as they evolved, they became increasingly intertwined. At the end of the 1990s, a new kind of regulation with significant implications for health care business relationships joined them. This was the protection of patient privacy under the Health Insurance Portability and Accountability Act of 1996 (HIPAA).[16]

The health care industry has been slower than many others in adopting information technology.[17] A customer can obtain comprehensive information on a bank account over the Internet or through an automated teller machine, but a patient can rarely accomplish more electronically than scheduling an appointment. Many physicians and hospitals still rely mostly on paper records for documenting patient care.

Standardization of protocols for electronic medical information exchange could do much to promote the use of information technology in health care, but no single entity has enough of a national presence to lead the industry. Through HIPAA, Congress directed the Department of Health and Human Services (DHHS) to develop a common format for the transmission of medical information among providers and payers. Electronic exchange, however, poses a serious risk in its vulnerability to unauthorized access by determined computer hackers or through simple carelessness. Once security has been breached, information can be disseminated quickly and widely to an extent not possible with paper records. This threat could, paradoxically, lead computerization to undermine the basis of care, because without sufficient guarantees of privacy, patients may be reluctant to disclose confidential information that providers need to treat them.

Since an information system would be worthless without the confidence of patients and providers, Congress also directed DHHS to develop privacy standards for computerized medical data. These were to take the form of regulations that limit the release of confidential patient information without the patient's consent. The result was a new layer of oversight of transactions between health care entities.

The Structure of Health Care Business Regulation

The growth of business complexity and corresponding government regulation brought several legal programs to bear in health care that were tailored to the structures of very different kinds of industries. One result was a mismatch between legal doctrines and the business practices to which they were now being applied. This led to a mushrooming of legal and regulatory complexity to accommodate the discordance. Health care may behave in the same way as other businesses in some respects, but in many others, it is very different.

Applying Antitrust to Health Care

The policy premises behind antitrust enforcement assume a traditional market for goods and services in which free and fair competition is presumed to be the best way to ensure efficiency.[18] Although no industry functions in a market that meets the traditional model in all respects, there is none that deviates to the extent of health care. The Sherman Act was passed by Congress in 1890 in the midst of the era of industrial robber barons who dominated much of American industry.[19] Monopolies or oligopolies characterized many important markets, including oil, coal, banking, and railroads.[20] Buyers often suffered as industrial giants were able to extract exorbitant prices in the absence of competition. An example was the plight of family farms, which needed to move their goods to market. In regions covering much of the country, only a single railroad provided shipping services, resulting in rates that stretched the means of many.

The market dynamics of health care today are quite different from those of railroads and other major industries of the 1890s. The consumers of health care services, who are patients, are usually not the actual buyers. Most health care is paid for by insurance companies, including HMOs and other kinds of managed care organizations that negotiate prices and pay the bills, with consumers rarely even knowing what each service costs. Managed care organizations even decide in many cases what services health care consumers will receive. Even without the intervention of an insurance company, patients rarely make purchasing decisions on their own but rather rely on their physicians to decide what products and services they need.

The distribution of supply in the health care industry, moreover, is determined to a large extent not by the market but by government programs. The Hill-Burton Act of 1946, for example, expanded the supply of hospital beds by funding hospital construction and expansion, particularly in rural areas.[21] Certificate-of-need laws in many states restrict the supply of hospital beds and services by requiring state approval before new ones may be provided. The supply of physicians is shaped on the one hand by government programs that fund medical school enrollments and on the other by programs that limit access to some specialties by manipulating Medicare reimbursement. (These programs are discussed in more detail in chapters 2 and 3 on the regulation of professionals and institutions and in chapter 4 on the regulation of health care finance.) It is an unusual form of market competition when consumers do not actually buy the service and the government determines what services are available.

The Effects of Antitrust Law
on Health Care Business Practices

In four areas, the antitrust laws have exerted a profound influence on the structure of health care business relationships.[22] The most significant has been the application of section 1 of the Sherman Act to negotiations between payers and providers. HMOs try to reduce their costs by extracting price concessions from physicians and hospitals. However, courts have consistently held that providers such as these may not bargain collectively with HMOs so long as they function as separate business entities, for example, as distinct medical practices.[23] To do so represents a form of illegal price-fixing.

How can providers try to legally level the playing field, when there are many of them against a single HMO that seeks to maximize its bargaining clout? The clearest way is to cease acting as competitors by merging their businesses. If a group of physicians combine into a joint practice that shares revenues and expenses, they are no longer competing but have become a single, integrated entity. Business integration similarly protects hospitals that merge with one another or that acquire physician practices and then bargain with an HMO as a unit. Partly as a result of this legal imperative, a wave of mergers swept the health care industry during the 1990s, with the formation in many markets of large physician group practices, health systems composed of multiple hospitals, and hospital-owned physician practice networks.[24] The days of the solo physician practice and stand-alone hospital would probably have ended regardless of the regulatory setting; however, strict application of the antitrust laws clearly hastened the end of this era.

Success by providers at business integration solves only part of their antitrust challenge. The second major effect of the antitrust laws on the business of health care has been to limit the size to which provider networks can grow. While an integrated network avoids prosecution under section 1 of the Sherman Act as a conspiracy among competitors, it runs directly into the prohibition of section 2 against willfully acquiring monopoly power. It also risks contravening the prohibition in section 7 of the Clayton Act against mergers and acquisitions that may substantially lessen competition or create a monopoly.[25] Most health care networks, therefore, suspend further growth when they reach the verge of market dominance.

The federal Department of Justice (DOJ) and the FTC provide prospective guidance on avoiding antitrust liability under sections 1 and 2 of the Sherman Act for physician joint ventures that takes the form of defined "safety zones," types of activities that will be considered exempt from prosecution.[26] The safety zones describe in detail the key features of business arrangements that make them benign in the eyes of law enforcers.[27] They are structured as regulations, although they do not actually prescribe behavior. Rather, they outline how to immunize business arrangements from suspicion. The safety zones are similar in legal effect to the "safe-harbor" regulations that apply to prosecution under the antikickback statute, which are described later.

The third effect of the antitrust laws is on the composition of organizations that combine physician practices, such as hospital-owned practice networks, HMO networks, and hospital medical staffs. Exclusion of a physician in any of these settings can deal a crushing blow to his or her practice. A physician may not be able to compete on a solo basis against others who have the resources of a provider network behind them. Practice may also be difficult without access to HMO patients or the ability to admit patients to a local hospital. A physician who is excluded from any of these organizations may claim to be the victim of a boycott. If the boycott involves more than one entity, for example, a hospital and its physicians working in combination, it could be characterized as a prohibited conspiracy under section 1 of the Sherman Act. If it involves a single large market player, it can form the basis for a charge of abuse of monopoly power under section 2.

To avoid antitrust liability, organizations of physicians must carefully establish procedures and criteria for selecting or terminating members, since arbitrary decision-making can lend credence to a boycott allegation.[28] Hospital-owned networks generally work with guidelines for physician selection that include such factors as quality indicators and utilization measures. HMOs have similar rules, unless they are non-exclusive and let all physicians join. Hospital medical staffs are required under accreditation rules to follow clear procedures for judging physician quality and for permitting appeals of adverse actions such as suspensions or terminations of membership.[29] One result of these procedures is a set of legal protections for private practice physicians that exceeds those available to professionals who work as employees.

The final major effect of the antitrust laws is on the operations of organizations through which physicians regulate their own profession, such as private medical societies that certify physicians as competent to specialize in an area of practice. (See chapter 2 for a discussion of the role of specialty societies in regulating clinical practice.) Viewed from an economic perspective, these societies consist of competitors with the power to decide whether new businesses can enter the market. An excluded physician can claim, therefore, that a collusive boycott to restrict the market rather than a legitimate judgment on quality was at work. Specialty boards and other kinds of medical societies can protect themselves from such claims in the same manner as hospital networks, HMOs, and medical staffs by using clear criteria for judging the quality of applicants and for ongoing review of existing members. To avoid antitrust liability, therefore, most professional organizations that certify health care professionals implement intricate procedures for determining membership.

Enforcement of the Antitrust Laws

The web of antitrust enforcement is particularly far reaching.[30] In addition to the government agencies discussed later, another set of enforcers is of special concern to potential violators. Under the Sherman Act, any private party that claims injury from an anticompetitive activity can sue on its own.[31] If successful, the plaintiff automatically collects treble damages as a penalty, that is, three times the amount of actual damages. The government has a limited amount of resources to devote to antitrust enforcement, but there may be hundreds of potential private plaintiffs. A health system with a network of physician practices, for example, faces a potential lawsuit from any physician denied membership. With a possible verdict of three times the actual economic harm to any excluded practice, the deterrent effect of the Sherman Act can be substantial.

On the government side, the Sherman and Clayton Act are enforced by DOJ and the FTC. Either agency can bring an action against a suspected antitrust violator for civil penalties, such as fines or injunctions, but DOJ has responsibility when criminal penalties are sought. Moreover, the FTC is limited in its jurisdiction over nonprofit businesses, which include many hospitals. Antitrust actions can also be brought by state attorneys general under laws that mirror the federal Sherman Act in most states.

Agency Structure in Antitrust Enforcement

Federal Trade Commission (FTC). The FTC is headed by five commissioners, who are appointed by the president subject to Senate confirmation. The president also designates the chairman. Commissioners serve for seven-year terms, and no more than three may be from the same political party. The FTC's headquarters is located in Washington, D.C., and there are regional offices throughout the country.[32]

The agency operates through three bureaus, which have responsibility for consumer protection, competition, and economics, and an office of inspector general. The Bureau of Competition investigates suspected antitrust violations and recommends FTC action in response. It also conducts research on competition issues. Because of overlapping jurisdiction, enforcement actions are coordinated with the Antitrust Division of DOJ, as discussed later. The Bureau of Economics provides economic analyses to support agency investigations and enforcement actions, some of which is delivered as testimony in court cases. It also consults on the crafting of remedies to deter anticompetitive behavior and publishes more general analyses of the impact of government regulation on competition.[33]

Department of Justice (DOJ). DOJ is the federal government's primary law enforcement agency. It houses the Federal Bureau of Investigation (FBI), the Drug Enforcement Administration (DEA), and other agencies that prosecute criminal laws. The department is headed by the attorney general, who is the nation's top law enforcement official and is appointed by the president subject to Senate confirmation. DOJ includes many divisions that enforce laws in specific areas, including natural resources, civil rights, and tax. There is also a division for antitrust.[34]

The Antitrust Division prosecutes civil and criminal cases involving violations of the Sherman Act.[35] As discussed previously, much of this work is carried out in coordination with the FTC. Prosecutors work out of the department's headquarters in Washington, D.C., and out of many regional offices around the country.

The Enforcement of Fraud and Abuse

The 1977 amendments to the Medicare Act concerning fraud and abuse were sweeping in their scope, but the health care industry was left to wonder how vigorously the courts would enforce such a broad standard. Resourceful entrepreneurs had become adept at disguising payments to induce referrals behind complex financial arrangements. Under one type of scheme, mobile diagnostic equipment, such as portable X-ray machines, was placed in physicians' offices on a temporary basis. The equipment provider paid the physicians rent for the space that the machine occupied based on the number of patients on whom it was used. The effect was that the more patients who received X-rays, the greater the financial reward for the physicians who referred them. Until the courts had spoken, the health care industry could wonder whether this and similar schemes could be used to circumvent the law.

The answer came in 1985 in the case of *United States v. Greber,* in which a federal appeals court upheld the felony conviction of a cardiologist for paying fees to referring physicians.[36] The defendant characterized the payments as reasonable "interpretation fees" for help in analyzing medical tests, but the court found an implicit motive to reward referrals. The underlying principle that was enunciated reflected a vigorous enforcement attitude. Payments made to a referring physician from a recipient of referrals violate the law if any purpose behind them is to influence referrals, even if a legitimate motive could also be attached.

In the wake of the *Greber* decision, it was clear that the law against fraud and abuse had teeth.[37] However, the broad ruling left health care enterprises uncertain of how to structure any kind of legitimate business relationships with providers with whom they exchanged referrals. From a policy perspective, many such arrangements are completely appropriate. For example, hospitals accept admissions from physician employees who work in their emergency rooms and receive salaries. The fraud and abuse statute would produce an absurd result if an emergency room physician could not admit a patient to the same hospital. Similarly, hospitals routinely rent office space to staff physicians in adjacent buildings. All concerned, including patients, would suffer substantial inconvenience if physicians could not locate their offices close to the hospitals where they practice. Literal enforcement of the law could undermine these and other beneficial health care business dealings.[38]

Separating Good Business from Bad:
The Fraud and Abuse Safe Harbors

Congress resolved the dilemma by amending the law again in 1987 to permit exceptions to the prohibition.[39] The amendments specifically exempted employment compensation to permit all health care providers, including hospitals, to pay salaries to physicians who refer them patients. They also directed DHHS to issue regulations identifying other kinds of business arrangements that would be considered legitimate and immune from prosecution.

The regulations, which were issued in 1991, exempted eleven kinds of business relationships from enforcement.[40] If structured according to the regulatory prescriptions, these arrangements would be considered as "safe harbors" from prosecution. The relationships included many of the most common arrangements in health care commerce, such as rental of office space, professional services rendered by physicians as independent contractors, group purchasing of supplies by hospitals, and investment interests. For each arrangement, the regulations listed with considerable specificity the necessary elements to qualify for safe-harbor status. For example, the rental of hospital office space by a staff physician could create a financial inducement for referrals, if the rent were extremely favorable or if it varied with the number of patients admitted. To qualify for immunity, the rent charged was required to reflect a fair market value, to be set in advance, to reflect neither the volume nor the value of referrals, to remain constant for at least one year at a time to avoid adjustments that reflect referrals, and to be documented in writing to facilitate outside audits. Similar sets of rules apply to rentals of medical equipment and contracts under which physicians provide professional services.

The safe harbors for investment interests draw a particularly fine line.[41] The rules for investments in large corporations, those with at least $50 million in net tangible assets, are fairly lax. The rationale is that a single physician's referrals could have little actual effect on the value of any stock that he or she owns. However, investments in smaller entities are more strictly limited. No more than 40 percent of any class of stock in a company may be owned by health care practitioners who are in a position to refer patients, and no more than 40 percent of the company's revenues may result from referrals by investors. Prior to the law, abusive investment schemes had proliferated through which physician investors in smaller health care facilities received returns that were proportionate to the number of patients referred.

The safe-harbor regulations occupy an anomalous legal position similar to that of the antitrust safety zones. While they protect business dealings that meet their standards, they do not prohibit arrangements that do not. They create a presumption of legitimacy for complying arrangements while raising no implications for others. For instance, an office lease that falls outside of the applicable safe-harbor because the rent varies every six months, rather than every year, does not necessarily violate the law. However, if challenged in court, the participants would not enjoy an automatic assumption of innocence, and they would bear the burden of proving their lack of intent to induce referrals. In essence, the government has provided a road map for immunizing legitimate health care business arrangements but not an invariable prescription.

In the years since 1991, DHHS has issued regulations creating safe harbors for an additional twelve kinds of business dealings to bring the total to twenty-three.[42] These include the sale of physician practices, recruitment incentives offered to physicians by hospitals, investments in ambulatory surgical facilities, and risk-sharing arrangements with managed care organizations. In each case, the underlying kind of arrangement serves a beneficial purpose, if it is structured without clear financial inducements to refer patients.

Adding a New Line of Regulatory Attack:
The Stark Amendments

Despite its rigor, the law prohibiting referral payments leaves a large gap. Research indicates that even in the absence of explicit inducements, physicians are more likely to refer patients to medical facilities in which they have a financial interest than to those in which they do not.[43] For example, one study found that Medicare beneficiaries receive more tests when they are treated by physicians who have invested in the laboratories involved, regardless of whether there is actual remuneration in return for the referrals.[44] In other words, when physicians have a general interest in the financial success of a venture, their clinical decision making seems to be affected. The fraud and abuse statute does not reach such general financial relationships.

Congress responded with two companion amendments to the Medicare law, one enacted in 1989 and one in 1993.[45] While formally titled the Ethics in Patient Referrals Act, they are commonly known as the Stark Amendments after Congressman Fortney Stark of California, who sponsored them. The first amendment denied Medicare reimbursement for clinical laboratory services when the patient was referred by a physician who had a financial relationship with the facility. The prohibition covers referrals not only by physicians with investment interests in the laboratory but also by physicians with any other kind of financial dealings. Exceptions are permitted for legitimate business arrangements similar to those addressed in the fraud and abuse safe harbors, such as employment, contracts for services, rental of office space, and group practices.

The 1993 amendment extended the scope of the prohibition beyond laboratory tests to nine additional "designated" health services, including radiology, physical therapy, occupational therapy, and hospital services. In each case, Medicare reimbursement is denied when the patient is referred by a physician who has a financial relationship with the facility rendering the service, unless one of the specified exceptions is met. The relationship need not reflect any actual intent to steer referrals.

The combination of the Stark Amendments and fraud and abuse statute cast a wide net in circumscribing financial dealings between health care providers. However, the two regulatory schemes are not entirely consistent in their approach and effect. Under the Stark law, Medicare referrals may not be exchanged even in the absence of an intention to promote them, but there is no prohibition of the underlying business relationship. Under the fraud and abuse law, the business relationship is outlawed, but only if prosecutors can prove that the parties intended to steer referrals. The effect of each law is to discourage financial arrangements that may encourage referrals, but the task of deciding when a violation has occurred differs between them.

With two legal schemes addressing the same issue, the Centers for Medicare & Medicaid Services (CMS), the agency that administers the Medicare program, has issued two sets of regulations governing financial dealings between health care providers that exchange referrals. As discussed, one set creates "safe harbors" from enforcement under the fraud and abuse law. The other guides compliance with the Stark Amendments, specifying when a business arrangement qualifies as an exception to the broad prohibition contained in the law.[46] Navigating this maze of regulations can present a significant challenge for providers.

Referral Restrictions and the Future of Health Care

The practice of paying physicians to refer patients is widely considered to be a breach of medical ethics, since it can compromise the physician's obligation to put the interests of the patient first.[47] The promise of a kickback may cloud a physician's clinical judgment and induce referrals for services that are not needed or that are made to poor-quality providers. The business dynamic favoring referrals applies when health care services are reimbursed on a fee-for-service basis, that is, when the provider is paid a fee for each service rendered.[48] Under this arrangement, providers gain by seeing as many patients as possible. However, under managed care, some physicians are paid based on capitation, a set fee paid in advance for treating all of a patient's medical needs, regardless of how many services the physician actually renders. Moreover, referrals that physicians make under managed care are usually scrutinized by the payer, and penalties may be assessed if they are deemed to be excessive. Managed care payment arrangements, therefore, may obviate the need for regulation of referrals.[49]

The Stark Amendments acknowledge this shift in reimbursement paradigms with an exception to the definition of financial relationships that trigger the law's application for prepaid health plans.[50] If physicians are paid through a managed care arrangement on a prospective basis without regard to the number of services actually rendered, the economic relationship does not trigger the prohibition on referrals. However, the exception includes a proviso that addresses a different kind of possible abuse. The managed care arrangement may not encourage physicians to render too little care. This shift in focus of fraud and abuse concern may increase if capitation arrangements continue to proliferate.

Agency Structure for Fraud and Abuse Enforcement

Centers for Medicare & Medicaid Services (CMS) and DHHS Office of Inspector General (OIG). As the agency responsible for administering the Medicare program and the federal portion of the Medicaid program, CMS is charged with protecting the programs' integrity. CMS prides itself on its low administrative overhead rate of about 2 percent.[51] However, the combined budget for Medicare and Medicaid of more than $600 billion a year, most of which represents payments to providers, presents a temptation for fraud that requires enforcement attention. CMS issues regulations concerning all aspects of Medicare and Medicaid administration, including the safe-harbor rules under the antikickback statute and the details of exceptions to the Stark Amendments. The agency is a component of DHHS. (Its structure is described in more detail in chapter 4 on health care finance.) Actual enforcement is the job of the Office of Inspector General (OIG) in DHHS.

The OIG is the department's enforcement arm. It gathers data on suspected violations in several ways.[52] Audits of health care providers look for instances of fraud in billing or illegal financial arrangements. Fraud can be uncovered through actual evidence of billing for services that were not rendered or that were rendered at a lower level of intensity than was claimed. It can also be spotted as suspicious patterns of billing, for example, bills that seek payment for only one kind of procedure for all patients seen in a physician's practice over a long period of time. Illegal financial dealings can be revealed through documents, such as leases and contracts, that encourage referrals, or trails of unexplained payments exchanged between providers. Private parties can also bring violations to the OIG's attention, either directly or anonymously through a toll-free telephone number.

In response to evidence of suspected wrongdoing, the OIG can initiate a full investigation. This can lead to recommendations for penalties, including fines and exclusion of the provider from participation in Medicare and Medicaid. Exclusion from Medicare is the most commonly used and can deal a serious blow to a health care provider that treats a significant number of elderly patients.[53] Providers that are sanctioned can appeal to the Departmental Appeals Board within the OIG. From there, subsequent appeals are to the courts. When serious violations are found, the case may be referred to the DOJ for criminal prosecution.

Private citizens can also proceed against a suspect provider through a process known as a "qui tam" action.[54] Under this mechanism, the complaining party can directly file a lawsuit against the provider. The government has the option of taking over prosecution or letting the case proceed. If the government proceeds and prevails, the private party can receive between 15 and 25 percent of the recovery, at the discretion of the judge. If the complaining citizen proceeds and prevails, the reward is between 25 and 30 percent. Since the OIG and other government enforcement agencies have limited resources, the availability of qui tam actions brought by private parties enhances the threat of prosecution.

The OIG also has authority to issue advisory opinions that prospectively assess the legality of proposed business arrangements. A positive ruling provides an assurance of safety from prosecution but only as long as the actual arrangement follows the blueprint that the OIG approved. During 2001 and 2002, the OIG issued forty-two advisory opinions, most of which found the proposed transaction to be lawful.[55]

The OIG also provides advance guidance by publishing periodic "fraud alerts" that describe types of arrangements it considers suspect. These address trends of illegal conduct that the agency finds in its audits and investigations.[56] For example, a fraud alert issued in 2000 described rental arrangements between physicians and companies that provide medical supplies or diagnostic services.[57] It advised that if the companies use space in a physician's office and make rental payments to the physician that are unnecessary or that exceed fair market value, the OIG may consider the payments as kickbacks in return for the referral of the physician's patients. Other fraud alerts have dealt with joint ventures between providers,[58] and hospital discounts offered to patients.[59] These documents give providers a checklist of features to avoid in planning transactions.

The OIG is headed by the inspector general, who is appointed by the president subject to Senate confirmation. There are five operating offices within the agency, each headed by a deputy inspector general. These include offices for audit services, evaluation and inspections, management and policy, investigations, and chief counsel. There are eight regional offices and numerous field offices throughout the country.[60]

As the primary enforcement agency for health care fraud and abuse, the OIG exerts tremendous influence over business dealings in the industry. Its influence extends well beyond the parties that are directly subject to its prosecutions through a deterrent effect against improper conduct throughout health care.[61] The responsibility for enforcement carries with it the discretion to decide what kinds of conduct will be subject to prosecution and thereby most likely to be deterred. In wielding this power and in offering prospective guidance on how it will be used, the agency has become an important force in shaping health care commerce.

Other Enforcement Arms. The OIG's enforcement activities are supplemented by the heavier prosecutorial guns of DOJ. Attorneys at this agency handle cases that move beyond administrative proceedings to the courts. DOJ may initiate fraud and abuse investigations and prosecutions through its headquarters in Washington, DC, or through U.S. attorneys in one of the department's regional offices around the country. DOJ initiates actions when criminal and serious civil penalties are sought. The additional resources that this agency brings to bear bolster not only the prosecutorial reach of the OIG but also its ability to investigate suspected wrongdoing before charges are brought.

Providers must also beware of enforcement at the state level.[62] Since Medicaid is administered by the states, their law enforcement apparatus investigates and prosecutes suspected fraud and abuse in this and other state-level public health programs, including State Children's Health Insurance Programs (SCHIP). State departments of health and of welfare are most likely to take the lead in these activities. Officials in most states, usually in departments of insurance, also administer laws against fraud and abuse in private health insurance. The office of the state attorney general usually plays a role that corresponds to that of the federal DOJ in initiating, investigating, and prosecuting fraud and abuse cases involving state laws.

The Regulation of Tax-Exempt Status

America's private hospitals were once all nonprofit charitable organizations.[63] Starting with the first one, Pennsylvania Hospital, founded in Philadelphia by Benjamin Franklin and Dr. Thomas Bond in 1751, early hospitals cared primarily for poor patients who lacked the financial means to afford care at home. (For a discussion of the regulation of hospitals, see chapter 3.) Some grew from almshouses and others from religious missions. Hospitals could provide few, if any, actual medical treatments other than rest and comfort, so there was little to bill for, even if patients had the ability to pay. With few services, indigent customers, and no third-party reimbursement, these institutions subsisted largely on donations. They became known as voluntary hospitals because of their reliance on discretionary giving. They were true charities.

Over time, the business of hospitals has changed dramatically. During the late nineteenth and early twentieth centuries, new technologies transformed them into centers where medical procedures were performed. Anesthesia and antisepsis permitted an expansion of surgery, and X-ray machines facilitated advances in diagnosis. As the basis of their business changed, hospitals faced new cost pressures and also new opportunities to collect revenues. They began to attract patients who had financial means, and for the first time, they collected payments for their services.

The first for-profit hospitals were founded in the early decades of the twentieth century, mostly in southern and western states.[64] For the most part, they were smaller institutions created by physicians, and they tended to function as clinics. In the 1930s, the first Blue Cross and Blue Shield health insurance plans were established, largely as a way to help patients afford hospital and physician services during the Depression. (For a discussion of the regulation of health insurance, see chapter 4.) After World War II, private commercial insurers entered the market, and the availability of health insurance became widespread. At the same time, medical technology continued to advance and to bring a range of new services to hospitals' arsenals. As a result, America's hospitals had an array of services for which they could charge and a source of payment that extended beyond the financial means of most individual patients. With the implementation of Medicare and Medicaid in the mid-1960s, both trends accelerated dramatically.

Full-service hospitals that operated on a for-profit basis began to proliferate during the 1950s and through the decades that followed.[65] They gradually spread throughout the country from the south and west, so that by the 1990s, there were for-profit hospitals in most major cities. Many are part of larger regional or national chains. These institutions provide the same services as their nonprofit counterparts, but they derive their financial support from reimbursement for services and the sale of stock to investors. They do not receive donations, and they do not function as charities.

Despite the recent spread of for-profit hospitals, they remain in the minority.[66] Most American hospitals continue to function on a nonprofit basis and so are exempt from most taxes and can accept tax-deductible donations. Since both kinds of institutions provide similar sets of services and all of them collect reimbursement, this differential tax treatment is increasingly questioned. Why are some businesses subject to the full effect of the tax laws while their competitors are not?

The justification for the differential treatment lies in the regulatory scheme with which nonprofit, but not for-profit, hospitals must comply. Obtaining and maintaining tax-exempt status requires approval from revenue authorities at several levels of government, which set strict conditions. In return for a tax exemption, a hospital must serve a charitable mission that benefits its community in a way that the activities of a for-profit business would not. Commonly, this mission is reflected in the amount of uncompensated care that is provided to patients who lack insurance and other financial means to pay the bills.[67] It can also take the form of community outreach and public health efforts. Many for-profit hospitals also engage in these activities, but they do so to a large extent on their own initiative.[68] In essence, hospitals that remain nonprofit trade acceptance of an additional layer of regulatory oversight for a lower tax burden.

Tax-exempt status is available not just for stand-alone hospitals. The IRS has recognized entire health systems that include hospitals among their components as charities.[69] These systems often include integrated networks of hospitals, physician practices, and ancillary care providers that have become known as integrated delivery systems (IDSs). To qualify for a tax exemption, an IDS must meet a set of structural and operational criteria similar to those that apply to individual hospitals, including community representation on its governing board, reasonable limits on physician compensation, open emergency room access, adequate levels of indigent care, and participation in Medicaid and Medicare.[70]

In addition to hospitals and IDSs, other kinds of health care facilities commonly also operate as tax-exempt charities. These include nursing homes and free-standing clinics. America's original health insurers, Blue Cross and Blue Shield plans, were founded as nonprofit corporations at a time when the financing of health care was considered an ancillary function, rather than a profit-making opportunity in its own right. With this limited mission, Blue Cross and Blue Shield plans initially qualified for tax exemptions. As health insurance evolved into an enterprise that could be lucrative on its own, the IRS revoked its recognition of charitable status for nonprofit health insurers in the 1970s, and in the 1990s, many Blue Cross and Blue Shield plans converted into for-profit corporations.[71]

The Process of Gaining Tax-Exempt Status

To qualify for tax-exempt status, an organization begins by incorporating under the laws of its home state as a nonprofit corporation. While for-profit corporations are owned by stockholders who elect a board of directors to oversee operations, nonprofit corporations have no owners. They are controlled by a board that is either elected by voluntary members or is self-perpetuating and selects its own replacements. Members are commonly found in nonprofits that function as professional associations. Most nonprofit hospitals have boards that are self-perpetuating.

Since there are no actual owners, the assets of nonprofit corporations are, in theory, a form of public property, held in trust for the communal good.[72] Upon dissolution, any remaining assets must either be donated to another charitable entity, or they revert to the state. Without stockholders or other formal owners, there is no equity market and no securities regulators to oversee these corporations. Instead, they are subject to oversight by the attorney general in their state of incorporation, who conducts regular audits for compliance with standards for charitable operation. Enforcement actions are brought before special courts, known in many states as orphan's courts, which have authority over the nonprofit sector. Orphan's courts also oversee the dissolution of nonprofits to ensure that their assets are distributed appropriately.

Although it is a necessary first step, nonprofit incorporation is only the start of the process of gaining exemption from taxes. Exemption from state taxes is usually automatic, at least initially. This permits the organization to avoid a range of levies, including state income tax, state and local sales tax, and local real estate tax. However, in many states, maintenance of the exemption can be challenged.[73] State and local taxing authorities can proceed against nonprofit organizations, including hospitals, for failing to serve a community purpose, for example, by providing too little indigent care.[74] To avoid such challenges, hospitals in many localities make voluntary payments in lieu of property taxes. While less than the amount they would owe were actual taxes to be imposed, these sums can be substantial and can include free services in addition to monetary payments.[75] Programs to administer these payments are often known as payment in lieu of taxes (PILOT) and services in lieu of taxes (SILOT).

The most important step in becoming federally tax exempt is to obtain recognition of charitable status by the IRS. This is a substantial administrative burden and requires a lengthy application process. The federal Internal Revenue Code (IRC), which was last subject to substantial overhaul in 1986, recognizes several bases for exemption from federal taxes in section 501(c).[76] The most comprehensive exemption, and the one that applies to most hospitals, is contained in section 501(c)(3).[77] It permits not only exemption from taxes paid by the organization but also tax deductions for contributors who give it donations.

Under the IRC, tax exemption under section 501(c)(3) is reserved for organizations that are "operated exclusively" for a charitable purpose.[78] The code specifically mentions several kinds of organizations as meeting this standard, including those that serve religious, scientific, literary, or educational purposes. However, the list does not include health care. Therefore, hospitals and other health care organizations must offer a justification for why their provision of health care should qualify as charitable. As discussed, hospitals usually accomplish this by providing ample amounts of indigent care and other community services, but they must set forth their charitable activities in an initial application for a tax exemption and must be prepared to document them in response to subsequent IRS oversight.

Once charitable status has been recognized by the IRS, nonprofit hospitals have a tremendous amount at stake in maintaining it. In addition to avoiding tax payments, federal tax-exempt status forms the basis of their capital financing structure. Private hospitals can raise capital for expansion or other major expenses by selling stock, either directly or through a parent corporation. Since nonprofit corporations have no stock to sell, they must turn to the bond market instead, but with a special advantage. Interest earned on the bonds of a federally tax-exempt organization is tax deductible for the bondholders. As a result, the organization can sell its bonds at a lower rate of interest. Were a nonprofit hospital to lose its tax-exempt status, this benefit would be lost and with it the underpinning of its main source of capital financing.

Federal tax exemption also confers many other, less visible, benefits. Most research grants from government agencies and foundations are available only to tax-exempt organizations. Grant funding for education and training often has similar limitations. Recognition of charitable status can also confer an aura of prestige on a hospital by engendering a public perception that it functions as a community asset rather than a self-interested business.

The Process of Maintaining Tax-Exempt Status

After it grants tax-exempt status, the IRS enforces strict rules for maintaining it, a role that effectively makes it a major regulatory force for much of the health care industry. The three basic operational requirements for any 501(c)(3) organization are that no part of the earnings may "inure to the benefit" of private individuals, no substantial part of the activities may seek to influence legislation, and there may be no participation in any political campaign.[79] In addition, a health care organization must demonstrate that it provides a "community benefit." An IRS revenue ruling issued in 1969 listed the elements that evidence this commitment, including, as discussed, a board composed of members who are representative of the community, an open emergency room that treats indigent patients without charge, an open medical staff, and participation in Medicare and Medicaid.[80]

Of these operational restrictions, the one that generates the most IRS scrutiny is the proscription on letting the organization's earnings inure to the benefit of private individuals, commonly known as the prohibition on "private inurement." Hospitals most commonly run afoul of this rule in their dealings with staff physicians. Since hospitals rely on their physicians for patient admissions, they often find it advantageous to offer financial incentives for physician loyalty. These incentives can take the form of stipends for performing administrative tasks, salaries for employment, assistance in purchasing malpractice insurance, or funding for other practice enhancements. If the purpose behind the payments cannot be justified as legitimately related to the hospital's operations and the amount paid as reasonable, the IRS may see the arrangement as an impermissible diversion of hospital earnings to private individuals.

As discussed, aggressive financial arrangements between health care providers that exchange referrals can also contravene the antikickback law and Stark Amendments. Over and above these legal strictures, the IRS considers violation of the prohibitions against remuneration in return for referrals to be antithetical to a charitable mission and grounds in and of themselves for revocation of a tax exemption.[81] In effect, the prohibition on private inurement has positioned the IRS as an additional enforcer of the fraud and abuse laws.

Traditionally, hospitals and the physicians who practiced within their walls had no direct financial relationships. However, increases in the complexity of hospital operations have driven many to form closer economic ties with their physicians. Many hospitals now employ physicians to work in the hospital-based specialties of anesthesiology, radiology, pathology, and emergency medicine. Some have acquired the practices of community physicians to form regional networks in which the selling physicians remain as hospital employees. In some instances, hospitals pay the moving and initial practice expenses of physicians in needed specialties who relocate to join their staffs. Physicians may also be paid as consultants to chair hospital departments or to perform other administrative functions.

When these arrangements involve a tax-exempt hospital, remuneration to physicians that the IRS considers to be excessive may form the basis for a challenge to the institution's charitable status.[82] To assist hospitals in structuring financial relationships that avoid suspicion, the IRS offers guidance in the form of memoranda issued by the agency's general counsel. These are analyses of specific factual situations and the agency's position on whether private inurement is involved. The IRS also issues documents known as "private letter rulings" that prospectively adjudicate the propriety of proposed transactions. These pronouncements are similar in effect to the safety zones issued by the FTC and DOJ regarding antitrust enforcement and the safe harbors issued by the OIG concerning Medicare fraud and abuse in that they set the bounds of business activity through prospective enforcement policy.

In the view of the IRS, the key to legitimizing physician payments is to document that they reflect the fair market value of the services being performed.[83] Salaries should be consistent with those available in similar settings for similar activities, as should consulting payments. Purchase prices for physician practices should reflect the value of the practice as a business enterprise according to the analysis of an independent accountant. Moving and practice start-up expenses should cover legitimate costs, and the physicians receiving them should fill a clear clinical need in the hospital's community, which is easier to demonstrate when a physician is recruited to an underserved rural or inner-city area. In structuring any of these financial relationships with staff physicians, nonprofit hospitals commonly take great pains to document that the services obtained are necessary to the institution's mission and that the physicians involved are not overcompensated.

Penalties for Violating Charitable Standards

Violations of the restrictions on charitable operations usually come to the IRS's attention on routine audits. Large charitable organizations are subject to audit every few years, during which the agency may review all documents related to their financial dealings. In addition to routine reviews, IRS scrutiny may be prompted by information that charities are required to file each year on a form that substitutes for a tax return, known as a Form 990. It includes data on salaries of highly compensated executives and on major contractual relationships.[84]

When the IRS finds violations, it has two kinds of penalties available. The most extreme is to revoke the organization's tax-exempt status. This step can wreak havoc for most nonprofits and penalize parties beyond the organization itself, including bondholders who would owe taxes on the interest that they earn and donors who would no longer qualify for tax deductions. The hospital's entire financial foundation could be shaken, so revocation of tax-exempt status is usually employed more as a threat than an actual punishment, and is imposed only in egregious cases.

In the 1990s, Congress added new penalties to the IRS's arsenal that stop short of threatening an organization's economic base.[85] These penalties, known as "intermediate sanctions," include fines and reprimands. The agency can also advise the organization of corrective measures to maintain its tax-exempt status, with a follow-up audit to monitor compliance. The good news for tax-exempt organizations is that lesser penalties can now substitute for the drastic penalty of losing tax-exempt status altogether. The bad news is that the IRS is more likely to apply these lesser sanctions. However, under either set of penalties, tax-exempt hospitals face intense scrutiny of all aspects of their financial operations and a substantial compliance burden.

Leveling the Playing Field with Tax-Paying Competitors

For the majority of American hospitals, gaining the benefits of tax-exempt status in return for compliance with restrictions on financial dealings is worth the trade-off.

However, for-profit competitors often decry the uneven playing field that results. These hospitals provide the same services but do not receive special privileges that effectively amount to government subsidies. They particularly point to aspects of hospital operations that are extraneous to the underlying community mission and question whether the tax exemption should extend to these functions as well. The hospital's gift shop, cafeteria, and parking garage, for example, are not essential aspects of providing health care and are more like routine businesses. Why should the government subsidize these operations, when competitors that are not hospital owned receive no such largesse?

The IRC seeks to level the playing field between tax-exempt and for-profit businesses by taxing business income of tax-exempt organizations that is unrelated to their community mission. Component functions that are not a substantial component of a charitable purpose are subject to "unrelated business income tax" (UBIT) representing the tax that would apply if these activities were conducted by a for-profit enterprise.[86] Proceeds from the gift shop, cafeteria, and parking garage, therefore, as well as other activities that extend beyond the central charitable mission, are generally not tax-exempt. In one case, for example, the IRS denied shelter from federal taxation to an HMO owned by a nonprofit health system because it was not central to the mission of providing health care. The decision was eventually upheld in court.[87] The IRS can impose tax liability along with penalties if unreported unrelated business income is discovered in an audit.

Switching Sides: Hospital Conversions into For-Profit Businesses

The number of for-profit hospitals grew substantially through the 1990s, fueled mostly by conversions in the status of existing nonprofit hospitals rather than by the construction of new facilities.[88] Some institutions found the allure of investment capital worth the loss of tax-exempt status, while others were acquired by for-profit corporations that changed their financial footing in the process. The transition is complex in both conceptual and legal terms, since nonprofit organizations have no shareholders and therefore no owners from whom they can be acquired. To convert to for-profit status, a nonprofit corporation does not simply change its form. It must be transformed from a public trust into a private possession.

The law provides a procedure for accomplishing this change and creating a profit-making enterprise out of a nonprofit hospital.[89] To effectuate the transition, the original corporation continues to exist; however, it sells all its assets, including its physical plant, equipment, and value as an ongoing business, to the acquiring enterprise. The acquirer can be a new company set up for the purpose or an existing hospital chain. After the transaction, it owns all the hospital's assets and has the right to operate the institution. In return, it pays the nonprofit corporation a purchase price.

The old nonprofit hospital corporation now finds itself in an unusual situation. It has a sizable sum of money but no other assets and no ongoing business. What does a nonprofit corporation with a mission of providing health care in its community do without a business purpose? The answer in most cases is that it functions as a charitable foundation contributing a portion of its assets each year as grants to others who serve the purpose of promoting health. The grantees can be community outreach organizations, clinics, or other health-related charities, which can turn to the foundation as a new source of financial support. A similar procedure applies when nonprofit health insurers undergo the same kind of transformation.

The process of converting a nonprofit charitable health care enterprise into a conventional business is controversial. Critics see it as a giveaway of community assets to private parties for corporate gain without sufficient public benefit in return. Proponents counter that hospital assets are often put to more efficient and productive use in the for-profit sector and that the establishment of new grant-giving foundations enhances overall health care to a greater extent than the hospital in its old form could have done. Moreover, since the dissolution of nonprofit corporations is supervised by the state attorney general with oversight by the state's orphan's court, layers of government review and approval stand between conversions and disregard of the public's interest.

For-profit hospitals also acquire new kinds of regulatory oversight in return for the IRS and state attorney general review that they leave behind. Publicly traded companies must comply with numerous securities laws that are enforced by the federal Securities and Exchange Commission (SEC) and state regulators that require regular disclosure of substantial amounts of financial information.[90] For-profit corporations are also subject to the full jurisdiction of the FTC in antitrust enforcement.[91]

Controversies surrounding the conversion of nonprofit hospitals to for-profit status reflect larger issues of maintaining part of the health care industry as a charitable enterprise.[92] The days when hospitals subsisted entirely on charitable donations are long gone, and today all must face the financial pressures of the business world. However, the nature of a health care enterprise still distinguishes it in important ways from other kinds of commercial endeavors.[93] The lives and well-being of the customers are directly affected to a greater extent than in almost any other industry. Is a corporate structure that holds lives in the balance best left accountable to shareholders seeking financial value for their investment or to community boards that answer to the state? For-profit businesses are often seen as more prudent guardians of financial resources but nonprofits as more concerned with the public's well-being. To a large extent, the complexity of the government's regulatory oversight of the nonprofit health care sector reflects this societal uncertainty.

Agency Structure for Tax Exemption Enforcement:
Internal Revenue Service (IRS)

The origins of the IRS date to 1862, when Congress enacted an income tax to pay Civil War expenses at President Abraham Lincoln's request.[94] That tax was repealed ten years later. The income tax as we know it today was created in 1913, when the Sixteenth Amendment to the Constitution was ratified, giving Congress the authority to structure taxation in its present form.[95] The 1040 form for filing returns was first used the same year. The original tax rate was 1 percent of annual income above $3,000, with a surcharge of 6 percent on incomes above $500,000. Since then, tax rates have risen and fallen many times over the years.

The IRS is organized into four operating divisions. This structure is based on a reorganization that stemmed from the IRS Restructuring and Reform Act of 1998.[96] The Wage and Investment Division processes individual taxes; the Small Business/Self-Employed Division processes taxes for small businesses and self-employed taxpayers; the Large and Mid-Size Business Division processes taxes for corporations with assets of more the $10 million; and the Tax-Exempt and Government Entities Division oversees employee benefit plans, tax-exempt organizations, and government entities.[97] It is the last of these operating divisions that regulates nonprofit health care entities such as hospitals. There are also offices that handle appeals, communications, and criminal investigations.

The Tax Exempt and Government Entities Division oversees 3 million nonprofit organizations, including 1.6 million that are tax-exempt.[98] Although tax-exempt organizations pay no federal income tax themselves, they are still responsible for withholding income and payroll taxes for their employees. The division conducts audits and examinations to monitor compliance with the requirements for maintaining tax-exempt status, such as the prohibition against private inurement and the payment of tax on unrelated business income. Enforcement is coordinated with the Office of Chief Counsel. The division is headed by a deputy commissioner.

The IRS, itself, is a branch of the Department of Treasury. It is headed by a commissioner who, along with the chief counsel, is appointed by the president subject to Senate confirmation. The agency boasts that it deals with more Americans than any other public or private institution.[99] It has more than 99,000 employees, and each year it processes more than 222 million tax returns. The headquarters is located in Washington, DC, and there are eight field offices located around the country.

Protecting Patient Privacy While Promoting Information Technology

Medical information is inherently personal. A medical record contains intimate information that could bring embarrassment or even ridicule to its subject, if publicly disclosed. It could also cause economic hardship by making insurance more difficult or expensive to obtain or even jeopardizing employment. Clearly, patients have a strong interest in the confidentiality of their medical records. Clinicians have a stake, as well, since without adequate assurances of privacy, patients may be reluctant to share information that could be important to effective treatment.

Concerns about privacy are as old as medicine itself. The Hippocratic oath directs physicians to maintain patient confidences as an obligation of the profession.[100] However, the age-old worry that a clinician might misspeak or that a paper record might be misplaced is tremendously magnified when medical information is recorded in electronic form. Computers can store vast amounts of data and disseminate it instantly to any corner of the world. The opportunity for both intentional mischief and accidental disclosure is much greater.[101] Security lapses that compromised sensitive private information have been widely reported.[102]

Despite the risks, electronic medical records present significant opportunities to improve the quality and efficiency of care.[103] The positive side of easy dissemination is that data can be shared among clinicians, not only those involved in a course of treatment but those located around the world when a patient travels. Information can be transmitted instantly, obviating delays that accompany pulling, copying, and sending paper files.[104] Reimbursement requests can flow in bulk from providers to payers along with supporting documentation. Moreover, illegible handwriting, the bane of many who must decipher medical records, is no longer a concern.

To realize these benefits, both the sender and the receiver must be equipped to handle the information. Unfortunately, to accomplish this, more than just using the same computer equipment is required. Different formats have been devised for storing and sending medical data, and communication between them is not always possible. Implementation of an array of incompatible data platforms can significantly limit the usefulness of health care information technology. Industry-wide standards are needed, but often an external force is necessary to produce the required consensus.

In 1996, with computerization on the verge of revolutionizing medical record keeping, Congress addressed the twin concerns of facilitating technological advances while limiting the risks of unauthorized disclosures. The result was incorporated into HIPAA, a law that also added new protections for consumers of health insurance, as its name implies.[105] (For a description of HIPAA's health insurance provisions, see chapter 4 on health care finance.) HIPAA set standards to achieve uniformity in electronic medical claims submissions and, of more immediate concern to providers, imposed significant new restrictions on the handling and transmission of all patient information that is maintained in electronic form.

Standardizing Data Flow

In terms of standardization, HIPAA directed DHHS to develop rules for data transmission by health plans, data clearinghouses, and providers, with penalties for those that do not comply. Among the most significant aspects of the rules are protocols for identifying patients in data sets with unique and anonymous identifiers. DHHS developed the rules through a data council within the agency, which reports directly to the secretary. They are based on recommendations of the National Committee on Vital and Health Statistics (NCVHS), a public advisory body established by statute that is also housed within the department. The NCVHS has eighteen members, sixteen of whom are appointed by the secretary and two by Congress.[106]

Protecting Patient Confidences

HIPAA's directives to safeguard patient privacy are considerably more complex and controversial than those for data standardization.[107] They were formally implemented on 14 April 2003, after several years of debate over their scope.[108] The guiding principle behind them is that patients should have the ultimate say, whenever possible, over the dissemination of their records.

By the time of HIPAA's passage, concern over medical privacy had already prompted every state to adopt its own safeguards in one form or another.[109] However, the laws differed considerably.[110] Some applied only to physicians, some to institutions, some to insurers, and some to employers. The breadth of information protected varied from wide coverage of data on general public health data to a narrower focus on communicable diseases to a specific concern with sexually transmitted diseases. Similarly, penalties ranged broadly from criminal sanctions to civil liability to both. Many of these enactments imposed stricter standards than those that HIPAA contained. Congress chose to let states with more aggressive protections maintain them by designing HIPAA to preempt state privacy laws that are laxer but not those that are more stringent.

HIPAA's privacy regulations, often referred to as the HIPAA Privacy Rule, broadly define the kinds of health care organizations subject to their scope to include hospitals, physicians' offices, pharmacies, health plans, and other sites where clinical care is provided or through which it is financed.[111] These are known under the act as "covered entities" and include both private and governmental organizations. The Privacy Rule imposes both structural and process requirements. In terms of structure, institutions must appoint privacy officers with overall responsibility for the integrity of electronic patient data. They must also develop written privacy procedures that delineate which employees have access to which kinds of information, how medical information may be used, and to whom it may be disclosed. The privacy officer is responsible for enforcing the procedures, for employee training, and for discipline when procedures are ignored. Health care providers must make their privacy procedures available to patients and must collect a written acknowledgment from all patients that they have been made aware of the procedures.

Within this structure, medical data may be shared in a number of circumstances related to providing and financing a patient's care and operating a health care facility. Data may be accessed by other providers, such as consulting physicians and nurses, who are involved in treatment. It may also be sent to third-party payers. Beyond that, disclosure is severely restricted, with limited exceptions for emergencies and for government needs such as public health activities, judicial and administrative proceedings, law enforcement, and national defense. Any other disclosure of clinical information requires the patient's written consent in a form that the Privacy Rule explicitly prescribes. The consent must specify the information to be released, the provider authorized to release it, the provider authorized to receive it, a date on which the consent expires, and an acknowledgment that it may be revoked at any time prior to the disclosure.[112]

Even with the most stringent safeguards, some outside contact with patient information is unavoidable in any health care organization. Suppliers, service providers, and other external personnel must enter facilities where patients are treated and information on them is generated and stored. In a hospital, for example, outsiders deliver supplies and equipment, remove waste, and repair machinery. Since they do not work for the hospital, they are not employees of a "covered entity" and therefore are not directly subject to its patient privacy policies. However, they do work for entities that maintain ongoing commercial relationships with a covered entity. HIPAA refers to these organizations as "business associates." To continue their dealings with these partners, covered entities must enter into contracts with them that require adherence to the same data disclosure limitations.[113]

Disclosure of medical information can harm a patient only if the recipient of the data knows who he or she is. Anonymous data that cannot be traced to an individual poses little threat, but it can be instrumental to some health care activities. In particular, public health monitoring and health services research depend on such information to analyze medical treatments, understand disease trends, and monitor the performance of individual providers, but they do not require knowledge of which patients are involved. A rule that required patient consent for such disclosures would render these functions virtually impossible to perform while offering little benefit.[114]

To accommodate these broader health system needs, the Privacy Rule permits fairly broad access to clinical data when it is "deidentified," that is, when it has been stripped of any information that could link it to individual patients. To qualify as deidentified, the regulations require that data exclude several elements, including the patient's name, address, birth date, and other specific information such as occupation or income. Even with this patient-specific information removed, identification of identities still may be possible in small samples. The burden is on both the supplier and recipient of the data to ensure that inadvertent linkages of deidentified data with individual patients do not occur.[115]

The final piece of the HIPAA regulations put specific powers in the hands of patients themselves, by guaranteeing them access to their own medical information.[116] Prior to the passage of HIPAA, the right of patients to see their records was governed by the laws of each state, with many affording no right at all. Under HIPAA, patients must be permitted to see and obtain copies of their records and to ask for corrections when errors are discovered.[117] Limited exceptions are permitted when clinicians fear patient harm from revelations about their treatment or condition, primarily when mental health care is involved.

HIPAA Enforcement

HIPAA provides penalties for accidental violations that are fairly mild. Inadvertent disclosures are subject to fines of $100 each with a limit of $25,000 per year for any single requirement or prohibition that is violated.[118] Intentional violations, however, are subject to criminal sanctions, including significant fines and jail time that ranges up to ten years, if information is disclosed or obtained to be sold for personal gain, commercial advantage, or malicious harm. HIPAA does not include a private right of action, so the only recourse for patients who believe they have been harmed by an authorized disclosure or denied access to their medical records is to complain to the Office for Civil Rights (OCR) of DHHS, which enforces the law. They may not bring a lawsuit on their own.

Agency Structure for Medical Privacy Enforcement:
The Office for Civil Rights (OCR)

OCR enforces the privacy provisions of HIPAA and also oversees a range of civil rights laws as they apply to health care. These include the Civil Rights Act of 1964, which applies generally to discrimination based on race, religion, creed, or national origin; the Hill-Burton Act, which funded hospital construction in return for a non-discrimination commitment; portions of the Medicare and Medicaid programs, which prohibit discrimination as a condition of participation; and nondiscrimination provisions that accompany all of DHHS's other funding programs. Among OCR's primary activities are reviews of civil rights compliance in organizations that have received DHHS grants and pre-grant reviews of facilities that seek approval from CMS to participate in Medicare. Periodic ongoing reviews of grantees are also conducted. These enforcement activities apply to both private and governmental bodies. Under HIPAA, patient privacy is another civil right, which falls under the office's scope of responsibility.[119]

OCR is a relatively small component of DHHS. It consumes an annual budget of about $30 million out of a total department budget of more than $500 billion. The office has only about 260 employees, of whom about 185 are located in field offices scattered throughout the country. It is headed by a director, with a single deputy director who oversees most compliance and outreach activities. OCR is organized into divisions according to broad functions, with one for program, policy, and training and one for voluntary compliance and outreach, rather than according to the regulatory program involved. However, the deputy director has two senior advisers on HIPAA implementation, one for outreach and one for policy.[120]

In enforcing HIPAA and other civil rights laws, OCR conducts investigations both in response to complaints and on its own initiative. It also implements public education efforts. Civil enforcement actions are handled by its Office of General Counsel, and criminal enforcement is handled by DOJ. HIPAA issues consume a large portion of the OCR's resources, with about one-quarter of its compliance staff devoted to medical privacy violations, most of which involve denials of patient access to medical records.[121]

Overall Policy Issues: Can Health Care Be Like Any Other Business?

The proper place of health care in America's economy is a subject of perennial debate. Is it a business like any other in which market forces can ultimately determine supply and demand, or is it an essential public service that should be provided with more government direction? Historically, different regulatory programs have proceeded under each assumption.

There is no question that the consumption of health care services is subject to factors that are not at work to the same extent in other industries. A vast gulf in knowledge separates buyers and sellers, a phenomenon that economists call "asymmetry of information."[122] Physicians know much more about their patients' medical needs than the patients themselves, so it is extremely difficult for the consumers of health care to decide on their own what services they should purchase. They also have little data with which to compare the quality of competing providers. The emergence of quality scorecards, clinical guidelines, and Internet access to information is bringing some change, but a large gap remains. Consumers of health care services also face purchasing decisions in which the stakes are extremely high. These are decisions that can determine health and well-being and can literally be matters of life and death.

Even if perfect information were available, patients in many situations must acquire services immediately regardless of cost. Trauma victims, for example, do not have the luxury of comparison shopping. Economists characterize this imperative to acquire a good or service regardless of cost as an example of "inelasticity of demand," and it greatly attenuates the laws of supply and demand.[123]

The most notable factor of all in differentiating health care from other industries is the presence of third-party payment. Insurance of one sort or another pays for most health care services, with patients contributing only a small portion through deductibles and copayments. Insulated from the actual cost of their consumption decisions, patients have little incentive to heed the economic consequences. Economists refer to this phenomenon as "moral hazard," the risk that buyers of a good or service will ignore costs to others.[124] Moreover, in health care the inversion of rational purchasing incentives extends even further. Physicians who guide purchasing decisions of their patients usually face no negative economic repercussions from excessive spending and may even realize financial rewards. This is a long way from a conventional market.

Although a traditional market structure does not guide health care consumption, underlying economic forces are always at work. Providers, as sellers of services, generally seek to maximize their revenue, and purchasers, whether they are third-party payers or patients, generally seek to minimize their cost. While they may be attenuated in health care, these forces constantly shape the industry's business dynamics in one way or another. However, without the discipline of a traditional market, the result may not always encourage the highest quality at the lowest price. Health care business regulation seeks to compensate for the market's failings or to modify health care business structures to better accommodate market principles.

The challenge of fitting health care into a market model has been substantial. Antitrust laws must acknowledge an unconventional relationship between buyers and sellers. Fraud and abuse laws must police the narrow line between providers acting as patient advocates and as self-interested enterprises. Tax-exemption rules must distinguish between the charitable health care industry for which they were developed and the increasingly for-profit business structures that exist today. Privacy regulations must create incentives to respect confidentiality in an industry that is increasingly driven by the use of information.[125] Each regulatory scheme faces a delicate balancing act.

Is it possible that health care can adapt its economic structure to one that is similar enough to other industries to permit a traditional market model to apply? Efforts have begun on several fronts to move it in that direction. The emerging field of quality measurement seeks to generate data with which patients can compare providers. New insurance models permit beneficiaries to accumulate funds in tax-free accounts that can be used to pay providers directly, making patients more sensitive to prices. The Internet offers a wealth of information on diseases and treatments that patients can use to better query their physicians. These efforts constitute the movement toward "consumer-driven" health care, in which the patient is better able to act as a conventional consumer.[126]

A more fundamental question is whether America's health care system would serve patients more effectively if it emulated a market-based structure. Some see an industry made more efficient through market forces, but others fear that a small segment of sophisticated consumers would benefit at the expense of those who are less savvy with medical information. Most other industrialized countries see health care as a necessity whose provision is primarily a government concern to ensure widespread and equitable access. The United States is the only industrialized country that does not have a national health insurance system that covers all citizens.[127] This distinguishing feature of American health care reflects a strong historical preference for private market-based solutions to economic concerns. However, even the most aggressive efforts to incorporate conventional market forces cannot entirely overcome the factors that differentiate health care transactions from other kinds of business relationships. Health care business in America, therefore, will likely always face a combination of private market forces and regulatory restrictions, and business regulators will continue to struggle with incompatibilities between the health care industry and the oversight programs that they administer.

8

Regulation and Funding of Research

[T]he National Institutes of Health (NIH) have become the foremost biomedical research facility not only in the United States but in the world.
—Victoria A. Harden, *Inventing the NIH*

It would be difficult to identify an enterprise that has contributed more to the improvement of human lives than medical research. Imagine a world without vaccines to protect against dreaded childhood illnesses, antibiotics to cure life-threatening infections, or diagnostic imaging technologies to find signs of lethal diseases when they are still treatable. It would be a world with much lower life expectancies and much greater suffering from disease. It would be the world of just a hundred years ago.

It would also be difficult to identify a more significant driver of this research than government funding. While industry and foundation financial support play important roles, the channeling of public funds to medical research created this enterprise as we have come to know it. No other government has been as great a contributor to the advancement of medical knowledge over the past century as that of the United States.

Government research funding in America is unique in ways other than its size. For the most part, funded research projects are initiated by the investigator, not by the government funding agency. Within broad parameters, private researchers at universities and foundations determine what they wish to study and then try to convince reviewers that their project has merit. In most other countries that support research, the government generally decides what it wants to investigate and then finds scientists to follow through.[1] Publicly funded scientific research in America, therefore, represents a vast public-private partnership with a significant democratic element.

Three federal agencies provide the bulk of funding for medical and health-related research—the National Institutes of Health (NIH), the Agency for Healthcare Research and Quality (AHRQ), and the National Science Foundation (NSF). A small amount is also provided by a few other agencies, most notably the Veterans Administration (VA), the Health Resources and Services Administration (HRSA), the Centers for Medicare & Medicaid Services (CMS), the National Center for Health Statistics (NCHS), the U.S. Department of Agriculture (USDA), and the Department of Energy (DOE). Of the total of all government funding, more than three-quarters comes from NIH.[2] It is the largest government sponsor of medical research in the world, and it is often cited as a model of government policy for nurturing science.[3] In addition to extramural sponsorship of independent investigators at universities and foundations, it conducts a considerable amount of research within its own facilities through intramural programs.

Government policy also directs medical research in another significant way—through regulation. Despite its accomplishments, research has faced its share of scandals, and regulatory policy has responded. The most serious scandals have involved harm to subjects who participated in research in circumstances in which they were not fully informed of the risks or were not provided with adequate protections. NIH administers a program of institutional review boards (IRBs) that review research protocols at each institution that receives its research funding. The Food and Drug Administration (FDA) administers a similar program for clinical research that is part of the drug approval process. (FDA's other regulatory activities are discussed in chapter 5.)

The history of government regulation and funding of research is a story of a small and insignificant function that grew exponentially during the twentieth century as the applications of research discoveries in improving health and saving lives became increasingly apparent. However, despite the dramatic rise in significance and budgets, government research funding still exists in a world of limited resources. Not only must NIH and other science funding agencies compete with other users of federal revenues, but their internal components must compete among themselves. Greater funding for one disease can mean that less is available to study another. One result of this competitive environment is that federal research budgets have become matters of tremendous political interest. As in other areas of health care regulation, politics and science can make explosive bedfellows.

History and Structure of Government Funding and Regulation of Medical Research

Modest Beginnings

The massive research apparatus that is today's NIH traces its origins to the nineteenth century and a small obscure laboratory in Staten Island, New York.[4] In 1887, Dr. Joseph J. Kinyoun of the Marine Hospital Service, the predecessor to the Public

Health Service (PHS), used a room in a marine hospital as a laboratory to try to identify the strains of bacteria that cause common infectious diseases. He succeeded in identifying the cholera bacillus, which was then used to diagnose suspicious cases of this dreaded illness. Dr. Kinyoun's success was rewarded with a move to a new home in Washington, DC, in 1891 and a change in name for his endeavor to the Hygienic Laboratory. The office gained further political legitimacy in 1901 when Congress authorized $35,000 for a new building. This relatively modest sum can be seen in hindsight as the first NIH appropriation.

Dr. Kinyoun's efforts took another significant step forward in 1902, when Congress reorganized the Marine Hospital Service and created the Division of Pathology and Bacteriology to house the Hygienic Laboratory's research. This gave it a more formal bureaucratic home. The professional workforce was also expanded to add Ph.D.-trained researchers to the existing complement of physicians.[5]

The Hygienic Laboratory also took on a major new set of responsibilities the same year when Congress passed the Biologics Control Act. New technologies for producing vaccines and antitoxins, which resulted from the laboratory's research work, often produced products with serious side effects, sometimes including death. Under the Biologics Control Act, Congress charged the laboratory with setting standards and issuing licenses for the manufacture of these products by private companies. Along with new regulatory duties came an expanded mission of research to support them. The Hygienic Laboratory and its successor agencies retained responsibility for regulating biologics until 1972, when the FDA took over this role.[6] (The FDA's role in regulating drugs and other medical products is discussed in chapter 5.)

Medical Progress Shows the Value of Research

Over the next several decades, the Public Health and Marine Hospital Service that had been formed in 1902 contributed several significant advances to American public health. Its expanding role was recognized in 1912 with a name change to the Public Health Service. It was during this time that scientists who monitored and regulated research were first accepted as officials in the executive branch of government.[7] Among the advances of the newly renamed agency were the identification of a dietary deficiency as the cause of pellagra and enforcement of sanitation near military bases during World War I. (The PHS's role in American public health regulation is discussed in chapter 6.) As the powerful effects of public health interventions became increasingly evident, the research that made them possible gained new respect, and greater responsibility and larger budgets followed.

The government's role in funding research grew significantly in the years following World War I. Ironically, the enhanced government presence grew out of an effort that initially sought to encourage a larger role for private companies. After the conclusion of the war, several chemists from the Chemical Warfare Service, an agency established during the war effort, saw the potential for private chemical companies to fund research on a large scale into uses of chemistry in medicine.[8] They tried to encourage interest for several years, but with no success. In 1926, they redirected their quest to seek funding from the government. They found a friend in Louisiana senator Joseph E. Ransdell, whose efforts led to the enactment in 1930 of legislation establishing and funding fellowships for basic research into biology and medicine within the Hygienic Laboratory.[9] The Ransdell Act also changed the Laboratory's name to the National Institute of Health. (The recognition of multiple institutes did not follow until 1948.) The initial funding was modest, with the nation recently having entered the Great Depression, but the change in public policy was not. The era of public funding as the foundation for basic scientific research in America had arrived.

In 1937, Congress took another major step in building the federal research apparatus by establishing the National Cancer Institute (NCI). This agency was not formally linked to NIH until 1944, but its creation brought about two significant new policy directions that guided NIH's future development. NCI was the first research agency focused on a specific category of diseases, forming the model for NIH's subsequent structure. It was also the first to fund a significant amount of research by scientists outside of the government.

The structure of disease-specific institutes funding extramural scientists has drawn praise but also criticism.[10] Congress gave the institutes disease-specific names partly in the belief that it would be politically easier to justify funding than if they were identified with more technical names. On an administrative level, however, the separate institutes have sometimes functioned as independent fiefdoms under directors seeking bureaucratic advantage. Perhaps most significantly, while the emphasis on specific diseases has nurtured public acceptance of high levels of funding, it has also facilitated a key role for politics in determining funding allocations and in setting the nation's scientific research agenda. This conflict between a more democratic and more expert-oriented approach to setting research priorities continues to this day. Over the decades, political pressures have influenced many congressional decisions on the NIH budget in a decision-making process that some would call fair but others would term uninformed.

NIH took another giant step forward in 1940 with the opening of its sprawling campus in Bethesda, Maryland.[11] The land had comprised a private estate owned by Mr. and Mrs. Luke Wilson, who donated it for government use.[12] The complex of research and administrative buildings that was constructed on the grounds is today one of the largest in the world dedicated to biomedical research, and it serves as an icon for the importance of the research enterprise. The campus was dedicated on 31 October 1940, as World War II was raging in Europe and the United States was looking to improve its national defense. In his dedication speech,

President Franklin Roosevelt linked health and national security in a theme with poignant echoes today:

> The total defense that we have heard so much about of late, that total defense which this nation seeks, involves a great deal more than building airplanes, and ships and guns and bombs, but we cannot be a strong nation unless we are a healthy nation. We must recruit not only men and materials but also knowledge and science in the service of national strength and that is what we are doing here.[13]

Explosive Growth after World War II

Science and technology provided the keys to winning World War II. In the words of one observer, the successful war effort "had mobilized a concerted government effort—unprecedented to date—in applying research to practical use."[14] Radar, jet engines, and the atomic bomb were just a few of the discoveries that helped to determine the war's outcome and left indelible changes on life afterward. Medical breakthroughs during World War II were no less astounding and were responsible for saving hundreds of thousands of lives, not to mention countless more in the years that followed. They included penicillin for staphylococcus infections, sulfonamide drugs for wounds and burns, blood derivatives such as gamma globulin for measles and hepatitis, cortisone for inflammation, synthetic quinine for malaria, vaccines against typhus and yellow fever, and DDT for delousing clothing.[15] World War II demonstrated that the most advanced countries in science and technology tend to be the strongest militarily and economically.

NIH, America's gateway to financing advancement in medical science, was transformed with tremendous growth in the years after World War II, as the power of science made itself evident to politicians and the public. This growth coincided with wider acceptance of a larger government role in many other aspects of domestic life as well.[16] NIH's position as the key to promoting science began to take shape when it received responsibility for the government's wartime research contracts with universities to provide an orderly process for phaseout. Soon after the war ended, however, Congress changed direction and decided to continue to support these contracts instead of phasing them out. Their administration was kept within NIH, which was given more funding and staff for the job. Some contracts were later transferred to the National Science Foundation (NSF), which was created a few years later. Wartime research, apparently, had not exhausted its usefulness. In fact, the real dividend from the research effort was only about to be earned through countless discoveries in the following decades. The change of course in the treatment of postwar science funding has been characterized as "probably the most influential and far-reaching in the history of federal support for university research."[17]

The postwar expansion of NIH actually dates to the final years of the war and Congress's passage of the Public Health Service Act in 1944.[18] That law generalized the NCI model of disease-specific research funding for private scientists to areas beyond cancer. Under the law, a succession of dramatic budget increases began in 1946 that expanded NIH research funding from about $4 million in 1947 to $100 million in 1957 to $1 billion in 1974 to more than $27 billion in 2004.[19] A succession of new institutes joined the agency starting in 1946 as well, leading to the pluralization of its name in 1948 to the National Institutes of Health. Between 1946 and 1949, institutes that focused on mental health, dental health, and heart disease were added. Two existing NIH divisions were promoted to become institutes as the National Microbiological Institute (later renamed the National Institute of Arthritis and Metabolic Diseases) and the Experimental Biology and Medicine Institute (later renamed the National Institute of Allergy and Infectious Diseases). By 1998, NIH had grown to include twenty institutes and ten research centers.

The Public Health Service Act of 1944 also permitted NIH to conduct its own clinical research on-site with a staff of employee-investigators. This initiative included the creation in 1953 of a large hospital on the NIH campus at which research could be conducted, the Warren Grant Magnuson Clinical Center. While most NIH research continues to be conducted through extramural grants to private investigators, a significant amount of work is intramural, taking advantage of the agency's substantial facilities and resources.[20]

The remarkable growth of the NIH during the postwar years followed recognition of dramatic advances that flowed from NIH-funded medical research during the war. In addition to those already mentioned, these included many others that provided invaluable support for the war effort, for example, by identifying toxic hazards for workers in war-related industries, developing vaccines for tropical diseases, and improving the visual acuity of pilots.[21] Policy makers became aware of a new calculus under which public funding produced advances in medical knowledge, which in turn produced improvements in health in fairly short order. In particular, they saw returns from the unique process of funding private scientists with public money. As one observer noted of this period, "Never in the nation's history had public funds in such amounts been placed at the disposal of individuals working in support of their own objectives outside the framework of federal institutions."[22]

The 1950s have been described as a "golden era" for the NIH.[23] In addition to the favorable political climate, a major push came from two women who worked behind the scenes to convince Congress of the need for ever higher levels of funding. Mary Lasker, the wife of a prominent advertising executive, and Florence Mahoney, a social advocate, used powerful political connections to lobby continuously over the course of several decades, adding a significant impetus to the overall push for increased federal involvement in research funding.[24] Had it not been for their efforts, NIH would likely be very different, and much smaller, today.

The Steady Parade of Budget Increases

In terms of the magnitude of funding, NIH represents an unparalleled success in the maze of Washington politics. Budget increases have been relentless in part because of the perceived success of biomedical research and in part because of adroit manipulation of the political process. In what has been called a "stylized kabuki dance" between the agency, the president, and Congress, NIH budgets are sent each year from the president to the House of Representatives, which usually requests input from each institute, generally resulting in calls for larger amounts.[25] When the budget reaches the Senate, that body requests input from outside experts, who then usually call for even larger sums. During the 1950s and 1960s, this sequence led to compromises between the House and Senate that invariably exceeded the president's initial proposal.

Enhanced funding was followed closely by more contentious politics as the congressional budget process took on growing importance in the agency's operations. As one former NIH director described it, "The politics of the budgetary process is one of the first civics lessons to be learned by a new director."[26] The establishment of many of the disease-specific institutes reflected the political influence of voluntary health organizations seeking investment in their areas of concern. Over the years, numerous groups representing patients and their family members have lobbied for a share of the NIH budget to be devoted to their areas of interest, and members of Congress have realized that the NIH research budget can be a powerful political force.

Another significant growth spurt occurred in the late 1960s and early 1970s. In 1968, Congress placed the National Library of Medicine, the largest medical library in the world, under the NIH umbrella.[27] In 1971, Congress passed the National Cancer Act, which substantially expanded funding for research and training in the fight against cancer.[28] In 1972, it passed the National Heart, Blood Vessel, Lung, and Blood Act to fund programs related to heart disease.[29] These two conditions, the largest killers of Americans at that time and today, were the focus of considerable political attention, including a "war on cancer" declared by the administration of President Richard Nixon.

Yet another growth spurt took place in the 1980s, again fueled in part by politics. In 1979, the first case of acquired immune deficiency syndrome (AIDS) was identified. Its course of relentlessly destroying the immune system of victims leading to inevitable death baffled physicians for several years.[30] In 1983, researchers at NIH identified a virus, which they named human immunodeficiency virus (HIV), as the cause. With this discovery, there was the possibility of prevention and treatment, and subsequent lobbying by activist groups led Congress to substantially increase funding for AIDS research to bring this about. One result of the funding devoted to AIDS has been the development of medications that permit many of its victims to live with the disease for years as a chronic condition rather than facing almost certain rapid death. Increased government investment in research had again produced dramatic public health returns. (The role of the Centers for Disease Control and Prevention [CDC] in early research on AIDS is discussed in chapter 6.)

Groups representing victims of numerous other diseases have lobbied Congress to increase funding in areas of interest to them. In 1997, supporters of funding for Parkinson's disease research successfully lobbied for $100 million in additional NIH funding, but aware of the issues raised by public lobbying for disease-specific funding, the Senate also approved a study by the Institute of Medicine of the National Academy of Sciences to examine the NIH's budgetary priority-setting process.[31] The resulting report found the process fundamentally sound but recommended better systemization of input to the agency and constraints on congressional involvement.

Significant growth in NIH's budget since then has become almost a matter of course. (Recent NIH budgets are presented in table 8.1.) In 1995, Congress for the first time considered substantial cuts in the NIH budget, but a concerted lobbying campaign by a collection of scientific organizations led it to reconsider.[32] In 1997, with the proposed cuts apparently forgotten, Congress made a commitment to double the agency's budget over the next five years. As a result, the budget rose from $12.7 billion that year to just under $25 billion in 2002. Overall, the NIH budget rose by 80 percent between 1990 and 1998, in contrast to 48 percent for all other

Table 8.1
Recent NIH Budget Appropriations

Fiscal Year	Amount
1990	$7,576,352
1991	$8,276,739
1992	$8,921,687
1993	$10,335,996
1994	$10,955,773
1995	$11,299,522
1996	$11,927,562
1997	$12,740,843
1998	$13,674,843
1999	$15,629,156
2000	$17,820,587
2001	$20,458,130
2002	$23,296,382
2003	$27,066,782
2004	$27,887,512
2005	$28,495,157
2006	$28,461,417

Source: National Institutes of Health, Office of Budget (http://officeofbudget.od.nih.gov)

nondefense discretionary spending.[33] However, the years since 2002 have seen a leveling off of this budget growth.

The number of institutes and centers has grown over the years as well, with some of the new units leading the agency in new directions. For example, in 1992 NIH recognized a growing interest in developing a scientific understanding of nontraditional health care by establishing the National Center for Complementary and Alternative Medicine, and in 1993 it recognized the role of social and economic factors in health and disease by creating the National Center on Minority Health and Health Disparities. These broadened the agency's scope well beyond traditional biomedical investigations.[34]

While the overall growth of NIH continues, politics has also intervened to oppose some of its activities, most prominently in the politically sensitive area of research using embryonic stem cells.[35] Scientists have found that certain cells produced by human embryos in the earliest stages of development have the capacity to develop into almost any organ in the body. These are known as "stem cells." Although they are present in adults as well as in embryos, they do not appear to be as malleable after the early embryonic stage. A cell that can create any human organ can, in theory, be used to regenerate damaged tissue that otherwise could not be repaired. Scientists have been intrigued by the possibility of using stem cells to treat diseases and injuries that damage the brain and spinal cord, such as Alzheimer's disease, Parkinson's disease, and paraplegia, and to treat juvenile diabetes, which results from damage to the pancreas.

Under existing technology, scientists generally obtain embryonic stem cells by destroying embryos that are left over after attempts at in vitro fertilization. Opponents of abortion see this technology as tantamount to that practice and have lobbied to halt federal funding for research into its use. In 2001, President George W. Bush announced a policy to permit federal funding for research using the progeny of stem cells that had already been developed as of the date of the announcement but not for research using any lines of stem cells created subsequently.[36] Neither side was fully satisfied with this approach. Regulatory activity has moved to the states, with some, such as Louisiana, outlawing embryonic stem cell research entirely, and others, such as California and New Jersey, implementing their own funding programs to make up for lost federal support.[37]

NIH's Regulatory Role in Disseminating Research

Although the NIH's primary mission is funding, its expertise and reputation led Congress to grant it regulatory responsibilities as well. The agency's role in protecting human subjects in research that it funds is described later in this chapter. It also has a role in fostering the dissemination of research findings through the Government Patent Policy Act, commonly known as the Bayh-Dole Act, which was passed in 1980.[38] That law strengthened patent protections for inventions that result from research conducted with NIH funding in order to encourage the development of practical applications. However, sometimes patents are used to delay innovation when patent holders decline to commercialize their product. To prevent such abuses of patent protection, the law also contains a "march-in" provision that gives NIH the authority to overrule a patent and permit a potentially life-saving drug or device to be marketed by another entity.

The march-in provision, however, has never been applied. NIH has been asked to use it only once, and it declined.[39] In 1997, a small biotechnology company sought access to a patented device for separating stem cells used to treat cancer for a personal rather than a commercial need.[40] Its CEO had been diagnosed with lymphoma, and the company sought to use the device in his treatment. The agency decided not to interfere with market forces on behalf of a single individual out of concern for the effect it might have on future investment in technologies developed with NIH funds.[41]

Government Support beyond Medical Research: The National Science Foundation

Another major initiative of the post–World War II period complemented that of NIH to broaden America's research base beyond medical science. Congress created the National Science Foundation (NSF) in 1950 to promote and fund research across all sciences and engineering.[42] The agency was directed "to promote the progress of science; to advance the national health, prosperity, and welfare; and to secure the national defense."[43] NSF has always been much smaller than NIH. Its annual budget today of about $5 billion, while substantial, pales in comparison.[44] Its mission is also broader than that of NIH. As a general science promotion agency, NSF spends a larger percentage of its resources on activities other than making research grants, placing particular emphasis on education and training. It seeks to make America a more scientifically capable nation overall.

Much of the impetus for the creation of NSF came from the head of an agency that promoted scientific research during World War II, the Office of Scientific Research and Development.[45] Vannevar Bush envisioned a program of large-scale government funding for basic scientific research after the war at universities across the country. He convinced President Roosevelt to commission a report on the need to increase America's scientific research infrastructure, which was issued in 1945. Based on the report, he advocated for the creation of a new funding agency, which came into existence as NSF five years later.[46]

After Congress debated creation of the NSF in the years following World War II, the value of science to social improvement and national defense became increasingly clear across a range of disciplines in both the natural and social sciences. As science advanced, America's policy-making apparatus needed more sophisticated technical input to respond. This was especially evident with the start of the cold war, as the atomic and then hydrogen bomb dominated national defense planning. In 1957, the successful launch of the Soviet *Sputnik* satellite brought the exploration of outer space from the world of science fiction to a major defense imperative. There was no apparent choice but to improve the country's scientific infrastructure. By 1997, the United States accounted for almost half of the world's research and development investment.[47]

President Harry Truman signed the National Science Foundation Act of 1950, which created NSF, from the rear platform of a railroad car in Pocatello, Idaho.[48] Ironically, this law helped to propel the country into the age of space travel. It broadly directed the agency to strengthen America's overall scientific and engineering research potential through grants, contracts, and education and to appraise the impact of research on industrial development and general welfare. The breadth of the NSF's mandate is evident in the list of its activities contained in table 8.2. About 10 percent of the overall budget today is devoted to biology and other life sciences. NSF today funds research projects at 2,000 sites, which include not only universities but also elementary and secondary schools, nonprofit institutions, and small businesses. The agency reviews 30,000 proposals and issues 10,000 new awards each year.[49]

From Funding to Regulation of Research

With biomedical research established as a significant part of America's health care enterprise, fictions and disputes arose over time that led to calls for greater regulatory oversight. To some extent, NIH oversees the conduct of its grant recipients prospectively when it reviews their applications for funding. However, revelations

Table 8.2
Key National Science Foundation Activities

Foster scientific interchange between American and foreign scientists

Promote the use of computers in research and education

Evaluate the country's scientific and engineering needs

Maintain a national register of scientists

Provide information for policy development in other federal agencies

Monitor the federal research funding of universities and the construction of research facilities

Initiate activities related to international cooperation, national security, and the effects of science on society

Initiate support for science at academic and other nonprofit institutions

Promote basic research and education

Increase the participation of women and minorities in science

Source: http://www.nsf.gov/about/glance.jsp (25 May 2006).

of abuses highlighted the perceived need for concurrent regulation as well, particularly regarding the treatment of research subjects.[50]

Initial concern over harm to subjects centered not on human patients but on the welfare of research animals. Early NIH pronouncements warned against cruelty toward those used in laboratories.[51] In 1963, the agency published a guide for the treatment of animals, and beginning in the 1970s, institutions receiving NIH funding were required to establish animal care committees. In 1985, NIH began to conduct unannounced site visits at laboratories using animals in agency-funded research.

Awareness of the potential for harm to human subjects followed revelations in the years after World War II of Nazi research abuses.[52] Among the atrocities committed in Nazi concentration camps during the 1930s and 1940s were medical experiments performed on inmates. These included observations of the physiological effects of extreme cold, extreme heat, and other brutal, and often lethal, conditions. Much of this research was conducted under the supervision of licensed physicians.[53] In the 1950s, an NIH medical board was established to review research protocols to ensure adequate protection for human subjects.[54] In the 1960s, the agency required institutional grant recipients to develop written guidelines. However, as in many other areas of health regulation, truly vigorous oversight did not follow until a scandal arose.

In 1970, news was first widely reported of an NIH-sponsored project dating from 1932 to observe the natural course of syphilis infections.[55] In what has become known as the Tuskegee study, a group of 600 African American men in Tuskegee, Alabama, 399 with the disease and 201 without, were recruited as subjects. Investigators promised free medical examinations for as long as the subjects would permit physicians to observe the progression of their symptoms, but the examinations did not include treatment. In the 1930s, treatments for syphilis were rudimentary, and regular monitoring was not too far from the actual standard of care. However, starting in the mid-1940s, penicillin became available as an extremely effective therapy and was widely used, but it was never offered to the men in the study. None of them—poor, uneducated, and unaware of medical advances—had any way to realize that a cure was available but not offered, even as the research progressed into the 1960s.

Press reports of the study engendered widespread outrage. What made the scandal particularly distressing to many was that its protagonists were among the most highly educated, and presumably well-intentioned, of America's professional elite. If they could ignore the fundamental medical ethical principle to "first, do not harm," who could be trusted to assure research safety?

Congress responded in 1974 by passing the National Research Act, which created the National Commission for the Protection of Human Subjects of Biomedical and Behavioral Research to identify principles for the ethical treatment of subjects.[56] The law also established a system of institutional review boards (IRBs) to oversee the protection of human subjects in research at every organization receiving federal funding.[57] A similar system addressed clinical trials of new drugs and devices that are supervised by the FDA although supported by private funding. IRBs review research protocols before they are implemented and oversee studies on an ongoing basis. NIH oversees their activities through its Office for Protection from Research Risks.

With their placement within each grant-receiving institution, IRBs apply regulatory control at a level close to the research rather than in a centralized bureaucracy. In addition to the institutions that host NIH-funded research, NIH itself operates at least one IRB in each of its component institutes to review intramural studies. Under federal regulations, IRBs must be composed of a combination of local scientists, administrators, and members of the public.[58] Their records are periodically reviewed by the supervising agency, either the NIH or FDA, for compliance with structural and organizational rules.

IRBs review the proposed protocols of local investigators with a mandate to minimize risks to subjects consistent with maintaining sound research design.[59] Recognizing that much medical research can present unavoidable risks, IRBs balance potential harm to subjects against the potential benefits of new knowledge that may be gained. In conducting their risk-benefit analyses, regulations of the NIH and FDA direct IRBs to pay particular attention to the possibility of coercion in the recruitment of subjects and to the circumstances of vulnerable populations, such as children, prisoners, and those with mental disabilities.[60]

Underlying the regulatory scheme that established IRBs is the bioethical analysis of an advisory committee to DHHS published in 1979 as *The Belmont Report.*[61] This document, compiled in response to the National Research Act of 1974, set forth the principle of respect for the individual autonomy of subjects as the philosophical foundation for conducting ethical research. At the core of this proposition is the notion that subjects must willingly agree to participate based on full knowledge of relevant risks. In other words, subjects must give "informed consent" before they can ethically be exposed to research risks.

IRBs focus much of their review of research protocols on the process of obtaining informed consent. They seek to ensure that the participation of subjects is truly voluntary and is based on clear explanations of potential harm. Researchers can obtain informed consent through written or oral means, and often they use both. IRB members spend much of their time reviewing written summaries of risks that will be presented to potential subjects for completeness and clarity. Consent that is obtained coercively or without full disclosure can lead the NIH to withdraw funding from the project involved, and in extreme cases to the entire institution that hosts it. It can also form the basis for legal liability of an investigator or institution, should a subject experience harm.

Regulation of Privately Funded Research:
Clinical Trials and the FDA

NIH and NSF spawned an American research enterprise that advances basic under-standing of the natural world on an almost daily basis. However, as funding sources they are now just players on larger team. A sizable portion of medical research has historically been conducted to meet the shorter-term needs of private corporations that produce medical products and provide health care services. In particular, the pharmaceutical industry commits substantial resources to developing and testing new drugs. Over the past five years, private pharmaceutical research has overtaken NIH grant programs as the largest source of medical research funding in America, even with a recent acceleration in the growth of NIH's budgets.[62]

While the funding is private, pharmaceutical research takes place in a heavily regulated environment. With the passage of the Food, Drug, and Cosmetic Act of 1938, the FDA assumed responsibility for overseeing the entire drug development process from the first tests for basic safety to the advertising claims that are made once a drug is on the market.[63] As part of this mission, the agency regulates the clinical testing that forms the scientific backbone of drug development. Given the magni-tude of pharmaceutical industry spending on research, this means that the FDA has taken a central role in regulating much of America's medical research enterprise. It now oversees, directly or indirectly, more scientific research than any other single agency.[64] (FDA regulation to protect the public from unsafe and ineffective drugs is discussed in chapter 5.)

The FDA's regulatory efforts to protect human subjects in clinical research began in earnest in 1971.[65] Like NIH, the agency requires that IRBs operate at each institu-tion hosting clinical trials.[66] FDA regulations dictate with considerable specificity the content of informed consent forms that are presented to research subjects.[67] For example, no consent form may include language waiving the subject's right to sue the investigator in the event of harm. The form may not include a certification by the subject that the disclosure of risks was complete and may not include unproven claims of effectiveness for an experimental medication. Subjects must also be in-formed of procedures for maintaining confidentiality of records and for receiving compensation for research-related injuries.

From Laboratory Bench to Bedside:
The Growth of Health Services Research

The bulk of NIH-sponsored research is conducted in laboratories and clinical settings, notwithstanding some of its recent initiatives into the social aspects of medicine. The findings of these studies have substantially broadened our scientific understanding of the mechanisms of health and disease, but the best science in the world will not help a single patient if medical practitioners do not know how to use it. By the late 1980s, health policy makers had become aware that the behavior of physicians could be as important in determining the health status of populations as the general level of scientific understanding. If the goal was to produce better health outcomes in practice, then the research picture was incomplete.

Of particular concern were findings of large variations in health care practices around the country.[68] Treatment for the same condition could vary widely depending on the region in which it was rendered. Physicians differed in the frequency of performing surgery, the length of hospital stays, the use of prescription drugs, and many other aspects of clinical practice. Contrary to expectations, however, variations in the intensity of care showed no correlation with health outcomes. If more care did not necessarily lead to better care, then medical resources were being wasted. Here was a fertile field to find not just quality enhancements but cost savings as well.

In 1989, Congress established the Agency for Health Care Policy and Research (AHCPR) to support health services research.[69] Included in this field are studies on ways to improve the scientific basis for medical practice and to control health care costs. Initial investigations sought to understand the causes and consequences of variations in medical practices and other possible ways to reduce costs. AHCPR was designed to complement the biomedical research mission of NIH, as a sister, although much smaller, agency within DHHS.

The agency began its mission by funding the development of clinical practice guidelines for a range of medical procedures. These guidelines, also known as clinical protocols, lead physicians through the decision-making process in treating an illness. They indicate which diagnostic tests to order, which medications to prescribe, and which procedures to perform over the course of a patient's treatment. Unlike conventional medical decision-making, which can vary with the happenstance of the physician's training, knowledge, and individual practice style, guidelines can reflect the expertise of the most prominent clinicians in each field.

Over the course of its first few years, AHCPR issued numerous guidelines in various medical specialties.[70] Advocates saw them as a way to replace variation in medical practices with uniformity at the level of top national experts. Opponents, however, feared that they would lead to standardization that could obliterate the clinical judgment of experienced practitioners. The debates surrounding the agency's efforts were often fierce. With the livelihood of hundreds of thousands of medical practitioners at stake, it had stumbled into a political hornet's nest.

In 1995, several political factors converged to threaten the new agency's existence.[71] Stiff resistance to guidelines for the treatment of lower back pain, which sought to minimize the use of surgery, led to vigorous lobbying of Congress to limit not just these guidelines but all of the agency's activities. In addition, several of its studies had contributed to the development of President Bill Clinton's health reform plan in 1993. When the plan failed to become law, the agency became associated with a politically unpopular cause. In addition, the new Republican leadership of Congress was looking for programs to cut, and the politically vulnerable agency was a likely target. AHCPR appeared to be on its last legs.

To the surprise of many, the agency did survive, but in the process, its mission changed.[72] Guidelines were gone as its primary focus and were replaced by support for practical research on improving health care quality, controlling costs, and improving access. Through its rescue and reauthorization in 1995, the agency also received a new name, the Agency for Healthcare Research and Quality (AHRQ). By deleting the reference to "policy," Congress sought to distance the agency's image from politics.

AHRQ was fortified again with a new sense of purpose a few years later. In late 1999, the Institute of Medicine of the National Academy of Sciences published a report on the prevalence of serious medical errors in America's hospitals.[73] The findings showed that serious errors were widespread, possibly resulting in as many as 98,000 excess patient deaths each year. After decades of policy concern focused on spiraling health care costs and limitations on access, the public spotlight quickly turned to lapses in quality. Congress gave AHRQ a leading role in funding research into this newly recognized public health threat.[74] Just five years after facing near-certain demise, AHRQ moved to the center of America's health policy agenda.

Today, AHRQ sponsors a wide range of research on health care quality, cost, and access, with an emphasis on reducing clinical errors. It also funds fellowships and training programs. Its annual budget, which has recently been in the range of $250 million, is a fraction of the size of NIH's, but it is the primary player in funding applied research to improve the practice of medicine.[75]

The Future of Medical Research: Exploring the Human Genome and Regulating the Results

In 1953, the door to a fundamentally new approach to scientific investigation in biology and medicine was opened. After years of trying and intense competition with other scientists, two researchers working in England, James Watson and Francis Crick, identified the molecular blueprint for life itself.[76] They described the structure of deoxyribonucleic acid, commonly known as DNA, the molecule that directs the functioning of living cells. It resides in the nucleus of every cell and determines the genetic characteristics of all living organisms, including humans. Through understanding and manipulating DNA, the nature of biomedical research can take a dramatically new form.

Initial progress in exploring human health and disease based on examination of DNA proceeded slowly over the two decades immediately following Watson and Crick's discovery. During that time, researchers expanded their basic understanding of the DNA molecule, its structure, and its function. The earliest significant applied breakthroughs occurred in the 1970s, when scientists first reported success at manipulating the genetic structure of microorganisms. The field of genetic engineering began with the artificial rearrangement of genetic material in bacteria to create a recombined DNA molecule, known as "recombinant DNA."[77] The custom-designed organisms that resulted were seen as potentially serving a range of purposes. New species could manufacture life-saving substances like insulin, consume unwanted substances like oil from ruptured tanker ships, and even glow at night. Research had made it possible to use the blueprint of life as a resource to exploit.

The excitement over these discoveries, however, was tempered by caution, because artificially constructed life-forms could have unintended consequences. Skeptics warned that designer bacteria could cause new forms of illness for which there would be no natural immunity. They could consume valuable resources, not just unwanted ones. They could be designed as pathogens for use by rogue governments as a means of warfare. Science was about to enter unknown territory.

Wider implications of designing microorganisms for commercial goals were also apparent. Since DNA determines the genetic makeup of humans, as well as of bacteria, the new field of genetic engineering could ultimately apply to people. Exciting prospects were in store to cure genetic diseases and improve human functioning but with long-term implications that could not be predicted.

With the prospect of revolutionary medical benefits but also the specter of catastrophic consequences, Congress in 1988 provided funding to enable NIH and the federal Department of Energy (DOE) to jointly establish an effort to map the structure of the entire complement of human genetic material.[78] In 1989, the National Center for Human Genome Research (NCHGR), later to become the National Human Genome Research Institute (NHGRI), was created to house this project. The following year, it initiated the Human Genome Project (HGP), the endeavor that completed the task. DOE's role stemmed from its interest in the effects of radiation on genetic mutations. NIH's role stemmed from its interest in advancing medical research. Various universities and other research organizations throughout the country also served as partners, along with research centers in other countries around the world.

The HGP completed its work ahead of schedule. Originally predicted to take fifteen years, a first draft containing 90 percent of the DNA map was published in February 2001, and the final version in 2002. A crucial step in the effort came in 1996, when the HGP took the unusual step of putting all findings in a public database within twenty-four hours of their disclosure without limits on their use. The project thereby facilitated competition from a private company seeking to reach the finish line first. Celera Corporation started work in 1998 but was able to catch up to and keep pace with the federal effort in a quest to find commercial uses for genetic knowledge. The HGP and Celera jointly announced that they had completed the initial sequencing of the human genome in 2000.[79]

The HGP is today regarded as "the crowning achievement of twentieth century biology."[80] Its impact on research within NIH was felt even before its map was complete. In 1993, NIH created the Division of Intramural Research within the NCHGR to study the application of genetic technologies to specific diseases. In 1996, eight NIH institutes jointly created the Center for Inherited Disease Research to further promote these investigations. The following year, the center achieved institute status. The final map of the human genome is just the start of the institute's work. Ahead lies the task of identifying the function of each gene and the actual effects on health and disease.

When it created the HGP, the NCHGR realized that its mission could not be limited to just facilitating laboratory research. Awareness of the profound social implications that would accompany genetic discoveries led it to establish a component program to investigate broader implications of genetic science for society. The Ethical, Legal and Social Implications (ELSI) Research Program was created within the HGP when it was founded in 1990 and was given a mission to fund research, workshops, and conferences in these areas.[81] Because of the size of the HGP, the program became the largest single federal funding source for bioethics research. It has focused particular attention on issues related to the privacy of genetic information, clinical uses of genetic technologies, the conduct of genetic research, and professional education about genetic research findings. Concerns raised by ELSI investigations over the possibility of discrimination against people based on their genetic profiles led to the issuance of a presidential executive order in 2000 protecting federal workers from such discrimination and to passage of legislation to the same effect in most states.[82]

ELSI is not a regulatory body. Its funding and educational programs seek to focus policy debates. However, ELSI's efforts are influencing the formation of new regulatory structures that will oversee the transformation of the health care landscape that genetics is bringing about.

Health Care Research beyond the Major Agencies

In addition to the major federal players that fund and regulate medical research, NIH, AHRQ, NSF, and FDA, several other federal agencies are involved to a lesser extent. These smaller programs diversify the reach of the government's role. The programs of two agencies are of particular significance. The Veterans Administration (VA), a cabinet-level department, supports studies into issues of importance to the health care needs of veterans. The Health Resources and Services Administration (HRSA), a component of DHHS, investigates health manpower needs.

Veterans Administration (VA)

Although it is a relatively small player, the VA is responsible for a considerable amount of research across a range of health care fields. Its role has grown steadily over the past several decades, branching out from clinical trials of medications used in its facilities to include health services research. This growth has mirrored on a smaller scale the types of research initiatives pursued by larger federal funding agencies. Although the VA focuses on issues of importance to veterans, many of its studies produce findings that are generalizable to health care in the broader population.

The VA was created in 1930 to coordinate medical and other services for veterans. In 1989, it was elevated in status to become a cabinet-level department. Of the services that it coordinates, the provision of health care is the most prominent. The VA's original network of 54 hospitals has grown to 157 medical centers, more than 800 outpatient clinics, and 130 nursing home units. While supporting research has never been the VA's primary objective, it has increasingly focused on investigations into ways of improving its services and promoting the overall health of its constituency.[83] (The VA's role in providing health care services is described in more detail in chapter 3.)

Most of the VA's research is conducted within the agency rather than through extramural support. It sponsored significant medical research as early as the 1940s, when 10,000 veterans with tuberculosis were enrolled in trials of new medications. Clinical trials have been a major focus of the Cooperative Studies Program, which coordinates research across the VA's many medical centers. As many as sixty such studies are ongoing at any one time. The Health Services Research and Development Service funds intramural investigations of patient outcomes, quality of care, access to care, delivery models, and new research methods and development tools. Its mission of studying health care services for veterans parallels that of AHRQ for the general population. The Rehabilitation Research and Development Service conducts an intramural program to study rehabilitation and to develop and disseminate technology for disabled veterans. The Medical Research Service sponsors most of the VA's extramural research, which primarily includes studies of diseases and conditions that affect veterans. It also conducts intramural projects.[84]

Health Resources and Services Administration (HRSA)

HRSA administers a collection of programs aimed at increasing access to health care and reducing health disparities. Its areas of focus include primary health care, maternal and child health, health professions and manpower needs, and rural health policy. It also administers the Ryan White CARE Act, which provides HIV/AIDS services for low-income patients; the federal Vaccine Injury Compensation Program, which pays no-fault compensation to children suffering adverse reactions from immunizations; federal support for the United Network for Organ Sharing (UNOS), which facilitates organ donations for transplants; and the National Practitioner Data Bank (NPDB), which compiles information on disciplinary and malpractice actions against physicians.[85] (HRSA's role in managing the national health care workforce is discussed in chapter 2.)

Research is only one of several activities that HRSA supports, along with training of health professionals and public outreach. Nevertheless, the agency has a fairly active research program in each of its areas of focus. It also publishes large amounts of data and statistics. Of particular importance to policy makers, HRSA's statistical reports include identification of designated Health Professional Shortage Areas, which are eligible for enhanced support under some federal funding programs, maintenance of a drug pricing database, creation of state health workforce profiles, and updated data on the operations of the Vaccine Injury Compensation Program and UNOS.[86]

Other Agencies with Research Programs

Several other federal and state agencies also fund research related to health and medicine but at lower levels than the agencies discussed earlier. Despite their size, however, these smaller programs can play important roles in specific fields of investigation. Among those of most prominence, the Centers for Medicare & Medicaid Services (CMS), which administers Medicare and the federal portion of Medicaid, conducts some internal research and funds extramural investigators on issues related to those programs.[87] (Medicare and Medicaid are discussed in more detail in chapter 4.) CMS's research budgets vary considerably from year to year, as does the focus of its interests. Generally, the agency is interested in questions related to the methods through which it reimburses providers for rendering services.

The National Center for Health Statistics (NCHS), a component of the Centers for Disease Control and Prevention (CDC), is the government's principle health statistics agency.[88] It compiles large amounts of statistical information on which it conducts analyses. The center performs its own research rather than funding extramural investigators. Its data are collected from a range of sources, including birth and death records, medical records, interview surveys, physical examinations, and laboratory testing. The information and analyses are particularly important in supporting CDC's health surveillance activities. They are also used by government policy makers and made available to the public.

The Department of Agriculture (USDA) conducts research and analyses on issues related to nutrition and food safety through several of its component agencies.[89] The Economic Research Service conducts economic analyses of regulatory issues, including estimates of the cost of foodborne illness, cost-benefit analyses of food safety programs, and risk-benefit analyses of the use of pesticides. The service also funds some external research on nutritional needs and on the effectiveness of USDA nutritional programs, such as food assistance and mandatory labeling. Among other research components of USDA, the Center for Nutrition Policy and Promotion publishes nutritional information and recommendations, including the Food Guide Pyramid, which graphically displays recommended daily intakes of different food groups.[90] The National Research Initiative Competitive Grants Program, which is part of the Cooperative State Research, Education, and Extension Service, funds external research on issues related to agriculture, food, and the environment.

Agency Structure

National Institutes of Health (NIH)

NIH's mission of supporting extramural studies and conducting intramural research is carried out through the agency's twenty-seven institutes and centers, each of which functions with a substantial amount of autonomy.[91] The institutes are described in table 8.3. Sitting atop the vast enterprise is the Office of the Director, which has several key supervisory responsibilities. It compiles the overall agency budget each year, and it contains the office that oversees human subjects safety. In administering the largest single scientific research budget in the world and regulating the conduct of a sizable portion of the world's biomedical research, the NIH director wields unparalleled influence in American health care.

The NIH Funding Process

The bulk of NIH's budget, more than 80 percent, is devoted to the support of extramural research.[92] With a total budget of about $25 billion a year, this gives the agency a huge amount of influence over the nation's medical research agenda. Some funding is earmarked by Congress for specific research areas, but the allocation of much of it is at the agency's discretion.

The guiding principle behind NIH's stewardship of its huge extramural research budget is that scientific proposals are best evaluated by those who are most expert in the field to be studied. These are the professional peers of the investigator. A system of peer review to evaluate the scientific merits of research proposals is mandated by law and underlies virtually all NIH funding decisions. It is intended to evaluate each proposal on its own merits, rather than on personal characteristics of the investigator. Personal biases of reviewers can still intrude, but for the most part scientists consider the NIH peer review process to be rational and impartial.

A large number of research proposals go through the NIH review process each year. In 1999, the agency received more than 26,000 applications for research funding, of which it approved about 32 percent. More than 50,000 principle investigators from every state and from several foreign countries conduct funded projects that are ongoing at any one time. NIH-sponsored studies explore every medical specialty and are conducted at every major American university and medical school. To support its work, the agency has almost 18,000 employees of whom more than 4,000 hold doctorates or other professional research degrees. As a measure of the

Table 8.3
NIH Component Institutes and Centers

Institute	Focus of Mission
National Cancer Institute	Cancer and the care of cancer patients and their families
National Eye Institute	Eye and visual system disorders
National Health, Lung, and Blood Institute	Diseases of the heart, blood vessels, lungs, and blood; also administers the Women's Health Initiative
National Human Genome Research Institute	Funding for Human Genome Project; also develops technologies to treat inherited diseases
National Institute on Aging	Aging processes and diseases and the special problems and needs of the aged
National Institute on Alcohol Abuse and Alcoholism	Alcohol-related problems
National Institute of Allergy and Infectious Diseases	Allergic, immunologic, and infectious diseases
National Institute of Arthritis and Musculoskeletal and Skin Diseases	Chronic diseases, including arthritis, musculoskeletal, and skin disorders
National Institute of Biomedical Imaging and Bioengineering	Promotes new technological capabilities and coordinates biomedical imaging and bioengineering programs in NIH
National Institute of Child Health and Human Development	Reproductive, neurobiological, developmental, and behavioral processes
National Institute on Deafness and Other Communication Disorders	Hearing and communications processes
National Institute of Dental and Craniofacial Research	Craniofacial, oral, and dental health
National Institute of Diabetes and Digestive and Kidney Diseases	Diseases of internal medicine and related subspecialty fields
National Institute on Drug Abuse	Drug abuse and addictions
National Institute of Environmental Health Sciences	Human illness and dysfunction from environmental exposures
National Institute of General Medical Sciences	Research and research training not targeted to specific diseases
National Institute of Mental Health	Disorders of mind, brain, and behavior
National Institute of Neurological Disorders and Stroke	Neurological diseases and stroke
National Institute of Nursing Research	Establish a scientific basis for the care of individuals across the life span
National Library of Medicine	Collection, organization, and provision of biomedical information
John E. Fogarty International Center for Advanced Study in the Health Sciences	Reduce disparities in global health
National Center for Complementary and Alternative Medicine	Complementary and alternative medicine
National Center on Minority Health and Health Disparities	Reduce and eliminate health disparities
National Center for Research Resources	General support for researchers across institutes

Source: http://www.nih.gov/icd/ (25 May 2006).

success of this effort, the agency boasts of 104 scientists who have won Nobel prizes for NIH-supported research.[93]

NIH grants support research projects and career development of new investigators. Major research grants are divided into two main categories. R01 grants provide support of several hundred thousand dollars, although some are as large as several million. The studies that are funded last up to five years, and the grants are renewable. R03 grants provide funding in the range of tens of thousands of dollars for up to two years and are not renewable.[94]

The review process for grant proposals begins with evaluation of scientific merit by a panel of sixteen to twenty experts, primarily from outside of the government, known as a scientific research group (SRG) or study section. This step is managed by the agency's Center for Scientific Review, or in some cases by the individual institutes. Based on preliminary reviews, about half of the proposals submitted are chosen for full discussion by the group, which assigns a priority score based on scientific merit. Next, National Advisory Boards (sometimes known as National Advisory Councils) composed of twelve to eighteen scientists and members of the public review projects to assess their value to the institute involved. At this stage, the availability of funds is weighed as a consideration and the appropriateness of the SRG's prior review can be reconsidered.[95]

While considerably smaller, NIH's intramural research effort nevertheless represents an important part of the agency's overall mission. With about 10 percent of an annual $25 billion budget at its disposal, it is a significant enterprise. NIH-employed scientists pursue their research interests, often as part of collaborations across institutes, using NIH's laboratories and other resources. They can study patients at the Warren Grant Magnuson Clinical Center, the hospital that serves inpatients and outpatients on the agency's campus in Bethesda, Maryland, perform experiments in the campus's extensive laboratory facilities, and use the National Library of Medicine. NIH also maintains research facilities across the United States and abroad. Five Nobel prizes have resulted from this work.[96]

Proposals for intramural projects are reviewed by boards of scientific counselors, which are comprised of scientists from outside of the government. These bodies also evaluate research in progress and the performance of the agency's staff scientists. In addition, they provide general oversight for each institute's overall intramural program.[97]

Agency for Healthcare Research and Quality (AHRQ)

AHRQ is structured in a similar manner to NIH, with the Office of the Director overseeing centers, the equivalent of small institutes, which grant extramural funding in specific research areas. The centers are described in table 8.4. As of 2005, there were eight of them focusing on different aspects of the improvement of health care in practice.

Table 8.4
AHRQ Component Centers

Center	Focus of Mission
Center for Cost and Financing Studies	Cost and financing of health care and data to support policy, research, and analysis
Center for Organization and Delivery Studies	Health care markets, delivery systems, and organizations
Center for Outcomes and Effectiveness Research	Outcomes and effectiveness of diagnostic, therapeutic, and preventive health care services and procedures
Center for Primary Care Research	Primary care, and clinical, preventive, and public health policies and systems
Center for Practice and Technology Assessment	Narrow the gap between research and practice
Center for Quality Improvement and Patient Safety	Measurement and improvement of the quality of health care and enhancement of patient safety

Source: http://www.ahrq.gov/about/organix.htm (25 May 2006).

National Science Foundation (NSF)

NSF receives overall direction from a twenty-four-member National Science Board composed of prominent scientists and engineers. The board, the agency's director, and its deputy director are all appointed by the president subject to Senate confirmation. There are also eight assistant directors. The size and political visibility of this governance arrangement suggest the prominence that Congress originally attached to the agency.[98]

Funding of NSF research is divided into eleven program areas.[99] They are described in table 8.5. Their range reflects the agency's broad mission. The breadth of programs creates unique opportunities for projects to cross disciplinary boundaries between medicine and other areas of science, including not only natural sciences but also social and behavioral fields. NSF is better positioned than the NIH, therefore, to promote interdisciplinary research in its most expansive sense.

Food and Drug Administration (FDA)

The FDA oversees the conduct of clinical trials through the Bioresearch Monitoring Program, which was established in 1977. Its mission is "to ensure the quality and integrity of data submitted to FDA for regulatory decisions, as well as to protect human subjects of research."[100] It has authority to oversee clinical investigators, research sponsors, animal laboratories, and the IRBs that review human subjects protection. The program's reach extends to research supporting all products that the FDA regulates, which in addition to drugs to treat human diseases

Table 8.5
NSF Program Areas

Biology
Computer and Information Sciences
Crosscutting Programs
Education
Engineering
Geosciences
International
Math, Physical Sciences
Polar Research
Science Statistics
Social, Behavioral Sciences

Source: http://www.nsf.gov/funding/
aboutfunding.jsp (7 August 2006)

include biologic products, medical devices, radiological products, foods, and veterinary drugs.

The focus of the program's efforts is on inspections of research sites that conduct studies that form the basis for FDA product evaluations. A special kind of inspection called a "bioequivalence study inspection" is conducted when a single study supplies all the data for a product approval. In conducting inspections, FDA investigators examine the research process that is followed and look at original records and data. To review the process, they consider the roles played by different personnel, the amount of authority that was delegated, the ways in which data were recorded, and the ways in which study sponsors monitored the behavior of the clinical researchers who administered the experimental product to subjects. Reviewers also compare the data submitted to the agency with records maintained at clinical sites where the drug or product was actually studied. These sites can include physicians' offices, hospitals, and laboratories. FDA investigators may also examine patient records predating the study to determine whether the patients who participated were properly diagnosed, and they may examine records of treatment after the study was concluded to check for appropriate follow-up and late-appearing side effects.[101]

In addition to reviewing the sponsors of multisite clinical trials, the FDA can also inspect the records of individual investigators. Numerous red flags can bring a researcher to the agency's attention. These include direct signs of trouble reported by research sponsors or subjects and indirect indicia such as research that is conducted outside of a clinician's specialty area, results that are inconsistent with those of other investigators, inclusion of more subjects than would be expected based on the prevalence of the disease being studied, and suspicious laboratory results. When the FDA finds that an investigator has submitted false data, he or she can be disqualified from conducting further research that is eligible to be used to support new drug or product approval applications.[102]

Veterans Administration (VA)

Medical research at the VA is coordinated by the Office of Research and Development. There are several component services, the most significant of which are described in table 8.6: the Cooperative Health Studies Program, the Health Services Research and Development Service, the Clinical Science Research and Development Service, and the Rehabilitation Research and Development Service. The health care topics investigated by these components are extremely broad in scope within the common theme of addressing the concerns of veterans.[103]

Health Resources and Services Administration (HRSA)

HRSA is led by an administrator, and it operates through four bureaus covering each of its key focus areas. There are also several offices that report directly to the administrator, including two that administer programs in minority health and in rural health policy, and an office that administers the Vaccine Injury Compensation Program, UNOS, hospital construction funding, and other special programs. Each bureau and office administers its own research. Much of HRSA's internal research consists of analyses of data derived from administering operational programs related to improving health care access. In addition, data are made available publicly for use by investigators outside of government. Grants are also provided, although on a fairly small scale, to private researchers for studies in areas related to each bureau's and office's mission.[104]

HRSA's bureaus and key programmatic offices along with their missions are summarized in table 8.7. HRSA is a relatively small agency. Its annual budget is about $6 billion, but most of it is spent on grants for health professional training, facilities construction, and provision of health care services, rather than on research. The agency has about 1,300 employees in its Rockville, Maryland, headquarters and about 750 in field offices throughout the country.[105]

Table 8.6
Veterans Administration Research Agencies

Agency	Focus of Mission
Cooperative Studies Program	Effectiveness of new or unproven therapies
Health Services Research and Development Service	Organization, financing, and management of health care
Clinical Science Research and Development Service	Fundamental biological processes
Rehabilitation Research and Development Service	Maximize independence, minimize disability, and restore restore function

Source: http://www.research.va.gov/programs/default.cfm (7 August 2006).

Table 8.7
Health Resources and Services Administration Bureaus and Key
Programmatic Offices

Bureau/Office	Key Elements of Mission
Bureau of Primary Health Care	Support community health centers and other community-based programs
Bureau of Health Professions	Promote and fund training programs to increase diversity and improve the distribution of the health care workforce; also operates the National Practitioner Data Bank
Maternal and Child Health Bureau	Provide health services, training, and research for women, children, and children with special health care needs
HIV/AIDS Bureau	Administer Ryan White CARE Act programs, mostly involving ambulatory care, for low-income patients
Office of Minority Health	Develop strategies for addressing minority health issues and provide oversight and coordination within HRSA for minority health initiatives; also advise on data collection needs for monitoring minority health programs
Office of Rural Health Policy	Provide advice on rural hospitals and health care, coordinate agency activities relating to rural health, and maintain a national information clearinghouse
Office of Special Programs	Operate and support the Vaccine Injury Compensation Program and the United Network for Organ Sharing; also administer construction assistance to hospitals and state health planning grants

Source: http://www.hrsa.gov/about/orgchart.htm (25 May 2006).

Perennial Policy Issues

For most Americans, biomedical research is a precious resource. The pace of its progress in producing tools to relieve suffering and death has accelerated over the decades, and the dawning era of genetic technology promises an even faster rate of growth in the future. Budgets of government agencies, private foundations, and pharmaceutical companies for funding research have soared as an investment that seems to pay dividends many times over.

However, it is inevitable that controversy would accompany such high levels of government funding for a single enterprise. Any expenditure of public funds in one area, no matter how meritorious, reflects a decision not to spend them somewhere else, so political ramifications are unavoidable. Some policy issues surrounding biomedical research date back to the dawn of public funding, whereas others have arisen more recently.

Basic versus Applied Research

The debate over how to balance basic and applied research is almost as old as research itself. Basic research investigates underlying scientific principles. Such studies in a biomedical context might examine the mechanisms of cellular function, the biochemical structure of chromosomes, or the processes of biological metabolism. The results expand our understanding of fundamental biological processes that may or may not lead to practical applications. However, even when applications exist, they may not be realized for several decades. Many of the questions that basic biomedical researchers ask help to build theories that have no immediate impact on the lives of patients.

Applied research creates tools that are used in clinical practice. It is the effort that develops new drugs, devices, technologies, and procedures. This is work on the front lines of medicine, where the weapons to combat disease are created. However, scientists can only develop new medical applications based on the theoretical foundation that basic research has provided.

In an ideal world, there would be large amounts of each kind of research. Clearly, both are needed. The practical applications of today are possible only because of the basic research conducted decades ago. It took more than twenty years from the discovery of the DNA molecule to produce the first bacteria containing a recombinant genetic code. On the other hand, basic research by itself does not cure patients. Applied research is needed to fulfill its promise.

In practice, there are large amounts of each kind of research, but not without continual tension between them. NIH spends a large portion of its budget on basic research and is the primary funding source in America for scientists who look at underlying life processes. However, this long-term investment can require tremendous patience. The rewards will take years to reach fruition, if they ever do. Therefore, money is spent with little clear payback when more immediate practical needs abound. How does a member of Congress justify large budgets for theoretical research, when constituents are clamoring for advances in treating scourges like AIDS, breast cancer, and heart disease that will more immediately save lives?

As large as it is, however, NIH is only one component in a network of organizations that finance biomedical research.[106] Private industry has grown to become a major player, with the pharmaceutical industry alone now spending more each year than NIH. Private foundations, while spending much less in the aggregate, also represent an important part of the mix by funding research into specific diseases and into focused areas of concern that otherwise elude government and industry attention. Each of these sectors has its own place in supporting research along the spectrum from basic to applied.[107]

Nevertheless, the government is left as the only source that can fund basic biomedical research on a large scale. Private industry must respond to the demands of investors and the marketplace for more immediate financial returns, and the resources of foundations tend to be more limited. Over the years, NIH funding has led to such key basic discoveries as how neurotransmitters facilitate communication between neurons, how proteins create the building blocks of life processes, and how the sequence of bases in a DNA molecule form the blueprint for life.[108] Today, the practical applications of these discoveries permeate almost every aspect of medicine. NIH also funds an extensive amount of practical research, but it is the magnitude of support for advancing basic biomedical science that is truly unique.

Politics and Science: Allocating the NIH Budget

The task of allocating research funding within the NIH to produce the greatest overall health benefits is a seemingly impossible one. There is no way to know in advance what new knowledge will be produced and what diseases that knowledge will help to cure. There also is no way to know what new disease challenges lie ahead. In the mid-1990s, few people had heard of West Nile virus, and most thought of anthrax as a threat primarily to livestock. It is also often unclear where research into a specific disease should reside bureaucratically within the agency, since many conditions cut across disciplinary boundaries.

With large amounts of money at stake, the process of setting priorities for funding takes on tremendous importance. Who should be entrusted to allocate research dollars in a democratic society? Clearly, scientists know best which avenues of study make the most technical sense, but they face conflicts in decision making. At the most basic level, they have natural biases toward support for their own areas of interest. Moreover, democratic principles demand public accountability for government spending decisions that have such significant policy implications.

With public accountability, however, comes politics. Democratic oversight of science is accomplished through our elected officials, who must respond to constituents and to interest groups. Congressional debates bring to bear an array of interests and opinions, both informed and uninformed. Who knows best what to fund—those who will conduct the research or those who believe they will most directly benefit from it?

Politics aside, are there general principles for determining the fairest way to allocate research dollars? Some in Congress support a principle of spending the public's money where the burdens and costs of disease are greatest.[109] This is where funding can do the greatest immediate good. However, where does this leave those unfortunate enough to suffer from rare diseases? Should research funding seek the greatest good for the greatest number or protection of the most vulnerable? This debate, which is at the core of competing notions of a just society, promises to play itself out continually.

Overall Lessons for Public Policy

The dramatic growth of federal funding over the past several decades has been driven largely by the accomplishments that biomedical research has achieved. There are few government programs as visibly successful and few public causes as consistently popular. As interest groups representing patients and others have come to realize the significant contribution that medical research can make, the pressure for higher levels of funding has only accelerated. For the most part, this pressure has not forced Congress to make trade-offs in funding so much as it has led to a larger overall pot of money for everyone. Regulation has followed funding, but with fewer constraints than in many other aspects of health care. Private scientists in America still mostly determine what will be studied with public funds and how.

Will the honeymoon for medical research funding continue as a permanent state? Controversy may lie ahead on several fronts. In addition to areas such as stem cell research and clinical practice guidelines, the era of genetic medicine promises particularly difficult challenges. Highly emotional issues arise as scientists manipulate the blueprint of life, and bioethicists are only beginning to understand them.[110] Should constraints be placed on research that helps parents to select characteristics of their children? Should clinicians be allowed to investigate ways to alter genes that will be passed on from generation to generation?

Nothing determines the shape of an enterprise as effectively as control over its funding. Government funding agencies, therefore, will likely face growing visibility and scrutiny regarding the consequences of their decisions. The missions of supporting, regulating, and evaluating medical research promise to become increasingly entangled and to raise increasingly complex policy issues.

9

New Regulatory Horizons
and Old Policy Conflicts

The history of medicine has been written as an epic of progress, but it
is also a tale of social and economic conflict over the emergence of
new hierarchies of power and authority, new markets, and new
conditions of belief and experience.
—P. Starr, *The Social Transformation of American Medicine*

Health care's importance to the American economy continues to grow steadily.[1]
After decades of consistent increases, it now consumes more than 15 percent of
the gross domestic product and has become the country's largest industry.[2] It is
also the fastest-growing element of government spending. The Medicare budget
exceeds $290 billion annually, and the combined state and federal budget for
Medicaid exceeds $300 billion.[3] As the large cohort born during the baby boom
years of 1946 to 1962 reaches the age of Medicare eligibility, the rate of spending
growth will likely accelerate even faster.

Beyond its financial significance, health care has worked its way into an ever
more central place in the fabric of our society. Americans direct a tremendous
amount of their attention to health and wellness, perhaps more so than at any time
in the past. It would be difficult to pick up any issue of a daily newspaper or to
watch a news program on television without noticing at least one major health-
related story. A large amount of the advertising that Americans see—in print,
broadcast, billboards, and Internet settings—relates to health care products and
services. Health care is a major source of employment and the focus of much of
our educational structure. Whether due to the expanding array of effective treatments or the growing number of elderly citizens who need care, health and wellness
have come to command a prominent place in our national consciousness.

The Challenges Ahead

After a hundred years of regulation, our health care system has made tremendous strides in addressing the three basic policy imperatives, discussed in chapter 1—improving quality, fostering widespread access, and controlling costs. However, the challenges seem to be even greater today than when the regulatory programs that emerged to address these areas of concern were first enacted. In a recent report, the World Health Organization ranked the United States at no better than number 37 among the health systems of 191 nations.[4] This assessment resulted in large part from a comparison of medical outcomes, including infant mortality and life expectancy, on which the United States fared worse than many other industrialized countries. Yet, the United States spends substantially more on health care than any other country, as measured both in the aggregate and on a per capita basis.[5] Widespread medical errors and documented disparities in practice patterns between geographic regions also attest to significant gaps in the quality of care actually rendered. They also highlight the distance between the standard of quality that is possible and the one that many Americans receive.[6]

A perennial level of 15 percent of the population that lacks insurance reflects how far the promise of widespread access still has to go before it is fulfilled.[7] Most of the uninsured still receive care, mostly in hospital emergency rooms and public clinics, but continuity is lacking, and access to specialty services is extremely limited. Despite numerous programs enacted over the past several decades to encourage wider coverage, the number of uninsured has grown relentlessly.

Health care costs have also climbed steadily at rates consistently above those of overall inflation.[8] Employee health benefits represent a source of significant financial stress for many businesses. National spending on health care even threatens to create a drag on the overall economic productivity.

However, the failure of policy makers to tame the challenges of improving quality, enhancing access, and controlling costs does not mean that the effort has been in vain. Quite to the contrary, health care regulation has in many ways nurtured the system as it has grown ever more effective at improving and saving lives.[9] If American health care did not deliver tremendous value, concerns over access and cost would be irrelevant. The challenges of today are actually reflections of the successes of the past.[10] There is cause for optimism in the accumulated wisdom of more than a hundred years' experience with different forms of regulatory oversight, which guide health care as it continues to evolve.

Looking ahead, the scientific underpinnings of medicine may be on the verge of significant change that could dramatically improve care. Breakthroughs are about to alter the clinical landscape in important ways, and new regulatory responses will be needed. The next phase of health care regulation will have to confront this challenge and will likely do so according to the same patterns, values, and constraints as in the past.

New Clinical Terrain

Three trends are transforming medicine and will exert an increasing influence in the decades ahead. The most significant is a growing reliance on information technology. Health care, like most other industries, is becoming an information-based enterprise, and all aspects of its operations from finance to management to clinical care are affected. Claims for reimbursement are routinely submitted to payers in bulk as data files. Medical records are commonly maintained on computers. Physician and hospital performance measures are aggregated, tracked, and analyzed by payers. Patients easily gain expertise on their conditions and on treatment options through the Internet. The combined effect is reshaping patient care. Managing information is becoming as essential to treatment as actual patient contact.

The consequences of the information revolution are already widely felt in opportunities to improve the quality of care.[11] For example, teams of providers can access computerized records of treatments by different clinicians to facilitate more effective coordination. Lack of communication between providers has historically presented one of the greatest impediments to high-quality care. Many patients see multiple physicians who are often unaware of each other's recommendations. A patient's primary care physician, for example, may prescribe a drug with no knowledge that specialists have prescribed others with which it may interact. Paper medical records that fail to travel with the patient cannot alert a physician to past symptoms and treatments. If the patient is away from home, moreover, access to a medical history may be impossible in an emergency.

Many health systems now maintain all medical records in electronic form so that providers can have instant access to complete information on patients seen by colleagues. Private systems now exist to maintain medical records on secure Internet sites for access by any provider whom the patient may see in an emergency, anywhere in the world. Diagnostic data are transmitted by e-mail, enabling physicians to consult across large geographic distances.

Another important contribution of information technology is in standardizing treatment. Large variability in medical practices has been blamed for inconsistent quality across the country.[12] In response, professional organizations and academic researchers have developed guidelines to direct practitioners in treating specific conditions. These protocols recommend best practice standards that are derived from the opinions of experts in the medical specialties involved. Information technology permits their ready dissemination to physicians around the world. Protocols can even be integrated into electronic patient charts to guide clinicians as they weigh treatment options.

The behavior of physicians in adhering to protocols also lends a tool for judging their performance. Electronic records can reveal the extent to which recommended best practices are followed. What is more, data on actual outcomes of care can be measured based on information contained in computerized patient records for a more fundamental assessment of the quality of care provided. The results can form the basis for creating "report cards" on providers that afford patients the ability to choose among them based on quantitative performance measures.[13]

Information technology also permits patients to become more active partners in their own care through Internet research. Without ever visiting a medical library, they can review vast stores of medical information on conditions and treatment options. In some cases, effective use of the Internet may even give patients expertise surpassing that of their physicians. As a result, the horizons of physician knowledge can grow based on the collaboration of their own patients.

The second trend that is transforming medicine is the advance of genetic technologies. Since the Human Genome Project succeeded in decoding the human genetic map in 2002, a range of therapeutic uses have begun to emerge. (The Human Genome project is discussed in more detail in chapter 8 on the funding and regulation of medical research.) Most have involved diagnostic applications based on genetic markers that enable clinicians to predict patient responsiveness to drugs and other treatments.[14] On the horizon lies the possibility of actual gene therapy in which metabolic deficiencies can be corrected.

In the near future, for example, pharmaceutical firms may be able to design drugs for individual patients that will maximize effectiveness and avoid side effects.[15] Physicians may be able to predict physiological susceptibilities to environmental stresses, enabling them to differentiate between patients who face near certain harm from behaviors such as smoking and those who are genetically disposed to avoid ill effects.[16] Eventually, clinicians may be able to replace disease-causing genes in a patient's cells to eliminate deleterious genetic conditions altogether.

The final trend is demographic, and it will present a different kind of challenge. The large cohort of Americans born during the baby boom years will begin to enter old age in the coming decades, with a consequent rise in demand for health care services. In particular, a dramatic increase is likely in the need for services to treat chronic conditions that are characteristic of aging, such as heart disease, hypertension, and diabetes. These diseases require different, and often more expensive, treatment paradigms over extended periods of time than acute illnesses require. The elderly are also heavier users of long-term care. The resource pressures on the health care system that result from this spike in demand will be tremendous.

Health care will also continue to grow in its range of applications. Researchers regularly report finding new treatments for previously intractable diseases. New and powerful pharmaceutical products and devices continue to proliferate. A range of conditions that were once considered deficiencies in lifestyle can now be treated medically. Demand is expanding for these new health care services by all age-groups, further exacerbating pressures on the system.[17]

The challenge for regulators will be to protect the public interest in balancing quality, access, and costs in the face of these new trends. Information-based medicine can tremendously enhance the quality of care, if data are collected accurately and patients have confidence that information will not be misused. Genomic medicine will offer powerful new diagnostic and therapeutic tools, but they will be extremely expensive, and their promise will not be realized without an adequate source of funding. The anticipated increase in demand from the growing elderly population will likely dwarf the access challenges of today. Health care regulation is about to enter new terrain.

New Regulatory Responses

On the immediate horizon lie a new set of regulatory responses. The Health Insurance Portability and Accountability Act (HIPAA), passed in 1996, was the first federal enactment directly regulating health care information technology.[18] It authorized the Department of Health and Human Services (DHHS) to develop standards for transmitting electronic claims and to devise regulations to protect the privacy of patient information stored in electronic form. (HIPAA is discussed in more detail in chapter 7 on health care business relationships.) In 2004, the agency established the Office of National Technology Coordinator for Health Information Technology to promote widespread national use of this new tool.[19] With these steps, a new era of information regulation has arrived.

The initial concern of policy makers in regulating health care information has been largely over threats to patient privacy. In addition to HIPAA, several states have enacted laws to protect the confidentiality of genetic information or to limit its use in insurance underwriting and employment decisions.[20] Other state laws guarantee patients the right of access to their medical records and in some instances the right to insist on correction of errors. However, these safeguards will almost certainly bring higher costs for using information technology that will likely force difficult trade-offs down the road.[21]

Other recent regulatory initiatives seek to harness the power of information technology to promote policy goals.[22] Outcomes data can represent a potent weapon for encouraging better quality. In 2002, the state of Pennsylvania created a new Patient Safety Authority to collect and analyze reports of errors that the state's hospitals are required to file.[23] The intent of the law is to use the reports to understand systemic failings in order to promote structural improvement rather than to assess blame as a court would in a lawsuit. On the private side, a number of initiatives use data on provider performance to create publicly available comparisons based on standardized measures, which are included in provider report cards.[24] In 1998, a group of thirty-four large corporate employers, including General Motors, General Electric, and Verizon, created an association known as the Leapfrog Group to exert pressure on hospitals, physicians, and managed care organizations to reduce errors and improve quality.[25] To this end, the initiative encourages better use of information technology, data reporting, and data analysis. (Uses of information manipulation as a regulatory tool are also discussed in chapter 3 on the regulation of health care institutions.)

Other private and governmental efforts seek to reimburse providers at higher rates if they achieve higher scores on outcome measures, a practice known as "pay for performance."[26] The Centers for Medicare & Medicaid Services (CMS), the agency within DHHS that administers the Medicare and Medicaid programs, is experimenting with such a mechanism. That agency also publicly reports the performance of hundreds of hospitals on a range of measures on its Web site in an effort to inform consumer decision-making.[27]

Information can also be used as a regulatory tool to control costs. Under an approach known as "consumer-driven" health care, patients are encouraged to make purchasing decisions in a market-oriented environment in which they are not buffered from the financial consequences of their treatments by insurance.[28] The premise for this approach is that individual patient choice operating through market forces can do a better job of controlling prices and maintaining quality than group purchasing of health care services by large insurance companies and managed care organizations. To this end, consumer-driven plans permit patients to accumulate money in tax-preferred "health savings accounts" from which they can pay physicians and hospitals for routine care directly. Major expenses are still covered by insurance but only after a large annual deductible had been met and the expenses have reached a "catastrophic" level. Funds in the accounts may be contributed directly by the patient or by an employer. The portion of the account that is not spent on health care during one year is available for use in the future. Ideally, this system would encourage patients to base purchasing decisions on relative prices and on objective data-driven quality indicators. In 1997 and again in 2003, Congress authorized creation of these kinds of accounts.[29] This approach is still experimental, and it remains controversial. However, debates over its use reflect growing acknowledgment of the notion that information technology can be used as a health care cost control technique.

Despite the increasing level of information-related regulatory activity, policy makers have so far been remarkably silent in confronting what may present the greatest challenge of all. The Internet is fundamentally transforming health care in many ways; however, few regulatory or legal programs oversee this vast new frontier. Medical Web sites, for example, operate with little external monitoring of the accuracy of their content. Internet-based pharmacies that regularly fill orders for drugs without actual prescriptions have largely escaped oversight by the Food and Drug Administration (FDA) and state pharmacy boards, which lack clear regulatory authority to control them. Many Web sites widely advertise medical services of unproven safety.

Opportunities for abuses clearly abound. Federal, state, and private regulators will likely vie among each other until an effective oversight mechanism emerges.

Beyond these new initiatives, health care regulators will, of course, continue to concern themselves with the implementation of more traditional programs. Licensure of physicians, review and monitoring of drugs and devices, research funding, and oversight of private insurance, among other existing programs, will remain vital to protecting the public interest in health care for the foreseeable future. As developing trends in technology and demographics accelerate, however, the conduct of regulation will have to evolve along with them. The industry's pending transformation based on improved computer tools, clinical advances in genetics, and cost pressures resulting from rising demand will leave no choice.

How will the regulatory system of the next few decades take shape? The best guide to the future is to understand the past. The history of American health care regulation over the past hundred years teaches that responses to new challenges evolve through the competitive interplay of different forces in both the public and the private sector. It reflects the perennial policy conflicts between government oversight and private markets, between public and private regulators, and between different levels of government. These policy conflicts will take different forms in different contexts, but their influence will remain as they guide the continuing evolution of a system that will almost certainly remain as intricate as ever.

The Underlying Choreography of Public and Private Interests

Looking back over a century of health care regulation, two conflicting schools of thought have influenced public policy concerning what regulation should look like. One says that less regulation is always better. We should consolidate programs, pare them down, eliminate redundancy, and relegate as much authority as possible to private organizations and the market. The other assumes that government supervision is essential to protect the health and safety of America's citizens and that regulation of health care should be better coordinated and expanded to eliminate gaps and ensure consistent oversight. Our regulatory system contains elements that reflect both points of view.

Perhaps this complex, hybrid regulatory structure has emerged because it fits America's temperament. It may, in fact, be the only kind with which the country would be truly comfortable. The decentralization and complexity of health care regulation are distinctively American in the interplay of layers of government, different agencies within each level, and private forces.[30] It is a system of checks and balances that prevents any single regulatory authority from becoming too influential and that encourages diversity in programs and approaches. There is almost a "marketplace" of regulation, with a competitive harness that disciplines government policy in a similar manner to the discipline of a private market for goods and services. The system is unquestionably less efficient than one that is more centralized, but perhaps the inefficiency has its advantages. It may even enhance overall regulatory effectiveness.

The paradigm of public-private interaction creates a framework for much of health care regulation in which the government sets basic parameters and the private sector fills in the blanks. In few areas is public oversight exclusive; however, in none is it a silent partner. Similarly, in few areas is private involvement absent, but in none does it operate unchecked.

Examples of this public-private relationship permeate the regulatory system. In the oversight of professionals and institutions, for instance, state governments perform the basic function of licensing, but a maze of nongovernmental oversight surrounds this step. (The regulation of professionals and institutions is discussed in chapters 2 and 3.) Private organizations accredit the medical schools whose graduates are eligible to be licensed, and they write the examinations on which competency for licensure is assessed. They certify physicians who seek recognition as specialists and accredit hospitals that wish acknowledgment of superior quality. The government's licensing role in this regulatory structure is more analogous to the glue that holds the process together than to the process itself. It is crucial but not comprehensive.

In financing health care, the American "system" intertwines public and private roles to such an extent that it is difficult to tease apart their effects. (The regulation of health care finance is discussed in chapter 4.) The most visible element in the financing system is private insurance that is regulated by the states and administered primarily through employment. However, a web of federal and state rules governs its provision. They have objectives as diverse as encouraging employers to self-insure, promoting the use of managed care as a coverage arrangement, mandating coverage continuation after employment has ended, limiting the underwriting practices used by insurers, and prescribing the formulas used to determine rates. Even more significantly, private insurance is provided within the context of a massive tax subsidy exceeding $150 billion a year that actually makes the government, rather than the private market, the single most significant financial driver of the private health insurance system.[31]

Moreover, care for more than a third of the population is financed or delivered directly through government programs. These encompass a broad assortment that includes Medicare, Medicaid, State Children's Health Insurance Programs, Veterans Administration hospitals, and public clinics. Even when these public arrangements take the lead, moreover, the arrangements still reflect more of a partnership between the governmental and private sectors than exclusive authority by either one. Claims processing and other details of Medicare implementation are administered by private insurance companies in each state that act as intermediaries and carriers.

Medicaid is provided to beneficiaries in most states by private HMOs. The Medicare prescription drug benefit is administered primarily through private prescription drug plans and HMOs. In all these programs, the government sets parameters to structure the system, and the private sector plays key roles in managing it.

In public health, which has historically been the poor stepchild of health care, the system is guided by an implicit collaboration of public and private elements. (The regulation of public health is discussed in chapter 6.) The magnitude of the government investment in maintaining the overall health of the population has historically been microscopic compared with the sums spent on financing individual care.[32] Those public health activities that the government directly implements tend to arise in response to crises and then fade into the background.[33] In some respects, however, the private sector has picked up some of the slack. Several of the most aggressive efforts at disease prevention have actually been carried out not through public programs but through private HMOs, which encourage regular checkups and immunizations.[34] Care for indigent patients who lack private insurance is more likely to be rendered at a private hospital emergency room than at a public clinic. Reduction in the prevalence of smoking, one of the most significant public health accomplishments of the last fifty years, has been greatly assisted by prohibitions on smoking in private office buildings, theaters, restaurants, and other facilities. Although not always acknowledged as such, private sector efforts have been essential to meeting many of the nation's public health goals.

Nevertheless, governmental public health programs remain essential to the functioning of the system overall. CDC has been the key player in identifying the cause of several significant communicable diseases, including AIDS and Legionnaire's disease, and its data-gathering and surveillance programs offer the most reliable snapshots of national health and disease trends. The information and reports that CDC disseminates represent an essential resource for many private practice physicians. State and local health departments similarly provide data and investigative tools that manage the forest of population health while individual clinicians and facilities work with the trees of individual care. As in other aspects of health care, the government is the indispensable backbone for the public health system, but its structure relies on significant private contributions.

Health care business relationships are inherently private activities, but the massive regulatory apparatus that oversees their integrity serves as yet another example of a governmental framework that guides private implementation. (The regulation of health care business relationships is discussed in chapter 7.) The interplay is perhaps most apparent in the oversight of tax-exempt hospitals by the Internal Revenue Service (IRS). The American system of granting favorable tax treatment to private organizations that provide essential public services is unusual. In most other countries, the government operates or directly funds most community services such as welfare organizations, museums, and hospitals. In the United States, on the other hand, it is primarily the private nonprofit sector that develops and manages these operations with support from an indirect government subsidy in the form of a tax exemption. Federal laws, as well as the laws of each state, permit charitable organizations to avoid paying most taxes, if they can prove that they truly serve the public interest. However, to qualify for this support, these entities must submit to extensive IRS oversight that includes continual government supervision of their organizational structure and ongoing operations. After determining that a community organization, such as a hospital, truly fulfills a charitable purpose, the IRS regulates every element of its ongoing activities for consistency with this mission.

This system for providing community services places a tremendous amount of operational discretion in the hands of nongovernmental organizations. Nonprofit hospitals function under the immediate oversight of boards composed of members of the community rather than of government officials. However, public guidance and supervision of business operations constantly lurk in the background through the watchful eyes of the IRS. In other words, the government sets the rules for administering this sector of health care while private entities actually carry out the mission.

The funding and regulation of research is perhaps the ultimate model for America's public-private regulatory interplay. (The regulation and funding of research are discussed in chapter 8.) The largest single funder of biomedical research in the world, the National Institutes of Health (NIH), implements most of its projects in partnership with scientists who work in universities and institutes outside of the government. These private investigators initiate proposals for studies that the agency evaluates for funding through its extramural programs. It is a system in which government funding and direction permit private research to flourish.

Through this financing process, budget allocations for the various component institutes within NIH effectively set the overall agenda for the areas of biomedical research that American investigators will explore. NIH officials and Congress work to develop a budget each year that forms a blueprint for much of America's scientific inquiry. Nongovernmental investigators then submit proposals for projects that fall within the parameters that the blueprint delineates. Proposals that are approved for funding determine the actual details of which specific questions will be explored and how. Over the past several decades, this collaboration of public direction and private implementation has engendered a tremendously effective and productive machinery for scientific discovery and innovation.

The Fabric of Our Regulatory System:
Complexity, Confrontation, and Compromise

With its choreography of public and private interests and its balance between different levels of government, America's system of health care regulation can certainly be characterized as complex. In its continual evolution, it thrives on confrontation between competing interests but survives on its ability to engender compromise. Intertwining regulatory structures can be overwhelming in their intricacy, but a more direct system would not necessarily be fairer or more effective.

Confrontation between competing interests fuels the process at many levels, even between different levels of government.[35] State and federal public health regulators, for example, have struggled for supremacy since the earliest days of government health programs in the nineteenth century.[36] They did so when the first quarantine and immunization efforts to control the spread of infectious diseases were developed, when the licensure programs that control access to the health care professions were established, and when the initial regulation of health insurance was implemented. They continue to do so in many spheres, including the oversight of clinical practice, the regulation of insurance under the Employee Retirement Income Security Act (ERISA), the shared administrative structure of the Medicaid program, and the emerging regulatory apparatus to handle public health preparedness.

At the same time, private interests confront both federal and state regulators on several stages. Professional organizations representing various kinds of providers, for instance, lobby for and against government actions that impose restrictions on clinical practice and that set reimbursement rates under payment programs. The American Medical Association (AMA) has interjected itself into debates over administration of Medicare's prospective payment system and into disputes over payment rates for different medical specialties. The pharmaceutical industry consistently seeks to be heard in controversies surrounding reform of FDA procedures and administration of publicly financed drug benefit programs. Managed care companies seek to influence state and federal regulation of health care finance.

Fortunately, the process also engenders compromise. With few exceptions, individual constituents rarely achieve everything that they want, but they usually learn to live with what they can obtain. The system seems to maintain a dynamic equilibrium between different interests that keeps it in balance.[37] The list of past and present compromises permeates every area of regulation. The AMA, for example, vigorously opposed the creation of Medicare and Medicaid when those programs were debated in Congress in 1965.[38] It argued that government funding programs of the magnitude proposed could represent the first step toward socializing America's health care system, which in turn would empower the government to control clinical practice. The organization predicted that the costs of these initiatives would dwarf those predicted by their proponents.[39] Ironically, even the AMA's dire cost predictions fell well short of the actual mark.[40] Nevertheless, Medicare and Medicaid became law, and as the AMA feared, their administrative structure has grown increasingly intrusive into medical practice over the years to the point of promoting the use of protocols to guide physician practice. However, the medical profession's positions are continually heard as the program evolves, and the outcomes of policy debates have often been beneficial to it.

Moreover, the overall effect of Medicare and Medicaid on the prominence of the medical profession has been quite positive. By injecting new funding into the health care system, these programs have facilitated substantial expansion in the size of the profession and in the incomes of its members. Both rose precipitously in the decades after the programs were enacted.[41] Without Medicare and Medicaid as significant funding sources, far fewer patients would be able to afford care, and opportunities for physician practice would, consequently, be more limited.

Pharmaceutical companies often complain about the cumbersome and inefficient FDA approval process. They contend that it is slower and more bureaucratic than necessary, and that it adds substantial costs and delays to the process of bringing beneficial new drugs to market. These criticisms led to passage of the Prescription Drug User Fee Act of 1992 (PDUFA), which shortened the time frame for FDA review of new drug applications (NDAs).[42] However, the process of drug testing that leads up to filing an NDA is still long, costly, and complex. The FDA supervises many aspects of the clinical trials that must be performed before approval for marketing is sought, which introduces opportunities for substantial bureaucratic delay even before an NDA is filed. The process can take up to ten years, at a cost that can approach a billion dollars.[43]

Nevertheless, the perception of vigorous government oversight is an essential ingredient in generating public trust in pharmaceutical products. If patients had no reason to believe that the drugs their physicians prescribed had been subject to rigorous review by impartial regulators, they would be less likely to comply with prescriptions, and fewer would be written. The arduous regulatory scheme to which drugs are subjected can actually be seen as one of the most effective marketing tools that pharmaceutical firms have. It differentiates their products from the untested and often dangerous folk remedies that proliferated before drug regulation went into effect. The industry continually seeks reforms to streamline the process, but at the same time, it benefits from the overall structure.

States jealously guard their prerogative of licensing physicians and other health care professionals but accept a growing federal coordination role to maintain key aspects of the system's integrity. Licensure laws were enacted at the state level during the late nineteenth and early twentieth centuries. Other professions, for example, nursing, podiatry, psychology, and pharmacy, are also regulated exclusively by the states.[44] Despite occasional calls to federalize the system, state governments have remained eager to retain primary control over access to clinical practice. However, the past hundred years have presented numerous examples of the need for national coordination. Early voluntary coordinating efforts of the Federation of State Medical Boards (FSMB) and other groups turned out to be largely ineffective.

Today, federal involvement in overseeing clinical practice takes several forms. The National Practitioner Data Bank (NPDB), which is administered by the Health Resources and Services Administration (HRSA), compiles information on physician discipline, medical staff sanctions, and malpractice payments across states. The Medicare program credentials participating practitioners and reviews their performance through Quality Improvement Organizations (QIOs) and other means. The Drug Enforcement Administration (DEA) regulates prescribing of controlled substances. State licensure remains the gateway to entering a health care profession, but federal oversight regulates many aspects of ongoing practice. In this aspect of regulation, it is different levels of government, rather than governmental and private interests, that have reached compromises in structuring a system that respects the concerns of each.

A Proper Role for Each Kind of Regulator

The interplay among the different kinds of regulators and interests remains forceful because each contributes in a unique way. Every layer of regulation has a role and a purpose. If any of these elements were missing, the system would be deficient.

The federal government provides coordination and consistency in the oversight of an industry that is national in scope. Regulation at the state level alone would be fragmented and disjointed. As the experience with physician licensure revealed, physicians are mobile across the country, so the integrity of their oversight requires at least some elements of national management. Drugs are sold nationwide, and regulation on a state-by-state basis would be chaotic and, in all likelihood, unmanageable. Biomedical research benefits the entire nation, so the responsibility for its support is appropriately at the federal level with NIH. Moreover, few states have the resources to create the kind of research support infrastructure that is possible with federal funding. National coordination is also essential for infectious disease monitoring and control, since germs readily cross state boundaries, and for prevention of chronic diseases, which follow national trends. The same applies to the regulatory efforts of the Environmental Protection Agency (EPA) to limit population exposures to hazardous pollutants, which travel across regions through air and water.

State-level regulation is important because it is closer to provision of care. State governments, for example, bring regional knowledge and values to bear in overseeing medical practice and determining the acceptable bounds of clinical behavior. Health planning through state-level certificate-of-need programs, which determine the geographic allocation of hospital services, is a regional rather than a national concern. Rapid responses and prevention efforts for many public health threats are most effective at the local level. Regulators who have the greatest familiarity with regional conditions are likely to have the greatest effectiveness at addressing concerns such as restaurant hygiene, drinking water contamination, and toxic chemical spills.

Private professional organizations bring the highest level of expertise to bear on regulatory issues. Medical specialty boards can call on the most prominent clinicians in the country to design certification programs. The Joint Commission on Accreditation of Healthcare Organizations (JCAHO) compiles knowledge from many of America's most experienced hospital executives and health care researchers in designing its surveys of hospital quality. The Liaison Committee on Medical Education (LCME), a joint program of the Association of American Medical Colleges (AAMC) and the AMA, relies on the judgment of top leaders in medical education to design curriculum requirements for physician training and to assess the competence of the institutions that implement them.[45]

This set of roles and competences for different kinds of health care regulators should not belie serious conflicts that remain. Each player can overstep its bounds, leaving gaps and inconsistencies in oversight, as the history of American health care regulation amply reveals. Critics charge, for instance, that state medical boards and allied health professional licensure boards are often dominated by local practitioners who seek to hide professional incompetence from public view.[46] As an organization controlled by the member hospitals that it regulates, skeptics view the JCAHO as perennially soft on violations.[47] Wayward institutions rarely, if ever, lose accreditation completely. The EPA is often criticized as insensitive to local economic concerns when it restricts industrial activities that pollute. CMS has several times adjusted its safe-harbor regulations, which govern financial relationships between physicians and hospitals, to reflect unique needs of rural and inner-city health care providers that state officials might have spotted more readily.

Moreover, a lack of clear delineation between different authorities has left some major areas of regulation in a confused state. The most prominent among these is private health care finance, in which states regulate insurance, but ERISA exempts employer-based coverage from many state-level rules. Under this law, managed care organizations answer to the states for some aspects of their operations and to the federal government for others. A private organization, the National Committee for Quality Assurance (NCQA), is seeking to fill part of the void with an accreditation system, but its program has not yet been universally adopted.

While gaps and contradictions such as these persist, the system nevertheless reflects an underlying logic that relies on distinct regulators with varying perspectives and different kinds of expertise. The interplay among them forms the framework within which a comprehensive, albeit complex, regulatory structure can and does operate. The multiplicity of players, moreover, maintains a constant flow of input that helps the system to adapt as circumstances change.

Regulation and Health Care Evolution

American health care regulation is indeed a system of complexity, confrontation, and compromise. However, what appears to be an overly complex web of rules and enforcing organizations is actually the outcome of an intricate process that strives to meet many needs. Expertise and opinions from across a spectrum of perspectives offer guidance and provide for balance among participants. Interests from all sides have a chance to be heard, and their rights are protected in numerous ways; however, no single element goes unchallenged, at least not indefinitely.

American health care has flourished over the past hundred years. Rather than holding it back, our complex regulatory system that balances interests, values, and goals may have, in fact, provided much of the support that has nurtured the overall enterprise.[48] As health care has grown more complex, its regulation has evolved with it through a structure that facilitates diverse input and innovation. In the years ahead, the pattern will likely repeat, as America faces the challenge of protecting the public interest in an industry that has woven itself into the fabric of our economy and our society.

Appendices

Appendix A

Major Health Care Regulatory Agencies and Organizations

Level of Regulation	Agency	Primary Health Regulatory Function	Chapters in which Primary Functions are Discussed
Federal Agencies	Department of Health and Human Services (DHHS) (formerly Department of Health, Education and Welfare [DHEW])	Implements most of the federal health care regulatory infrastructure though component agencies	1 8
Components of DHHS	Agency for Healthcare Research and Quality (AHRQ)	Funds research on health services	
	Centers for Disease Control and Prevention (CDC)	Compiles and disseminates national health care data, investigates disease outbreaks, researches public health threats	6
	Centers for Medicare & Medicaid Services (CMS) (formerly Health Care Finance Administration [HCFA])	Administers the Medicare program and the federal portion of the Medicaid program and State Children's Health Insurance Program	4

Level of Regulation	Agency	Primary Health Regulatory Function	Chapters in which Primary Functions are Discussed
	Food and Drug Administration (FDA)	Oversees the safety of drugs, medical devices, biologic products, food, and cosmetics	5
	Health Resources and Services Administration (HRSA)	Administers funding programs for health care training, the National Practitioner Data Bank for physician disciplinary actions, and coordinates the organ donation network (UNOS)	2, 8
	Indian Health Service (IHS)	Operates hospitals and provides other health care services for Native Americans	3
	National Institutes of Health (NIH)	Funds biomedical and related research at universities, institutes, and hospitals and conducts intramural research	8
	Substance Abuse and Mental Health Services Administration (SAMHSA)	Funds community mental health services	6
	Office for Civil Rights (DHHS)	Enforces privacy provisions of the Health Insurance Portability and Accountability Act of 1996 (HIPAA) and civil rights protections	3,7
	Office of Inspector General (DHHS)	Enforces prohibition against fraud in billing federal health care payment programs and against payments for referrals	7
Other Federal Agencies	Environmental Protection Agency (EPA)	Regulates the discharge of environmental pollutants	6
	Occupational Safety and Health Administration (OSHA)	Regulates workplace safety and health	6
	United States Department of Agriculture (USDA)	Regulates food safety, conducts research on food safety	6, 8
	Department of Defense (DOD)	Operates hospitals and provides other health care services for active-duty military personnel, their dependents, and retirees	3
	Department of Homeland Security (DHS)	Coordinates responses to natural disasters and bioterrorist attacks	6

Level of Regulation	Agency	Primary Health Regulatory Function	Chapters in which Primary Functions are Discussed
	Department of Justice (DOJ)	Enforces antitrust laws and prohibition on payments for referrals	7
	Department of Labor (DOL)	Administers Employee Retirement Income Security Act of 1974, which applies to employee health benefits arrangements	4
	Federal Trade Commission (FTC)	Enforces antitrust laws, regulates advertising of nonprescription drugs	5, 7
	Internal Revenue Service (IRS)	Regulates the structure and activities of nonprofit hospitals and other health care institutions that are recognized as tax-exempt	7
	National Science Foundation (NSF)	Funds basic science research	8
	Patent and Trademark Office (PTO)	Grants patents for new inventions and discoveries, including drugs and devices	5
	Veterans Administration (VA)	Operates hospitals and other health care services for veterans, conducts and funds research on health services	3, 8
State Agencies	Departments of health	Investigate public health threats, house licensure boards in some states, administer health planning and certificate-of-need programs in some states, regulate clinical operations of managed care organizations	2, 3, 6
	Boards of medicine	License and discipline physicians	2
	Boards (other health professions)	License and discipline allied health professionals	2
	Departments of welfare	Administer Medicaid programs in many states	4
	Departments of insurance	Regulate the sale and underwriting of private health insurance, including managed care arrangements, except when preempted by ERISA	4

Level of Regulation	Agency	Primary Health Regulatory Function	Chapters in which Primary Functions are Discussed
Local Agencies	Departments of health	Investigate public health threats, inspect restaurants and other public facilities	6
Private Organizations	Accreditation Council on Graduate Medical Education	Accredits medical residency programs	2
	American Board of Medical Specialties (ABMS)	Coordinates activities of medical specialty societies	2
	Association of Schools of Allied Health Professions (ASAHP)	Coordinates the certification of training programs for allied health professionals	2
	Educational Commission for Foreign Medical Graduates (ECFMG)	Certifies graduates of foreign medical schools to enter ACGME-accredited medical residencies and fellowships	2
	Federation of State Medical Boards (FSMB)	Coordinates some activities of state physician licensure agencies, including maintenance of records of physicians who have been disciplined	2
	Joint Commission on Accreditation of Healthcare Organizations (JCAHO)	Accredits hospitals and other kinds of health care facilities	3
	Liaison Committee on Medical Education (LCME)	Accredits medical schools	2
	Medical specialty societies	Certify physicians as qualified to practice in medical specialties	2
	National Board of Medical Examiners (NBME)	Develops and administers the examination for medical licensure that is used by all states	2
	National Committee on Quality Assurance (NCQA)	Accredits managed care plans and related organizations	4
	United Network for Organ Sharing (UNOS)	Administers system for allocating organs for transplantation	3

Appendix B

Chronology of Major Developments in Public Health Regulation

State and Local Health Departments

1790–1820	Some eastern port cities developed municipal agencies to fight epidemics; New York City advisory board of health established
1820–1840	Only five city boards of health are in existence
1840–1860	Louisiana experiments with state board of health, and it fails
1860–1880	First permanent state board of health established in Massachusetts
1920–1940	By 1928, 208 county health departments in 17 states; Social Security Act provides grants for state and local health departments

Centers for Disease Control and Prevention (CDC)

1940–1960	Malaria Control in War Areas becomes CDC; helps to develop polio and influenza vaccinations; Epidemic Intelligence Service created (EIS)
1960–1980	*Mortality and Morbidity Weekly Report* published; smallpox eradicated; last case of polio in United States
1980–present	First case of AIDS identified; CDC responds to first bioterrorism attack

Environmental Protection Agency (EPA)

1920–1940	Soil Conservation Service founded; state fish and wildlife programs established; Oil Pollution Act passed
1940–1960	Clean Air Act passed; Clean Water Act passed
1960–1980	National Environmental Protection Act; EPA opens its doors

Occupational Safety and Health Administration (OSHA)

1960–1980	Occupational Safety and Health Act passed; OSHA created; first standards developed to protect Americans at work

Agency for Toxic Substance and Disease Registry (ATSDR)

1960–1980	Resource Conservation Recovery Act passed
1980–present	CERCLA (Superfund Act) passed; ATSDR created

Department of Agriculture (USDA)

1790–1820	New York State Board of Agriculture (first state board) created
1820–1840	First committees on agriculture in Congress
1860–1880	USDA set up with focus on the science of agriculture; a few states inspect dairy products
1880–1900	Meat Inspection Acts of 1890 and 1891 passed; USDA raised to cabinet level; first state agriculture department established in Georgia
1900–1920	Meat Inspection Act of 1906 passed; Insecticide Act passed
1940–1960	Poultry Products Inspection Act passed

Health Resources and Services Administration (HRSA)

1960–1980	HRSA created to hire National Health Service Corps personnel, manage community health centers, and administer national health care workforce management programs

Other Significant Developments

1790–1820	First dispensaries established to care for health of the poor
1860–1880	Quarantine Act of 1873 passed; National Board of Health created (and dismantled four years later)
1880–1900	Bacteria discovered; germ theory proposed; Act to Establish a Hospital Corps passed
1900–1920	Development of epidemiology and biostatistics as scientific disciplines; first Food and Drug Act passed
1920–1940	Social Security Act passed; Food, Drug and Cosmetic Act passed; Nurse Training Act passed
1940–1960	Hill-Burton Act passed to promote hospital construction; Mental Health Act passed
1960–1980	Medicare and Medicaid enacted; Civil Rights Act passed; Health Professions Education Assistance Act passed; Lead Based Paint Poisoning Prevention Act passed
1980–present	Managed care begins to proliferate; Americans with Disabilities Act passed; Health Insurance Portability and Accountability Act passed

Appendix C

List of Acronyms

AACOM	American Association of Colleges of Osteopathic Medicine
AAMC	Association of American Medical Colleges
ABMS	American Board of Medical Specialties
ACGME	Accreditation Council for Graduate Medical Education
ACS	American College of Surgery
AHRQ	Agency for Healthcare Research and Quality (in DHHS)
AIDS	acquired immune deficiency syndrome
ALF	assisted living facility
ALJ	administrative law judge
AMA	American Medical Association
ANA	American Nurses Association
AOA	American Osteopathic Association
AOTA	American Occupational Therapy Association
APC	ambulatory payment classification group
APhA	American Pharmacists Association
APTA	American Physical Therapy Association
APA	American Psychological Association
ASAHP	Association of Schools of Allied Health Professions
ATSDR	Agency for Toxic Substances and Disease Registry (in EPA)
BBA	Balanced Budget Act of 1997
BPHC	Bureau of Primary Health Care (in HRSA)
BHPr	Bureau of Health Professions (in HRSA)
CARF	Commission on Accreditation of Rehabilitation Facilities
CDC	Centers for Disease Control and Prevention (in DHHS)
CERCLA	Comprehensive Environmental Response, Compensation and Liability Act of 1980
CMHS	Center for Mental Health Services (in SAMHSA)
CDER	Center for Drug Evaluation and Research (in FDA)

CLIA	Clinical Laboratory Improvement Amendments
CMS	Centers for Medicare & Medicaid Services (in DHHS) (formerly HCFA)
CNPP	Center for Nutrition Policy and Promotion (in USDA)
COBRA	Comprehensive Omnibus Budget Reconciliation Act of 1986
COGME	Council on Graduate Medical Education
CON	certificate-of-need
CPSC	Consumer Product Safety Commission (United States)
CSAP	Center for Substance Abuse Prevention (in SAMHSA)
CSAT	Center for Substance Abuse Treatment (in SAMHSA)
DESI	drug efficacy study implementation
DOJ	Department of Justice (United States)
DHS	Department of Homeland Security (United States)
DHS	Department of Health Services (California)
DHEW	Department of Health, Education, and Welfare (United States) (now DHHS)
DHHS	Department of Health and Human Services (United States) (formerly DHEW)
DOD	Department of Defense (United States)
DOE	Department of Energy (United States)
DOL	Department of Labor (United States)
DRG	diagnosis-related group
DSHEA	Dietary Supplement Health and Education Act of 1994
DTC	direct-to-consumer advertising
EBSA	Employee Benefits Security Administration (in DOL) (formerly PWBA)
ECFMG	Educational Commission for Foreign Medical Graduates
EEOC	Equal Employment Opportunity Commission (United States)
ELSI	Ethical, Legal, and Social Issues research program (in HGP)
EMCRO	experimental medical care review organization (in HCFA)
EMS	emergency medical services
EMTALA	Emergency Medical Treatment and Active Labor Act of 1986
EPA	Environmental Protection Agency (United States)
EPSDT	Early Periodic Screening, Diagnosis, and Treatment (in Medicaid)
ERISA	Employee Retirement Income Security Act of 1974
ERS	Economic Research Service (in USDA)
ESRD	end-stage renal disease
FDA	Food and Drug Administration (in DHHS)
FDAMA	Food and Drug Administration Modernization Act of 1997
FEHBP	Federal Employee Health Benefit Plan
FEMA	Federal Emergency Management Agency (in DHS)
FNS	Food and Nutrition Service (in USDA)
FSIS	Food Safety and Inspection Service (in USDA)
FSMB	Federation of State Medical Boards
FTC	Federal Trade Commission (United States)
GAO	Government Accountability Office (formerly General Accounting Office)
HCFA	Health Care Finance Administration (in DHHS) (now CMS)
HCQIA	Health Care Quality Improvement Act of 1986
HEDIS	health plan employer data and information set
HGP	Human Genome Project (in NIH)
HIBAC	Health Insurance Benefits Advisory Council (in SSA)
HIP	Health Insurance Plan of New York
HIPAA	Health Insurance Portability and Accountability Act of 1996
HMO	health maintenance organization
HRSA	Health Resources and Services Administration (in DHHS)
HSA	health systems agency
HSCRC	Health Services Cost Review Commission (Maryland)
ICF	intermediate care facility

IDS	integrated delivery system
IHS	Indian Health Service (in DHHS)
IND	investigational new drug exemption
IOM	Institute of Medicine (in the National Academy of Sciences)
IRB	institutional review board
IRC	Internal Revenue Code of 1986
IRS	Internal Revenue Service (United States)
JCAHO	Joint Commission on Accreditation of Healthcare Organizations
LCME	Liaison Committee on Medical Education
MCAC	Medicare Coverage Advisory Commission (in DHHS)
MCE	medical care evaluation study
MedPAC	Medicare Payment Advisory Commission (in DHHS)
MMA	Medicare Prescription Drug, Improvement, and Modernization Act of 2003
NAIC	National Association of Insurance Commissioners
NAPH	National Association of Public Hospitals
NBME	National Board of Medical Examiners
NCD	national coverage determination
NCHGR	National Center for Human Genome Research (in NIH)
NCI	National Cancer Institute (in NIH)
NCVHS	National Committee on Vital Health Statistics (in DHHS)
NEPA	National Environmental Policy Act
NCHS	National Center for Health Statistics (in CDC)
NCQA	National Committee on Quality Assurance
NDA	new drug application
NHTSA	National Highway Traffic Safety Administration (in the Department of transportation)
NIH	National Institutes of Health (in DHHS)
NIOSH	National Institute of Occupational Safety and Health (in CDC)
NPDB	National Practitioner Data Bank (in HRSA)
NSF	National Science Foundation (United States)
OAS	Office of Applied Studies (in SAMHSA)
OCR	Office for Civil Rights (in DHHS)
OIG	Office of Inspector General (in DHHS)
OPM	Office of Personnel Management
OPTN	Organ Procurement and Transplantation Network
OSCAR	On-Line Survey, Certification, and Reporting System
OSHA	Occupational Safety and Health Administration (in DOL)
OTC	over-the-counter drug
PBGC	Provider Reimbursement Review Board (in CMS)
PBGC	Pension Benefit Guarantee Corporation
PBM	pharmacy benefit manager
PDP	prescription drug plan
PDUFA	Prescription Drug User Fee Act of 1992
PHC4	Pennsylvania Health Care Cost Containment Council (Pennsylvania)
PHS	Public Health Service (in DHHS)
POS	point-of-service plan
PPO	preferred provider organization
PPRC	Physician Payment Review Commission (in HCFA)
PRO	professional review organization (in HCFA)
ProPAC	Prospective Payment Assessment Commission (in HCFA)
PRRB	Provider Reimbursement Review Board (in CMS)
PSO	patient safety organization
PSRO	professional standards review organization (in HCFA)
PTO	Patent and Trademark Office (United States)
PWBA	Pension and Welfare Benefits Administration (in DOL) (now EBSA)

QAPI	quality assessment and performance improvement
QIO	quality improvement organization (in CMS)
RBRVS	resource-based relative value scale
RUG	resource utilization group
SAMHSA	Substance Abuse and Mental Health Services Administration (in DHHS)
SCHIP	State Children's Health Insurance Program
SEC	Securities and Exchange Commission (United States)
SEOPF	Southeast Organ Procurement Foundation
SRG	Scientific Research Group (in NIH)
SNF	skilled nursing facility
SRS	Social and Rehabilitative Service Administration (in DHHS)
SSA	Social Security Administration (in DHHS)
SSI	Supplemental Security Income
TEFRA	Tax Equity and Fiscal Responsibility Act of 1982
UBIT	unrelated business income tax
UNOS	United Network for Organ Sharing
USDA	United States Department of Agriculture (United States)
VA	Veterans Administration (United States)

Notes

Chapter 1

1. See discussion in D. Haas-Wilson, *Managed Care and Monopoly Power: The Antitrust Challenge* (Cambridge, MA: Harvard University Press, 2003), 12–15.

2. See discussion in W. A. Zelman, *The Changing Health Care Marketplace* (San Francisco: Jossey-Bass, 1996), 8–9.

3. W. Kissick, *Medicine's Dilemmas* (New Haven, CT: Yale University Press, 1994), 1–22.

4. P. Torrens, and L. Breslow, "The Evolution of Public Health: A Joint Public-Private Responsibility," in S. Williams, and P. Torrens, eds., *Introduction to Health Services,* 5th ed. (Albany, NY: Delmar, 1999), 208–224.

5. W. Janssen, "The Story of the Laws behind the Labels," *FDA Consumer* 15, no. 5 (1981): 32–45.

6. The development of physician licensure laws and accreditation standards for medical education are discussed in P. Starr, *The Social Transformation of American Medicine* (New York: Basic Books, 1982), 112–144.

7. The development of health insurance is discussed in ibid., 295–310.

8. Committee on Quality of Health Care in America, Institute of Medicine, *To Err Is Human* (Washington, DC: National Academy Press, 1999).

9. D. Mechanic, "Policy Challenges in Addressing Racial Disparities and Improving Population Health," *Health Affairs* 24, no. 2 (2005): 335–352.

10. J. E. Wennberg, "Variation in the Delivery of Health Care: The Stakes Are High," *Annals of Internal Medicine* 128, no. 10 (1998): 866–868.

11. The Kaiser Commission on Medicaid and the Uninsured, *Health Insurance Coverage in America 2003 Data Update* (Washington, DC: Henry J. Kaiser Family Foundation, 2004).

12. G. F. Anderson, P. S. Hussey, B. K. Frogner, and H. R. Waters. "Health Spending in the United States and the Rest of the Industrialized World," *Health Affairs* 24, no. 4 (2005): 903–914.

13. Organization for Economic Cooperation and Development, *OECP Health Data 2004* (Paris: OECP, 2005).

14. See discussion in B. B. Longest, *Health Policy Making in the United States* (Chicago: Health Administration Press, 1998), 4–27.

15. Starr, *Social Transformation of American Medicine*, 102–123.

16. See discussion in Zelman, *Changing Health Care Marketplace*, 311–312.

17. See C. S. Weissert and W. G. Weissert, *Governing Health: The Politics of Health Policy* (Baltimore: Johns Hopkins University Press, 2002), 185–190.

18. U.S. Department of Health and Human Services [home page], Washington, DC: United States Department of Health and Human Services, HHS: What we do (25 February 2005) http://www.hhs.gov/about/whatwedo.html (1 April 2005).

19. For a description of the role of regulation in bureaucratic management of government policy, see Weissert and Weissert, *Governing Health*, 171–176.

20. For a detailed description of the legal context of the process, see J. S. Lubbers, *A Guide to Federal Agency Rulemaking*, 3rd ed. (Chicago: ABA Books, 1998).

21. L. D. Brown, "Political Evolution of Federal Health Care Regulation," *Health Affairs* 11, no. 4 (Winter 1992): 17–37.

22. See discussion in Longest, *Health Policymaking in the United States*, 4–27.

23. See discussion in ibid., 146–149.

24. U.S. Const. amend. V and XIV.

25. Administrative Procedures Act, 5 U.S.C. §§ 551 et seq.

26. Ibid.

27. The doctrine of judicial deference to the substance of regulatory agency decision making is discussed in M. C. Tolley, "Judicial Review of Agency Interpretation of Statutes: Deference Doctrines in Comparative Perspective," *Policy Studies Journal* 31, no. 3 (2003): 421–440.

28. Ibid.

29. Brown, "Political Evolution of Federal Health Care Regulation."

30. Haas-Wilson, *Managed Care and Monopoly Power*, 41–64.

31. See Zelman, *Changing Health Care Marketplace*, 305–311.

32. Medicare, Prescription Drug Improvement, and Modernization Act of 2003. P.L. 108-173.

33. For a description of the proposed Clinton health plan, see J. C. Robinson, *The Corporate Practice of Medicine* (Berkeley: University of California Press, 1999), 45–48.

34. For a discussion of federalism and health care, see P. Lee and A. E. Benjamin, "Health Policy and the Politics of Health Care," in S. J. Williams and P. R. Torrens, eds., *Introduction to Health Services*, 5th ed., 442–444.

35. Pennsylvania Medical Care Availability and Reduction of Error Act, 40 Pa. Stat. Ann. § 1303 (2002). States' efforts regarding patient safety are discussed in B. R. Furrow, "Regulating Patient Safety: Toward a Federal Model of Medical Error Reduction," *Widener Law Review* 12, no. 1 (2006): 1–38.

36. For a discussion of American attitudes toward government as they relate to health care, see V. Rodwin, "Comparative Analysis of Heath Systems: An International Perspective," in A. R. Kovner and S. Jonas, eds., *Health Care Delivery in the United States*, 6th ed. (New York: Springer, 1999), 133.

Chapter 2

1. P. Warren, "MH3: The Development of a Profession," University of Manitoba home page, 12 August 2002, http://www.umanitoba.ca/faculties/medicine/units/history/notes/profession (30 September 2005).

2. Royal College of Physicians, "About the College: The Oldest Medical Institution in England," 24 June 2004, http://www.rcplondon.ac.uk/college/about_history.htm (30 September 2005).

3. U.S. Department of Labor, Bureau of Labor Statistics, "Occupational Outlook Handbook, 2004–05 Edition," 29 June 2004, http://www.bls.gov/oco/home.htm (21 September 2005).

4. T. S. Jost, "Oversight of the Quality of Medical Care: Regulation, Management, or the Market?" *Arizona Law Review* 37 (Fall 1995): 828.

5. P. Starr, *The Social Transformation of American Medicine* (New York: Basic Books, 1982), 64.

6. Ibid., 102–127.

7. Ibid., 102–104.

8. K. C. Yohn, "The History and Role of the Federation of State Medical Boards of the United States," *Federation Bulletin* 75, no. 9 (1988): 275–277.

9. Jost, "Oversight of the Quality of Medical Care," 828.

10. Starr, *Social Transformation of American Medicine,* 117.

11. A. Flexner, *Medical Education in the United States and Canada: A Report to the Carnegie Foundation for the Advancement of Teaching* (New York: Carnegie Foundation for the Advancement of Teaching, 1910). The Flexner report is discussed in detail in Starr, *Social Transformation of American Medicine,* 116–123.

12. Starr, *Social Transformation of American Medicine,* 120–121.

13. Ibid., 121.

14. Ibid., 123–127.

15. See R. Stevens, *In Sickness and in Wealth: American Hospitals in the Twentieth Century* (New York: Basic Books, 1989), 52–79.

16. Starr, *Social Transformation of American Medicine,* 124.

17. For a discussion of the history of medical licensure and a survey of state licensing laws, see R. C. Derbyshire, *Medical Licensure and Discipline in the United States* (Westport, CT: Greenwood, 1978).

18. American Medical Association, *State Medical Licensure Requirements and Statistics* (Chicago: American Medical Association, 1999).

19. See T. S. Jost et al., "Consumers, Complaints and Professional Discipline: A Look at Medical Licensure Boards," *Health Matrix* 3 (1993): 309–338.

20. Health Research Group, "Ranking of State Medical Boards Serious Disciplinary Actions in 2002," HRG Publication No. 1658, 27 March 2003, http://www .citizen.org/publications/release.cfm?ID=7234&secID=1158&catID=126 (30 September 2005).

21. See Derbyshire, *Medical Licensure and Discipline in the United States.*

22. New York State Department of Health, "Professional Misconduct and Physician Discipline," June 2004, http://www.heatlh.state.ny.us/nysdoh/opmc/main.htm (30 September 2005).

23. Health Research Group, "20,125 Questionable Doctors: Pennsylvania," 2000, http://www.citizen.org/hrg/qdsite/STATES/pennsylvania.htm. 2000 (30 September 2005). See also Health Grades, http://www.healthgrades.com (30 September 2005).

24. J. S. Samkoff and R.W. McDermott, "Recognizing Physician Impairment," *Pennsylvania Medicine* 91, no. 4 (1988): 36–38.

25. See L. Prager, "Doctor Sanctions Level Off; Boards Try Preventative Tack," *American Medical News,* 1 May 2002.

26. U.S. Congress, Office of Technology Assessment, *Unconventional Cancer Treatments* (OTA-H-405). (Washington, DC: Government Printing Office, 1990).

27. Committee to Study the Role of Allied Health Personnel, Institute of Medicine, "Allied Health Services: Avoiding Crises" (Washington, DC: National Academy Press, 1989), 235–258.

28. See B. R. Furrow, "Regulating Patient Safety: Toward a Federal Model of Medical Error Reduction," *Widener Law Review* 12, no. 1 (2006): 1–38.

29. Health Research Group, "Protecting Health, Safety, & Democracy," 2005, http://www.citizen.org/hrg (30 September 2005).

30. Yohn, "History and Role of the Federation of State Medical Boards of the United States," 275–277; see also Federation of State Medical Boards, 2005, "History," http://www.fsmb.org/history.html (25 October 2005).

31. Federation of State Medical Boards, History.

32. Ibid.

33. Ibid.

34. National Board of Medical Examiners, "NBME Statement of Guiding Principles," http://www.nbme.org/about/about.asp (25 October 2005).

35. Liaison Committee on Medical Education, "Overview: Accreditation and the LCME," 7 July 2004, http://www.lcme.org/overview.htm (25 October 2005).

36. Accreditation Council for Graduate Medical Education, "Home," http://www.acgma.org (31 October 2005).

37. Educational Commission for Foreign Medical Graduates, "Home," 11 October 2005, http://www.ecfmg.org (31 October 2005).

38. Information on the AMA is available at http://www.ama-assn.org/ma/pub/category/1854.html (14 October 2005).

39. Jost, "Oversight of the Quality of Medical Care." 830.

40. American Medical Association, "Illustrated Highlights of AMA History: 1900 to 1939," 20 December 2004, http://www.ama-assn.org/ama/pub/category/1917.html (7 September 2005).

41. Starr, *Social Transformation of American Medicine,* 355.

42. T. A. Brennan, R. I. Horowitz, F. D. Duffy, C. K. Cassel, L. D. Goode, and R. S. Lipner, "The Role of Physician Specialty Board Certification Status in the Quality Movement," *Journal of the American Medical Association* 292, no. 9 (2004): 1038–1043.

43. American Board of Medical Specialties, "History of the ABMS: Development," 2005, http://www.abms.org/Development (9 September 2005).

44. Starr, *Social Transformation of American Medicine,* 357. See also American Board of Medical Specialties, "History for the ABMS: Development."

45. See discussion of managed care arrangements in D. Mechanic, "A Balanced Framework for Change," *Journal of Health Politics, Policy and Law* 24, no. 5 (1999): 1107–1114.

46. P. R. Torrens and S. J. Williams, "Managed Care: Restructuring the System," In Williams and Torrens, eds., *Introduction to Health Services,* 5th ed., 151–169.

47. D. van Amerongen, "Physician Credentialing in a Consumer-Centric World," *Health Affairs* 21, no. 5 (2002): 152–156.

48. For an example of an HMO quality initiative based on measurement of outcomes data, see B. Van Acker, G. McIntosh, and M. Gude, "Continuous Quality Improving Techniques Enhance HMO Member's Immunization Rates," *Journal of Healthcare Quality* 20, no. 2 (1998): 36–41.

49. J. C. Robinson and J. M. Yelgin, "Medical Management after Managed Care," *Health Affairs,* Web Exclusive, W4 (19 May 2004): 269–280.

50. Ibid., 156.

51. J. K. Igelhart, "The American Health Care System: Community Hospitals," *New England Journal of Medicine* 329, no. 5 (1993): 372–376.

52. See A. R. Kovner, "Hospitals," in A.R. Kovner and S. Jonas, *Health Care Delivery in the United States,* 6th ed. (New York: Springer, 1999), 157–182.

53. C. W. Rosenberg, *The Care of Strangers: The Rise of America's Hospital System* (Baltimore, MD: Johns Hopkins University Press, 1995), 166–189.

54. See *Darling v. Charleston Hospital,* 33 I11.2d 326, 211 N.E.2d 253, cert. den. 383 U.S. 946 (Ill. 1965).

55. Jost, "Oversight of the Quality of Medical Care," 833.

56. In one such incident, a New Jersey physician whose license was suspended for spreading hepatitis to patients through the use of unclean needles and syringes was able to continue to practice across the border in Pennsylvania; D. Janson, "Doctor Suspended in Hepatitis Dispute Is Practicing in Pennsylvania: Agreement by Board Questioned in Drug's Role," *New York Times,* 14 January 1977, 43. For a more recent report reflecting continuing shortcomings in the national coordination of physician discipline, see P. Davies, "A Doctor's Tale Shows Weaknesses in Medical Vetting," *Wall Street Journal,* 21 September 2005, A1.

57. *Patrick v. Burget,* 108 U.S. 1658 (1988).

58. Health Care Quality Improvement Act, 42 U.S.C. §§ 11101–11152 (1986). See discussion in J. K. Igelhart, "Congress Moves to Bolster Peer Review: The Health Care Quality Improvement Act of 1986," *New England Journal of Medicine* 316, no. 15 (1987): 960–964.

59. U.S. Department of Health and Human Services, Office of Inspector General, *Managed Care Organization Nonreporting to the National Practitioner Data Bank: A Signal for Broader Concern* (OEI-01–99–00690), May 2001, http://oig.hhs.gov/oei/reports/oei-01–99–00690.pdf (7 September 2005).

60. S. Landers, "Legislators Debate Opening Data Bank to Public Scrutiny: A Report on the House Commerce Committee's Oversight and Investigations Subcommittee Hearing on Public Access to the National Practitioner Data Bank," *American Medical News* 43, no. 1 (2000): 34.

61. This was implemented through the Higher Education Act of 1965, P.L. 89–329, 79 Stat. 1219 (1965), portions codified at 20 U.S.C. § 1088.

62. Starr, *Social Transformation of American Medicine,* 421.

63. R. L. Phillips, M. Dodoo, C. R. Jaen, and L. A. Green, "COGME's 16th Report to Congress: Too Many Physicians Could Be Worse Than Wasted," *Annals of Family Medicine* 3 (2005): 268–270.

64. Council on Graduate Medical Education, "About the Council," 17 August 2005, http://www.cogme.gov/whois.htm (25 October 2005).

65. Center for Medicare & Medicaid Services, "Medicare Information Resource," 9 February 2005, http://www.cms.hhs.gov/medicare/ (7 September 2005).

66. The RBRVS payment system is described in B. R. Furrow et al., *Health Law,* 5th ed. (St. Paul, MN: West, 2004), 750–753. See also J. K. Igelhart, "Medicare's Declining Payments to Physicians," *New England Journal of Medicine* 346, no. 24 (2002): 1924–1930.

67. See Furrow et al. *Health Law,* 751.

68. Balanced Budget Act of 1997, 105 P.L. 33, 111 Stat. 251 (1997).

69. Council on Graduate Medical Education, "Summary of Eleventh Report: International Medical Graduates, the Physician Workforce, and GME Payment Reform, March 1998," 20 November 2001, http://www.cogme.gov/rpt11.htm (7 September 2005).

70. M. Whitcomb, "Correcting the Oversupply of Specialists by Limiting Residencies for Graduates of Foreign Medical Schools," *New England Journal of Medicine* 333, no. 7 (1995): 454–456.

71. Ibid.

72. Educational Commission for Foreign Medical Graduates, "About ECFMG," 31 September 2005, http://www.ecfmg.org/about.html (14 October 2005).

73. See Kaiser Family Foundation, *Medicare Chart Book* (Washington, DC: Kaiser Family Foundation, 2005), 55, available at http://www.kff.org/medicare/7284.cfm.
Also see Kaiser Family Foundation, "Key Medicare and Medicaid Statistics," available at http://www.kff.org/medicaid/upload/Key%20Medicare%20and%20Medicaid%20Statistics .pdf.

74. Center for Medicare & Medicaid Services (2005), Medicare Information Resource, 9 February 2005, http://www.cms.hhs.gov/medicare (7 September 2005).

75. See Furrow et al. *Health Law,* 1010.

76. N. Gevitz, *The DOs: Osteopathic Medicine in America* (Baltimore: Johns Hopkins University Press, 2004).

77. American Association of Colleges of Osteopathic Medicine, 2005, http://www .aacom.org/colleges (27 October 2005).

78. American Association of Colleges of Osteopathic Medicine. *2004 Annual Report on Osteopathic Education* (Chevy Chase, MD: American Association of Colleges of Osteopathic Medicine), 23, 57, http://www.aacom.org/data/annualreport/AROME2004.pdf (25 May 2006).

79. Ibid.

80. *Weiss v. York Hospital,* 470 U.S. 1060 (1985).

81. American Osteopathic Association, "Specialty Affiliates," http://www.osteopathic .org/index.cfm?PageID=lcl_spclty (4 November 2005).

82. For a description of different kinds of allied health professionals, see H. A. Sultz and K. M. Young, *Health Care USA: Understanding Its Organization and Delivery* (Gaithersberg, MD: Aspen, 2001), 174–197.

83. U.S. Department of Health and Human Services, "National Center for Health Workforce Analysis: US Health Workforce Personnel Factbook," 9 June 2003, http://bhpr .hrsa.gov/healthworkforce/reports/factbook.htm (7 September 2005).

84. Committee to Study the Role of Allied Health Personnel, Institute of Medicine, "Allied Health Services," 235–258.

85. Ibid., 236.

86. Ibid., 252–253.

87. Pharmacists, for example, have the American Pharmacists Association (see http: //www.aphanet.org//AM/Template.cfm?Section=Home), the National Community Pharmacists Association (see http://www.ncpanet.org/), and the American Society of Health-System Pharmacists (see http://www.ashp.org/).

88. For example, the National Commission for Certifying Agencies sets standards for organizations that certify allied health professionals (see http://www.noca.org/about/about .htm). See also Committee to Study the Role of Allied Health Personnel, Institute of Medicine, "Allied Health Services," 252.

89. Allied Health Professions Personnel Training Act, P.L. 89–751, 80 Stat. 1222 (1966).

90. Jost, "Oversight of the Quality of Medical Care," 863.

91. Medical Board of California, "About the Medical Board of California," http://www .medbd.ca.gov/abouttheboard.htm (26 October 2005).

92. New Jersey Division of Consumer Affairs, "State Board of Medical Examiners," 25 October 2005, http://www.state.nj.us/lps/ca/bme/bme.htm (26 October 2005).

93. Health Resources and Services Administration, "About HRSA," http://www.hrsa .gov/about.htm (26 October 2005).

94. See Health Resources and Services Administration, Bureau of Primary Health Care, "Health Center Program," http://bphc.hrsa.gov/chc/ (26 October 2005).

95. See Health Resources and Services Administration, Bureau of Health Professionals, "National Center for Health Workforce Analysis," http://bhpr.hrsa.gov/healthworkforce/ (26 October 2005).

96. Health Resources and Services Administration, "Maternal and Child Health Bureau," http://mchb.hrsa.gov/about/default.htm (31 October 2005).

97. Health Resources and Services Administration, HIV/AIDS Bureau, "About HIV/ AIDS Bureau (HAB)," http://hab.hrsa.gov/aboutus.htm (26 October 2005).

98. American Board of Internal Medicine, "Who We Are," 2005, http://www.abim .org/about/index.shtm (26 October 2005).

99. For an argument against physician licensure, see S. V. Svorny. "Does Physician Licensure Serve a Useful Purpose?" on The Independent Institute "Newsroom," 10 July 2000, http://www.independent.org/newsroom/article.asp?id=266 (26 October 2005).

100. The possible role of data in enhancing market-based oversight of physicians is discussed in Jost, "Oversight of the Quality of Medical Care," 850–855.

Chapter 3

1. The early history of hospitals is discussed in G. Risse, *Mending Bodies, Saving Souls: A History of Hospitals* (New York: Oxford University Press, 1999), 15–230.

2. P. Starr, *The Social Transformation of American Medicine* (New York: Basic Books, 1982), 145–179.

3. University of Pennsylvania Health System, "About Pennsylvania Hospital," 2005, http://www.pennhealth.com/pahosp/about/, 17 October 2005.

4. C. E. Rosenberg, *The Care of Strangers: The Rise of America's Hospital System* (Baltimore, MD: Johns Hopkins University Press, 1995), 15–46.

5. J. Connor, *Doing Good* (Toronto: University of Toronto Press, 2000), 266.

6. R. Stevens, *In Sickness and in Wealth: American Hospitals in the Twentieth Century* (New York: Basic Books, 1989), 52–79.

7. See J. K. Igelhart, "The American Health Care System—Teaching Hospitals," *New England Journal of Medicine* 329, no. 14 (1993): 1052–1056.

8. Risse, *Mending Bodies, Saving Souls*, 366.

9. For a discussion of different kinds of hospitals, see A. R. Kovner, "Hospitals," in A. R. Kovner and S. Jonas, eds., *Health Care Delivery in the United States*, 6th ed. (New York: Springer, 1999), 158–181.

10. Museum of London, "Past Exhibitions: Bedlam—Custody, Care, and Cure 1247–1997," 11 July 2005, http://www.museumoflondon.org.uk/MOLsite/exhibits/bedlam/bedlam.htm (30 September 2005).

11. D. Ramchandani and D. M. Ellis, "Institute of Pennsylvania Hospital: Remembrances Past," *Psychiatric News* 2 January 1998, http://www.psych.org/pnews/98-01-02/hx.html (4 November 2005).

12. K. C. Fleming, J. M. Evans, and D. S. Chutka, "A Cultural and Economic History of Old Age in America," *Mayo Clinic Proceedings* 78, no. 10 (2003): 914–921.

13. K. Stevenson, "ElderWeb: LTC Backwards and Forwards 1800–1899," 28 July 2005, http://www.elderweb.com/history/?PageID=2816 (7 September 2005).

14. See Rosenberg, *The Care of Strangers*, 262–285.

15. See J. S. Roberts, J. G. Coale, and R. R. Redman, "A History of the Joint Commission on Accreditation of Hospitals," *Journal of the American Medical Association* 258, no. 7 (21 August 1987): 936–940. See also Joint Commission on Accreditation of Healthcare Organizations, "A Journey through the History of the Joint Commission," 2005, http://www.jcaho.org/about+us/history.htm (10 November 2005).

16. Joint Commission on Accreditation of Healthcare Organizations, "Joint Commission Welcome Page," 2005, http://www.jcaho.org (30 September 2005).

17. Ibid.

18. C. H. Patterson, "Joint Commission on Accreditation of Healthcare Organizations," *Infection Control and Hospital Epidemiology* 16, no. 1 (1995): 36–42.

19. Joint Commission on Accreditation of Healthcare Organizations, "A Journey through the History of the Joint Commission."

20. Joint Commission on Accreditation of Healthcare Organizations, "Accreditation Decisions," April 2005, http://www.jcaho.org/htba/hospitals/survey+process/accreditation+decisions.htm (30 September 2005).

21. See discussion in B. R. Furrow, "Regulating Patient Safety: Toward a Federal Model of Medical Error Reduction," *Widener Law Review* 12, no. 1 (2006): 1–38.

22. Criticisms of JCAHO are discussed in U.S. General Accounting Office, *CMS*

Needs Additional Authority to Adequately Oversee Patient Safety in Hospitals, Report No. GAO-04-850, 20 July 2004.

23. See A. Donabedian, "The Quality of Care: How Can It Be Assessed?" *Journal of the American Medical Association* 260, no. 12 (1998): 1743–1758; and J. Mant, "Process versus Outcome Indicators in Assessment of Quality of Health Care," *International Journal for Quality in Health Care* 13, no. 6 (2001): 475–480.

24. Committee on Quality of Health Care in America, Institute of Medicine, *To Err Is Human* (Washington, DC: National Academy Press, 2000).

25. Joint Commission on Accreditation of Healthcare Organizations, "Joint Commission Welcome Page," 2005, http://www.jcaho.org (30 September 2005).

26. Committee on Quality of Health Care in America, Institute of Medicine, *To Err Is Human.*

27. Committee on Quality of Health Care in America, Institute of Medicine, *Crossing the Quality Chasm: A New Health System for the Twenty-first Century* (Washington, DC: National Academy Press, 2001).

28. Act 13, 49 P.S. § 1303.301 et seq.

29. P.L. 109–41.

30. Regulations implementing these requirements are published at 42 C.F.R. Part 482.

31. See the discussion of medical error reduction approaches in Furrow, "Regulating Patient Safety."

32. See Committee on Quality of Health Care in America, *Crossing the Quality Chasm,* 173–174.

33. United Network for Organ Sharing, *Timeline of Key Events in U.S. Transplantation and UNOS History,* 2005, http://www.unos.org/whoWeAre/history.asp (3 October 2005).

34. Ibid.

35. P.L. 98–507.

36. U.S. General Accounting Office, *Organ Transplants: Increased Effort Needed to Boost Supply and Ensure Equitable Distribution of Organs,* Report GAO-HRD-93-56, 22 April 1993.

37. 42 C.F.R. Part 121.

38. U.S. Department of Health and Human Services, "Division of Transplantation," http://www.hrsa.gov/osp/dot/dotmain.htm (10 August 2005).

39. United Network for Organ Sharing, *What We Do: Organ Center,* 2005, http://www.unos.org/whatWeDo/organcenter.asp (3 August 2005).

40. S. D. Halpern, P. A. Ubel, and A. L. Caplan, "Solid-Organ Transplantation in HIV-Infected Patients," *New England Journal of Medicine* 347, no. 4 (2002): 284–287.

41. G. J. Bazzoli et al., "Progress in the Development of Trauma Systems in the United States: Results of a National Survey," *Journal of the American Medical Association* 273, no. 5 (1995): 395–401.

42. R. J. Mullins, "A Historical Perspective of Trauma System Development in the United States," *Journal of Trauma* 47, no. 3 (1999): S8–S14.

43. Committee on Trauma, and Committee on Shock, Division of Medical Sciences, National Academy of Sciences/National Research Council, *Accidental Death and Disability: The Neglected Disease of Modern Society* (Washington, DC: National Academy Press, 1966).

44. P.L. 89–564.

45. P.L. 93-154 and P.L. 94-573.

46. Committee on Trauma, American College of Surgeons, "Optimal Hospital Resources for Care of the Seriously Injured," *Bulletin of the American College of Surgeons* 61 (1976): 15–55.

47. Bazzoli et al., "Progress in the Development of Trauma Systems in the United States."

48. Ibid.

49. Mullins, "Historical Perspective of Trauma System Development in the United States."

50. U.S. Department of Transportation, National Highway Traffic Safety Administration, "Emergency Medical Services Division," http://www.nhtsa.dot.gov/portal/site/nhtsa/menuitem .2a0771e91315babbbf30811060008a0c/ (25 October 2005).

51. P.L. 101–590.

52. Health Resources and Services Administration, "Trauma Emergency Medical Services System," http://www.hrsa.gov/trauma/overview.htm (11 August 2005).

53. Ibid.

54. Ibid.

55. R. R. Bass, P. S. Gainer, and A. R. Carlini, "Update on Trauma System Development in the United States," *Journal of Trauma* 47, no. 3 (1999): S15–S21.

56. Ibid.

57. Ibid.

58. Bazzoli et al., "Progress in the Development of Trauma Systems in the United States."

59. Department of Health and Human Services, Office of Inspector General, "The External Review of Hospital Quality—the Role of Medicare Certification," Report No. OEI-01-97-00052, July 1999.

60. Ibid.

61. Ibid.

62. Emergency Medical Treatment and Active Labor Act, 42 U.S.C. § 1395dd (1986).

63. This law also included protections for employees who lose health insurance because of termination of employment, which are discussed in more detail in chapter 3.

64. R. L. Schiff et al., "Transfers to a Public Hospital," *New England Journal of Medicine,* 314 no. 9 (1986): 552.

65. *Childs v. Weis,* 440 S.W.2d (Ct. of Civil App., Texas 1969).

66. L. C. Baker and L. S. Baker, "Excess Cost of Emergency Department Visits for Nonurgent Care," *Health Affairs* 13, no. 5 (1994): 162–171.

67. B. R. Furrow et al., *Health Law,* 5th ed. (St. Paul, MN: West, 2004), 538.

68. 42 U.S.C. §§ 263a et seq.

69. Centers for Medicare & Medicaid Services, "General Program Description," 16 September 2004, http://www.cms.hhs.gov/clia/progdesc.asp (3 October 2005).

70. Centers for Medicare & Medicaid Services, "CLIA Data Base," August 2005, https://www.cms.hhs.gov/clia/statupda.pdf (3 October 2005).

71. Hill-Burton Act, 42 U.S.C. §§ 291 et seq. (1946).

72. Starr, *Social Transformation of American Medicine,* 350.

73. Until 1963, hospitals in the South were permitted to meet the nondiscrimination requirement by providing services that were separated by race but of equal quality. This was

a vestige of the doctrine of "separate but equal" that had permitted states to maintain public facilities, including schools, that were segregated by race but that was overturned by the Supreme Court in 1954 in the case of *Brown v. Board of Education*, 347 U.S. 483 (1954).

74. Starr, *Social Transformation of American Medicine*, 349–350.

75. See discussion in Stevens, *In Sickness and in Wealth*, 200–226.

76. Comprehensive Health Planning and Services Act, 42 U.S.C. § 246 (1966).

77. National Health Planning and Resources Development Act of 1974, P.L. 93–641, 88 Stat. 2225 (4 January 1975) codified at 42 U.S.C. subchapter XIII § 300k et seq. and 42 U.S.C. subchapter XIV §§ 3000 et. seq.

78. Starr, *Social Transformation of American Medicine*, 399.

79. P. J. McGinley, "Beyond Health Care Reform: Reconsidering Certificate of Need Laws in a Managed Competition System," 1995, http://www.law.fsu.edu/journals/lawreview/issues/231/mcginley.html (3 October 2005).

80. Those states with no CON programs at all include Arizona, California, Colorado, Idaho, Indiana, Kansas, Minnesota, New Mexico, North Dakota, Pennsylvania, South Dakota, Texas, Utah, and Wyoming. American Health Planning Association, "National Directory of Health Planning, Policy and Regulatory Agencies 16th edition," January 2005, http://ahpanet.org/images/ahpadirectoryinfo.pdf (19 October 2005).

81. See C. Harrington et al., "Trends in State Certificate of Need and Moratoria Programs for Long-Term Care Providers," *Journal of Health and Social Policy* 19, no. 2 (2004): 31–58.

82. W. C. Hsiao et al., "Lessons of the New Jersey DRG Payment System," *Health Affairs* 5, no. 2 (1986): 32–45.

83. J. J. Baker, "Medicare Payment System for Hospital Inpatients: Diagnosis-Related Groups," *Journal of Health Care Finance* 28, no. 3 (2002): 1–13.

84. See D. Schactman, "Specialty Hospitals, Ambulatory Surgery Centers, and General Hospitals: Charting a Wise Public Policy Course," *Health Affairs* 24, no. 3 (2005): 868–873.

85. The prospective payment system for nursing home care was mandated by Congress in section 4432(a) of the Balanced Budget Act of 1997, P.L. 108-173, codified at 42 U.S.C. § 1395. The system is described at http://www.cms.hhs.gov/providers/snfpps/snfpps_overview.asp (25 October 2005). The system for ambulatory services was mandated by section 4523 of the same law. It is described at http://www.cms.hhs.gov/regulations/hopps/default .asp.

86. See K. E. Thorpe, "Health Care Cost Containment: Reflections and Future Directions," in A. R. Kovner and S. Jonas, eds., *Health Care Delivery in the United States*, 6th ed. (New York: Springer, 1999), 449.

87. D. W. Light and M. Widman, *Regulating Prospective Payment: An Analysis of the New Jersey Hospital Rate Setting Commission* (Ann Arbor, MI: Health Administration Press, 1988).

88. E. J. Schneiter, T. Riley, and J. Rosenthal, "Rising Health Care Costs: State Health Cost Containment Approaches," *National Academy for State Health Policy*, June 2002, http://nashp.org/Files/GNL46.pdf (3 October 2005).

89. J. E. McDonough, "Tracking the Demise of State Hospital Rate Setting," *Health Affairs* 16, no. 1 (1997): 142–149.

90. Schneiter, Riley, and Rosenthal, "Rising Health Care Costs."

91. McDonough, "Tracking the Demise of State Hospital Rate Setting."

92. Robert Wood Johnson Foundation, "Research to Monitor and Evaluate Massachusetts' Health Reform Law," January 2001, http://rwjf.org/reports/grr/023465.htm (3 October 2005).

93. R. E. Mechanic, S. Ginsburg, M. D. Williams, J. Kates, and H. T. Tu, "Health System Change in Newark, New Jersey: Case Study, September 1997," *Center for Studying Health System Change,* http://www.hschange.com/CONTENT/220 (7 September 2005).

94. New York State Department of Health, "Governor's Task Force Makes Recommendations on Reforming the State's Health Care Financing System," 5 December 1995, http://www.health.state.ny.su/nysdoh/consumer/pressrel/reform.htm (17 October 2005). See also the Public Policy Institute of New York State, Inc., "Misguided Money: A Health-Care System in Transition," http://www.bcnys.org/ppi/misgd1.htm (25 October 2005).

95. Maryland's Health Services Cost Review Commission, "About HSCRC," 14 September 2005, http://www.hscrc.state.md.us/about_hscrc/AboutHSCRC.htm (19 October 2005). See also Maryland Health Care Commission, "Maryland Hospital Evaluation Guide," http://hospitalguide.mhcc.state.md.us/ (19 October 2005).

96. 42 U.S.C. § 12101 et seq.

97. 29 U.S.C. § 749 et seq.

98. See, for example, *Bragdon v. Abbott,* 524 U.S. 624 (1998); and *Howe v. Hull,* 874 F.Supp. 779 (N.D. Ohio 1994).

99. Ibid.

100. For information regarding the role of the Office for Civil Rights in enforcing the Americans with Disabilities Act, see U.S. Department of Health and Human Services, "Office for Civil Rights: Your Rights under the Americans with Disabilities Act," 2005, http://www.hhs.gov/ocr/ada.html (6 October 2005).

101. For information regarding the role of the Equal Employment Opportunity Commission in enforcing the Americans with Disabilities Act and the Civil Rights Act, see U.S. Equal Opportunity Commission, "Overview—Laws," 20 April 2004, http://www.eeoc.gov/abouteeo/overview_laws.html (6 October 2005).

102. The laws that the Equal Employment Opportunity Commission enforces include the Americans with Disabilities Act, the Civil Rights Act of 1964, the Rehabilitation Act of 1973, and the Equal Pay Act of 1963. See U.S. Equal Opportunity Commission, "Laws Enforced by the EEOC," 15 January 1997, http://www.eeoc.gov/policy/laws.html (6 October 2005).

103. 42 U.S.C. § 2000d et seq.

104. U. S. Department of Health and Human Services, Office for Civil Rights, "Welcome to the Office for Civil Rights," http://www.hhs.gov/ocr/ada.html (6 October 2005).

105. W. L. Dowling, "Hospitals and Health Systems," in S. J. Williams and P. R. Torrens, eds., *Introduction to Health Services,* 5th ed. (Albany, NY: Delmar, 1999), 271.

106. 26 U.S.C. § 501©(3).

107. See Internal Revenue Service, "Chapter 3—Section 501(c)(3) Organizations," in *Tax-Exempt Status for Your Organization,* Publication 557 (March 2005), http://www.unclefed.com/Tax-Help/HTML/p557/ch03.html.

108. See IRS Revenue Ruling 97–21 (1997) http://www.unclefed.com/Tax-Bulls/1997/ Rr97–21.pdf (17 October 2005).

109. See statistics summarized in Dowling, "Hospitals and Health Systems," 270.

110. N. J. Wilson and K. W. Kizer, "The VA Health Care System: An Unrecognized National Safety Net," *Health Affairs* 16, no. 4 (1997): 200–204.

111. http://www1.va.gov/opa/fact/vafacts.html (retrieved 12 September 2005).

112. Ibid.

113. Ibid.

114. Dowling, "Hospitals and Health Systems," 29–31.

115. R. Galvin, "The Complex World of Military Medicine: A Conversation with William Winkenwerder," *Health Affairs*, Web Exclusive W5 (4 August 2005): W353–W357.

116. TRICARE: U.S. Department of Military Health, "TRICARE Beneficiaries," 13 October 2005, http://www.tricare.osd.mil (17 October 2005).

117. U.S. Department of Health and Human Services, Indian Health Services, "Indian Health Service Introduction," 7 February 2005, http://www.ihs.gov/PublicInfo/PublicAffairs/ Welcome_Info/IHSintro.asp (19 October 2005).

118. Ibid.

119. P.L. 93–638.

120. See L. E. Kazis et al., "Health Status in VA Patients: Results from the Veterans Health Study," *American Journal of Medical Quality* 14, no. 1 (1999): 28–38. See also S. F. Khuri et al., "The Department of Veterans Affairs' NSQIP: The First National, Validated, Outcome-Based, Risk-Adjusted, and Peer-Controlled Program for the Measurement and Enhancement of the Quality of Surgical Care, National VA Surgical Quality Improvement Program." *Annals of Surgery* 228, no. 4 (1998): 491–507.

121. Dowling, "Hospitals and Health Systems," 272.

122. The National Association of Public Hospitals and Health Systems, "Home Page," 2005, http://www.naph.org (18 October 2005).

123. For a discussion of characteristics of different kinds of long-term care service providers, see H. Richardson, C. Raphael, and L. Barton, "Long-Term Care: Health, Social, and Housing Services for Those with Chronic Illness," in A. R. Kovner and S. Jonas (eds.). *Health Care Delivery in the United States*, 6th ed. (New York: Springer, 1999), 213–237.

124. C. J. Evashwick, "The Continuum of Long-Term Care," in S. J. Williams and P. R. Torrens, eds., *Introduction to Health Services*, 5th ed., 313–317.

125. See Richardson, Raphael, and Barton, "Long-Term Care," 225–226.

126. Evashwick, "Continuum of Long-Term Care," 328.

127. Ibid., 317–328.

128. Richardson, Raphael, and Barton, "Long-Term Care," 214.

129. Furrow et al. *Health Law*, 736. See 42 U.S.C. § 1395d(a)(4).

130. Kaiser Commission on Medicaid and the Uninsured, *The Medicaid Resource Book* (Washington, DC: Kaiser Family Foundation, 2002), 53.

131. Kaiser Commission on Medicaid and the Uninsured, *Medicaid: A Primer* (Washington, DC: Kaiser Family Foundation, 2005), 8.

132. Nursing Home Reform Act, 42 U.S.C.S. §§ 1396 et seq. (1987).

133. U.S. General Accounting Office, *Nursing Homes: Prevalence of Serious Quality Prob-*

lems Remains Unacceptably High Despite Some Decline, Report GAO-03–1016T, 17 July 2003.

134. U.S. General Accounting Office, *California Nursing Homes: Federal and State Oversight Inadequate to Protect Residents in Homes with Serious Care Violations,* Report GAOT–HEHS-98–219, 28 July 1998.

135. B. Wright, "Federal and State Enforcement of the 1987 Nursing Home Reform Act—Fact Sheet," American Association of Retired Persons Web site, February 2001, http://www .aarp.org/research/longtermcare/nursinghomes/aresearch-import-686–FS83.html (19 October 2005).

136. Ibid.

137. M. Hash, Deputy Administrator, HCFA. "Testimony on Improving Oversight and Quality of Nursing Home Care," before the Senate Special Committee on Aging, 4 November 1999, http://www.hhs.gov/asl/testify/t991104a.html (18 October 2005).

138. U.S. Government Accounting Office, *Nursing Homes.*

139. North Carolina Code, Chapter 114, Article 4, Section 114–19.10.

140. New Jersey Department of Health and Senior Services, "New Jersey Nursing Home Oversight Program—Who Regulates Nursing Homes?" 20 June 2005, http://www.state.nj.us/health/ltc/penalty/report.shtml (18 October 2005).

141. Centers for Medicare & Medicaid Services, "CMS at a Glance," http://www.cms .hhs .gov/?1=cmsg (18 October 2005).

142. Centers for Medicare & Medicaid Services, "Quality Initiatives," 23 September 2005, http://www.cms.hhs.gov/quality/ (18 October 2005).

143. Centers for Medicare & Medicaid Services, "Quality Improvement Organizations," 16 September 2004, http://www.cms.hhs.gov/qio (17 October 2005).

144. Joint Commission on Accreditation of Healthcare Organizations, "Facts about . . . ," July 2004 http://www.jcaho.com/about+us/jcaho_facts.htm (19 October 2005).

145. Joint Commission on Accreditation of Healthcare Organizations, "Facts about Joint Commission Advisory Groups," February 2005, http://www.jcaho.com/about+us/facts+ about+advisory+groups.htm (19 October 2005).

146. Ibid.

147. See discussion in M. K. Wynia et. al., "Medical Professionalism in Society," *New England Journal of Medicine* 341, no. 21 (1999): 1612–1617.

148. Reports of the Pennsylvania Health Care Cost Containment Council are available at http://www.phc4.org (18 October 2005).

149. A press report that discussed the potential value of reports of the Pennsylvania Health Care Cost Containment Council for patients in choosing among hospitals is J. Goldstein, "Report on Pa. Hospitals Can Help Patients Choose," *Philadelphia Inquirer,* 29 September 2005, C1.

150. A dispute over the meaning of hospital mortality statistics reported by the Pennsylvania Health Care Cost Containment Council is presented in S. Burling, "Penn Hospital Gets Low Marks in a Report on Mortality Rates—The Hospital of the University of Pennsylvania Had Higher Rates in Five Areas. Officials Said the Study Missed Key Factors," *Philadelphia Inquirer,* 19 December 2001, B1.

Chapter 4

1. U.S. Census Bureau, "Health Insurance Coverage: 2003," 16 February 2005, http://www. census.gov/hhes/www/hlthins/hlthin03.html (7 September 2005).

2. U.S. Office of Personnel Management, "Federal Employees Health Benefits Program," http://www.opm.gov/insure/health/index.asp (23 September 2005).

3. U.S. General Accounting Office, *DOD and VA Health Care: Incentives Programs for Sharing Resources*, Report GAO-04–495R, 27 February 2004, Indian Health Service, 26 November 2004, http://www.ihs.gov (7 October 2005).

4. S. Woolhandler and D. U. Himmelstein, "Paying for National Health Insurance—and Not Getting It," *Health Affairs* 21, no. 4 (2002): 88–98.

5. Employee Retirement Income Security Act of 1974, 29 U.S.C. § 1144 (1974).

6. For a description of the health care finance system in the United States, see K. E. Thorpe and J. R. Knickman, "Financing Health Care," in A. R. Kovner and S. Jonas, eds., *Health Care Delivery in the United States,* 6th ed. (New York: Springer, 1999), 32–63.

7. P. Starr, *The Social Transformation of American Medicine* (New York: Basic Books, 1982), 240–243.

8. J. Melling, "An Inspector Calls: Perspectives on the History of Occupational Diseases and Accident Compensation in the United Kingdom," *Medical History* 49, no. 1 (2005): 102–106.

9. For historical background on workers compensation, see P. V. Fishback and S. E. Kantor, *A Prelude to the Welfare States: The Origins of Workers Compensation* (Chicago: University of Chicago Press, 2000). See also J. Gruber and A. B. Kruegger, "The Incidence of the Mandated Employer-Provided Insurance: Lessons from Worker's Compensation Insurance," December 1990, NBER Working Paper W3557, http://ssrn.com/abstract=226842 (4 November 2005).

10. Starr, *Social Transformation of American* Medicine, 295–310.

11. Ibid., 295.

12. T. S. Bodenheimer and K. Grumbach, *Understanding Health Policy: A Clinical Approach* (New York: Lange Medical Books/McGraw-Hill, 2002), 7.

13. R. Cunningham and R. M. Cunningham, *The Blues: A History of the Blue Cross and Blue Shield System* (DeKalb: Northern Illinois University Press, 1997).

14. Starr, *Social Transformation of American Medicine,* 297.

15. Ibid.

16. Cunningham and Cunningham, *The Blues.*

17. Starr, *Social Transformation of American Medicine,* 307.

18. Ibid., 311.

19. Ibid.

20. Ibid., 320–322.

21. 26 U.S.C. § 3121.

22. Woolhandler and Himmelstein, "Paying for National Health Insurance," 88–98.

23. See Department of the Treasury, Internal Revenue Service, "IRS Publication 502—Medical and Dental Expenses," http://www.irs.gov/publications/p502/ (4 November 2005).

24. U.S. Census Bureau, "Health Insurance Coverage: 2003," 16 February 2005, www .census.gov/hhes/www/hlthins/hlthin03.html (7 September 2005).

25. 26 U.S.C. §125. These accounts are also described in Department of the Treasury, Internal Revenue Service, "IRS Publication 502"; and H. T. Saleem, "Health Spending Accounts," U.S. Department of Labor, Bureau of Labor Statistics, 19 December 2003, http:// www.bls.gov/opub/cwc/cm20031022ar01p1.htm (4 November 2005).

26. Starr, *Social Transformation of American Medicine,* 327–331.

27. For a discussion of the history and structure of HMOs, see A. A. Kovner, "Health Maintenance Organizations and Managed Care," in A. R. Kovner and S. Jonas, eds., *Health Care Delivery in the United States,* 6th ed. (New York: Springer, 1999), 280–300.

28. Ibid.

29. Health Maintenance Organization Act, 42 U.S.C. § 280c, 300c, et seq. (1973).

30. A. J. Rosoff, "The Business of Medicine: Problems with the Corporate Practice Doctrine," *Specialty Law Digest—Health Care Monthly* 9, no. 14 (1988): 7–25.

31. For a description of any willing provider laws, see A. Carroll and J. M. Ambrose, "Any-Willing-Provider Laws: Their Financial Effect on HMOs," *Journal of Health Politics, Policy and Law* 27, no. 6 (2002): 927–945.

32. M. Markovich, *The Rise of HMOs* (RGSD-172), Rand Corporation, March 2003, http://www.rand.org/publications/RGSD/RGSD172/index.html (7 October 2005).

33. J. C. Robinson, *The Corporate Practice of Medicine* (Berkeley: University of California Press, 1999), 42–45.

34. See W. A. Zelman, *The Changing Health Care Marketplace* (San Francisco: Jossey-Bass, 1996), 16.

35. McCarran-Ferguson Act, 15 U.S.C. §§ 1011–1014.

36. National Committee for Quality Assurance, "Measuring the Quality of America's Health Care," 2005, http://www.ncqa.org/Communications/Publications/overviewncqa.pdf (7 October 2005).

37. National Committee for Quality Assurance, "About NCQA," http://www.ncqa.org/ about/about.htm (27 October 2005).

38. McCarran-Ferguson Act, 15 U.S.C. §§ 1011–1014.

39. U.S. Office of Personnel Management, "The Federal Employees Health Benefits Program (FEHB)," 2002, http://www.opm.gov/pressrel/2002/fehb/FEHB_FAQ.asp (7 October 2005).

40. The health benefits program for federal personnel is described in U.S. Office of Personnel Management, "FEHB Handbook," http://www.opm.gov/insure/handbook/fehb01 .asp (27 October 2005).

41. C. Middleton, "How to Improve the Federal Employees Health Benefits Program," *Pacific Research Institute* 78, 12 December 2001, http://www.pacificrescarch.org/pub/act/ 2001/act_01–12–12.html (7 October 2005).

42. U.S. Office of Personnel Management, "The Federal Employees Health Benefits Program (FEHB)," 2002, http://www.opm.gov/pressrel/2002/fehb/FEHB_FAQ.asp (7 October 2005).

43. F. P. McArdle, "Opening Up the Federal Employee Benefits Program," *Health Affairs* 14, no. 2 (1995): 40–50; see also J. Breaux, "The Breaux Plan: A Radically Centrist

Approach to a New Health Care System," *Health Affairs,* Web Exclusive W3 (5 March 2003): W131–W134.

44. Employee Retirement Income Security Act of 1974, 29 U.S.C. § 1144(b)(2), et seq. (1974).

45. See U.S. Department of Labor, "Reporting and Disclosure Guide for Employee Benefit Plans," April 2004, http://www.dol.gov/ebsa/pdf/rdguide.pdf (27 October 2005).

46. For a discussion of conflicts caused by ERISA, see E. H. Morreim, *Holding Health Care Accountable* (New York: Oxford University Press, 2001), 160–186.

47. *Aetna Health v. Davila,* 542 U.S. 200 (2004).

48. Comprehensive Omnibus Budget Reconciliation Act, 26 U.S.C. § 9801 (1986).

49. Health Insurance Portability and Accountability Act, 42 U.S.C. §§ 300gg, et seq. (1996).

50. P.L. 104–204, 110 stat. 2944.

51. P.L. 104–204, Title VI, § 605 (a)(4) codified at 110 Stat. 2941, 42 U.S.C. § 300 gg-4.

52. P.L. 105–277, codified at 294 U.S.C. § 1185 et. seq.

53. P.L. 79–725.

54. Starr, *Social Transformation of American Medicine,* 349–350.

55. Ibid., 389.

56. Many hospitals in the South, however, were permitted until 1963 to provide services that were separated by race if equal quality could be demonstrated. See Starr, *Social Transformation of American Medicine,* 350.

57. Hill-Burton, 42 U.S.C. §§ 291 et seq. (1970).

58. Hill-Burton requirements for hospitals that received funding are contained in regulations of DHHS published at 42 C.F.R. Part 124. They are summarized in Office for Civil Rights, Department of Health and Human Services, "Your Rights under the Community Service Assurance Provision of the Hill-Burton Act," June 2000, http://hhs.gov/ocr.hburton .html (1 November 2005).

59. Starr, *Social Transformation of American Medicine,* 368.

60. Kerr-Mills Act, 86 P.L. 778, 74 Stat. 924 (1960).

61. Starr, *Social Transformation of American Medicine,* 369.

62. R. A. Culbertson and P. R. Lee, "Medicare and Physician Autonomy," *Health Care Financing Review* 18, no. 2 (1996): 115–130.

63. See E. D. Hoffman, B. S. Klees, and C. A. Curtis, "Overview of the Medicare and Medicaid Programs," *Health Care Financing Review* 22, no. 1 (2000): 175–193.

64. M. Gluck and V. Reno, eds., "Reflections on Implementing Medicare," National Academy of Social Insurance, January 2001, http://www.nasi.org/usr_doc/med_report_reflec tions.pdf (7 October 2005).

65. For a discussion of the administration of the Medicaid program, see B. R. Furrow et al. *Health Law,* 5th ed. (St. Paul, MN: West, 2004), 772–802.

66. For a description of the structure of Medicaid benefits, see Kaiser Commission on Medicaid and the Uninsured, *The Medicaid Resource Book* (Washington, DC: Kaiser Family Foundation, 2002), and material contained in the Kaiser Family Foundation Web site, http://www.kff.org.

67. Furrow et al., *Health Law,* 774.

68. See, for example, provisions regarding some types of ambulatory care and institutional care contained at 42 U.S.C. § 1396a(a)(10)(C)(iii).

69. See discussion of EPSDT in J. Perkins, "Medicaid Early and Periodic Screening, Diagnosis and Treatment as a Source of Funding Early Intervention Services," *National Health Law Program,* 20 June 2002, http://www.healthlaw.org/library.cfm?fa=download& resourceID=61027&appView=folder&print (26 September 2005).

70. See, for example, *Hern v. Beye,* 57 F.2d 906 (10th Cir. 1995), concerning the obligation of states to cover abortion under Medicaid.

71. P.L. 92–603, 42 U.S.C. § 1395 ss.

72. J. K. Iglehart, "The End-Stage Renal Disease Program," *New England Journal of Medicine* 328, no. 5 (1993): 366–371.

73. A. R. Nissenson and R. A. Rettig, "Renal Disease Program: Current Status and Future Prospects," *Health Affairs* 18, no. 1 (1999): 161–179.

74. P.L. 95–292.

75. ESRD Networks' Annual Reports, 2003.

76. P.L. 108–173, codified at 42 U.S.C. §1395.

77. See discussion in T. R. Oliver et al., "A Political History of Medicare and Prescription Drug Coverage," *Milbank Quarterly* 82, no. 2 (2004): 283–354.

78. The complex mechanism through which the Medicare prescription drug benefit is implemented under the Medicare Modernization Act is described in T. S. Jost, "The Most Important Health Care Legislation of the Millennium (So Far): The Medicare Modernization Act," *Yale Journal of Health Policy, Law, and Ethics,* 2005, http://ssrn.com/abstract= 661081; and in B. M. Meyer and K. M. Cantwell, "The Medicare Prescription Drug, Improvement, and Modernization Act of 2003: Implications for Health-System Pharmacy," *American Journal of Health-System Pharmacy* 61 (2004): 1042–1051. The effects on Medicaid are discussed in detail in Kaiser Family Foundation, *Implications of the Medicare Modernization Act for States: Observations from a Focus Group Discussion with Medicaid Directors* (Washington, DC: Kaiser Family Foundation, 2005), available at http://www.kff.org/medicaid/ uploadImplications-of-the-Medicare-Modernization-Act-for-States-Observations-from-a-Focus-Group-Discussion-with-Medicaid-Director-Report.pdf.

79. One approach to reforming Medicare that is frequently discussed would transform it into a mechanism that provides financial support for the purchase of insurance policies from private companies, most of which would provide coverage through managed care arrangements. See G. R. Wilensky and J. P. Newhouse, "Medicare: What's Right? What's Wrong? What's Next?" *Health Affairs* 18, no. 1(1999): 92–106.

80. See National Academy of Social Insurance (NASI), Study Panel on Medicare's Management and Governance, *Reflections on Implementing Medicare* (Washington, DC: National Academy of Social Insurance, 2001).

81. See L. D. Schaeffer, "Turning Medicare and Medicaid into Health Programs: The Role of Organizational Culture," *Health Affairs* Web Exclusive W5(2005): 329–330.

82. National Academy of Social Insurance, *Reflections on Implementing Medicare,* v.

83. Ibid.

84. Ibid.

85. Ibid.

86. S. Duff, "Drop in the Bucket: Newly Seen Surplus Not Encouraging," *Modern Healthcare* 32, no. 10 (2002): 16.

87. *Medicare Chart Book 2005* (Washington, DC: Kaiser Family Foundation, 2005), available at http://www.kff.org/medicare/upload/Medicare-Chart-Book-3rd-Edition-Summer-2005–Report.pdf (25 October 2005).

88. Kaiser Family Foundation, "Medicaid Enrollment and Spending Trends" (Washington, DC: Kaiser Family Foundation, 2005), available at http://www.kff.org/medicaid/upload/Medicaid-Enrollment-and-Spending-Trends-Fact-Sheet.pdf (25 October 2005).

89. A. J. Bhatia et al., "Evolution of Quality Review Programs for Medicare: Quality Assurance to Quality Improvement," *Health Care Financing Review* 22, no. 1 (2000): 69–75.

90. Background on the PSRO program is discussed in Committee on PSRO Disclosure Policy, Institute of Medicine, *Access to Medical Review Data: Disclosure Policy for Professional Standards Review Organizations* (Washington, DC: National Academy Press, 1981).

91. Peer Review Improvement Act of 1982, 42 U.S.C. §§ 1305, 1320c et seq. (1982).

92. Research indicates that QIOs have not been effective in improving hospital quality. See C. Snyder and G. Anderson, "Do Quality Improvement Organizations Improve the Quality of Hospital Care for Medicare Beneficiaries?" *Journal of the American Medical Association* 293, no. 23 (2005): 2900–2907.

93. See J. J. Baker, "Medicare Payment System for Hospital Inpatients Diagnosis-Related Groups," *Journal of Health Care Finance* 28, no. 3 (2002): 1–13.

94. See L. L. Keough, "DSH Adjustment Controversies Continue," *Healthcare Financial Management* 56, no. 11 (2002): 84–86.

95. Tax Equity and Fiscal Responsibility Act of 1982, 42 U.S.C. §§ 1395, 1395x, 1396a (1982).

96. S. Suthummanon and V. K. Omachonu, "DRG-Based Cost Minimization Models: Applications in a Hospital Environment," *Health Care Management Science* 7, no. 3 (2004): 197–205.

97. Kaiser Family Foundation, *Medicare Chart Book*, 3rd ed. (Washington, DC: Kaiser Family Foundation, Summer 2005), 55, available at http://www.kff.org/medicare/upload/Medicare-Chart-Book-3rd-Edition-Summer-2005–Section-6.pdf (25 October 2005).

98. For background on the development of the RBRVS system, see Culbertson and Lee, "Medicare and Physician Autonomy," 124–126.

99. For a discussion of the relationship between RBRBS and physician autonomy, see ibid.

100. C. White, "Rehabilitation Therapy in Skilled Nursing Facilities: Effects of Medicare's New Prospective Payment System," *Health Affairs* 22, no. 3 (2003): 214–223.

101. J. S. Lee, R. A. Berenson, R. Mayes, and A. K. Gauthier, "Medicare Payment Policy: Does Cost-Shifting Matter?" *Health Affairs,* Web Exclusive W3 (8 October 2003): W480–W488.

102. Medicare Act, 74 P.L. 271, 49 Stat. 620 (1965).

103. Medicare Payment Advisory Commission, "Payment for New Technologies in Medicare's Prospective Payment Systems," in *Report to the Congress: Medicare Payment Policy* (Washington, DC: Medicare Payment Advisory Commission, 2003), 177–192.

104. 42 U.S.C. § 217(a).

105. Centers for Medicare & Medicaid Services, "Medicare Coverage—Medicare Coverage Advisory Committee (MCAC)," http://www.cms.hhs.gov/mcac/ (7 October 2005).

106. Medicare Payment Advisory Commission (MedPAC), "Advising the Congress on Medicare Issues," http://www.medpac.gov/ (7 October 2005).

107. Centers for Medicare & Medicaid Services, "The Provider Reimbursement Review Board," 28 February 2005, http://www.cms.hhs.gov/providers/prrb/prrb.asp (7 November 2005).

108. Omnibus Budget Reconciliation Act of 1981, P.L. 97–35. The development and early experience with waivers that permitted states to use managed care to deliver Medicaid services is discussed in A. Dobson, D. Moran, and G. Young, "The Role of Federal Waivers in the Health Policy Process," *Health Affairs* 11, no. 4 (1992): 72–94.

109. D. Rowland and R. Garfield, "Health Care for the Poor: Medicaid at 35," *Health Care Financing Review* 22, no. 1 (2000): 23–34.

110. See J. Holahan et al., "Medicaid Managed Care in Thirteen States," *Health Affairs* 17, no. 3 (1998): 43–63.

111. A. E. Benjamin, "Health Policy and the Politics of Health Care," in S. J. Williams and P. R. Torrens, eds., *Introduction to Health Services,* 5th ed. (Albany, NY: Delmar, 1999), 457.

112. M. Gold, "Medicare+Choice: An Interim Report Card," *Health Affairs* 20, no. 4 (2001): 120–138.

113. For a description of one such proposal, see Wilensky and Newhouse, "Medicare."

114. The Oregon Medicaid plan is discussed in C. Ham, "Retracing the Oregon Trail: The Experience of Rationing and the Oregon Health Plan," *British Medical Journal* 316, no. 7149 (1998): 1965–1969.

115. Gail R. Wilensky, Chair, Medicare Payment Advisory Commission, "The Balanced Budget Act of 1997: A Current Look at Its Impact on Patients and Providers," statement before the Subcommittee on Health and Environment, Committee on Commerce, U.S. House of Representatives, 19 July 2000, 5–11, available at http://www .medpac.gov/publications/congressional_testimony/071900.pdf (25 October 2005).

116. Ibid., 2.

117. R. Tannenwald, "Implications for the Balanced Budget Act of 1997 for the 'Devolution Revolution,'" *Publius* 28, no. 1 (1998): 23–28.

118. A. Weil, "Chipping Away at the Uninsured," *Health Affairs* 23, no. 5 (2004): 153–154.

119. J. K. Ingelhart, "The Centers for Medicare and Medicaid Services," *New England Journal of Medicine* 345, no. 26 (2001): 1920–1924.

120. Ibid.

121. Ingelhart, "Centers for Medicare and Medicaid Services," 1920–1924.

122. Ibid.

123. Ibid.

124. CMS still has a responsibility to oversee various aspects of the operations of Medicare HMOs, such as beneficiary appeals procedures, marketing materials, and the composition of provider networks.

125. J. K. Ingelhart, "The American Health Care System—Medicare," *New England Journal of Medicine* 340, no. 4 (1999): 317–332.

126. Ingelhart, "Centers for Medicare and Medicaid Services," 1920–1924.

127. Ibid.

128. U.S. Department of Labor, Employee Benefits Security Administration, "Employee Benefits Security Administration Main Page: EBSA in the 21st Century," 2005, http://www.dol.gov/ebsa (7 October 2005).

129. Ibid.

130. See U.S. General Accounting Office, *Private Health Insurance: Wide Variation in State Insurance Departments' Regulatory Authority, Oversight, and Resources,* Report GAO-T-HRD-93-25, 27 May 1993.

131. Background on the National Association of Insurance Commissioners is available at http://www.naic.org/index_about.htm (7 November 2005).

132. For a discussion of the effects of Medicare on physician autonomy, see Culbertson and Lee, "Medicare and Physician Autonomy."

133. D. J. Palmisano, D. W. Emmons, and G. D. Wozniak, "Expanding Insurance Coverage through Tax Credits, Consumer Choice, and Market Enhancements: The American Medical Association Proposal for Health Insurance Reform," *Journal of the American Medical Association* 291, no. 18 (2004): 2237–2242.

134. Woolhandler and Himmelstein, "Paying for National Health Insurance," 88–98.

Chapter 5

1. Kaiser Family Foundation, "Prescription Drug Trends: Fact Sheet #3057–02," May 2003, http://www.kff.org/rxdrugs/upload/Prescription-Drug-Trends-October-2004-update.pdf (October 2004).

2. P. B. Hutt and P. B. Hutt II, "A History of Government Regulation of Adulteration and Misbranding of Food," *Food, Drug, and Cosmetic Law Journal* 39 (1984): 2–73.

3. Ibid., 9.

4. P. Hutt, "Transformation of United States Food and Drug Law," *Journal of the Association of Food and Drug Officials* 68, no. 3 (1996): 1–9.

5. U.S. Food and Drug Administration, "Milestones in US Food and Drug History," August 2005, http://www.fda.gov/opacom/backgrounders/miles.html (1 October 2005).

6. J. H. Young, "Food and Drug Administration (FDA)," in D. R. Whitnah, ed., *Government Agencies* (Westport, CT: Greenwood Press, 1983), 251.

7. See W. J. Heath, "America's First Drug Regulation Regime: The Rise and Fall of the Import Drug Act of 1848," *Food Drug Law Journal* 59, no. 1 (2004): 169–199.

8. W. Janssen, "The Story of the Laws behind the Labels," *FDA Consumer* 15, no. 5 (1981): 32–45.

9. P. Hilts, *Protecting America's Health: The FDA, Business, and One Hundred Years of Regulation* (New York: Knopf, 2003), 28.

10. W. Janssen, "Outline of the History of US Drug Regulation and Labeling," *Food, Drug, Cosmetic Law Journal* 36, no. 8 (1981): 420–441.

11. Ibid.

12. Ibid.

13. J. P. Swann, "Food and Drug Administration," in G. Kurian, ed., *A Historical Guide to US Government* (New York: Oxford University Press, 1998), 248.

14. U.S. Food and Drug Administration, "Milestones in US Food and Drug History," August 2005, http://www.fda.gov/opacom/backgrounders/miles.html (1 October 2005).

15. Hilts, *Protecting America's Health,* 69.

16. J. H. Young, *Pure Food: Securing the Federal Food and Drugs Act of 1906* (Princeton, NJ: Princeton University Press, 1989), 148.

17. 32 Stat. 728

18. Hilts, *Protecting America's Health,* 69.

19. Janssen, "The Story of the Laws behind the Labels," 32–45.

20. Hilts, *Protecting America's Health,* 49.

21. For background on the Pure Food and Drug Act of 1906, see ibid., and Young, *Pure Food.*

22. Pure Food and Drug Act of 1906, 30 June 1906, ch. 3915, 34 Stat. 768.

23. Federal Meat Inspection Act, Act 4 March 1907, ch. 2907, titles I to IV, 34 Stat. 1260, codified at 21 U.S.C. § 601 et seq.

24. Young, "Food and Drug Administration (FDA)," 253.

25. The United States Pharmacopoeia was established in 1820, when eleven physicians, three of whom were congressmen, met in the Senate chambers to establish principles for the preparation of the *Pharmacopoeia,* a book of drug standards. Since the passage of the 1906 act, the FDA has enforced its standards. See W. M. Heller, "The United States Pharmacopeia: Its Value to the Professions," *Journal of the American Medical Association* 213, no. 4 (1970): 576–579. See also Anonymous, "The United States Pharmacopeia 1820–1970," *American Journal of Hospital Pharmacy* 27 (1970): 223–227.

26. *United States v. Johnson,* 221 U.S. 448 (1911).

27. Swann, "Food and Drug Administration," 250.

28. Harrison Narcotics Tax Act of 1914, P.L. 223, 38 Stat. 785 (1914).

29. McNary-Mapes Amendment, P.L. 538, 46 Stat. 1019 (1930).

30. The scandal involving elixir of sulfanilamide and its effect in promoting passage of enhanced drug safety legislation is described in C. Crossen, "How Elixir Deaths Led U.S. to Require Proof of New Drugs' Safety," *Wall Street Journal,* 3 October 2005, B1.

31. C. Ballentine, "Taste of Raspberries, Taste of Death: The 1938 Elixir Sulfanilamide Incident," *FDA Consumer* 31, no. 6 (1981): 18–21; see also A. H. Hayes, "Food and Drug Regulation after 75 Years," *Journal of the American Medical Association,* 246, no. 11 (1981): 1223–1226; see also Hilts, *Protecting America's Health.*

32. Federal Food, Drug, and Cosmetic Act, 21 U.S.C. § 355c (1938).

33. Wheeler-Lea Act, 15 U.S.C. § 45 (1938).

34. 21 C.F.R. Part 300.

35. Background on the new drug approval process is presented in M. Mathieu, *New Drug Development: A Regulatory Overview* (Waltham, MA: Parexel International, 1994), 1–14.

36. Background on the process of clinical trials is available at ibid., 10–11.

37. Ibid., 12–14.

38. 21 C.F.R. Part 201 et seq.

39. 21 C.F.R. Part 17.

40. 21 C.F.R. § 314.80.

41. Issues raised by the FDA new drug approval process are discussed in S. L. Nightingale, "Drug Regulation and Policy Formulation," *Milbank Memorial Fund Quarterly* 59, no. 3 (1981): 412–444.

42. P. B. Fontanarosa, D. Rennie, and C. D. DeAngelis, "Postmarketing Surveillance—Lack of Vigilance, Lack of Trust," *Journal of the American Medical Association* 292, no. 21 (2004): 2647–2650.

43. Ibid.

44. Hayes, "Food and Drug Regulation after 75 Years," 1223–1226.

45. A. H. Kaplan, "Fifty Years of Drug Amendments Revisited in Easy-to-Swallow Capsule Form," *Food and Drug Law Journal* 50, no. 5 (1995): 179–197. See also Janssen, "The Story of the Laws behind the Labels," 32–45.

46. Delaney Amendment, 21 U.S.C. § 348 (1958).

47. Color Additive Amendment of 1960, 21 U.S.C. § 379e (1960).

48. See W. Lepkowski, "The Saccharin Debate: Regulation and the Public Taste," *Hastings Center Report* 7, no. 6 (1977): 5–7.

49. Saccharin Study and Labeling Act, 21 U.S.C. § 348 (1977).

50. P.L. 104–170.

51. Perhaps the most remarkable feature of the midcentury Kefauver hearings is how little the arguments on both sides have changed. Today, high prices are still defended on the basis of high research costs, politicians still point to Canada for cheaper drug prices, and the industry is still constantly criticized for excessive marketing activities.

52. T. D. Stephens, *Dark Remedy: The Impact of Thalidomide and Its Revival as a Vital Medicine* (Cambridge, MA: Perseus, 2001).

53. R. McFadyen, "Estes Kefauver and the Drug Industry" (Ph.D. diss., Emory University, 1973), abstract in *Dissertation Abstracts International,* 34, no. 5 (1973): 2524. See also Hilts, *Protecting America's Health.*

54. Janssen, "The Story of the Laws behind the Labels," 32–45.

55. Kaplan, "Fifty Years of Drug Amendments."

56. Hayes, "Food and Drug Regulation after 75 Years," 1223–1226.

57. Swann, "Food and Drug Administration," 253.

58. P.L. 94–295, 90 Stat. 539, codified at 21 U.S.C. §§ 360 et seq.

59. Janssen, "The Story of the Laws behind the Labels," 40.

60. See G. R. Higson, *Medical Device Safety: The Regulation of Medical Devices for Public Health and Safety* (Philadelphia: Institute of Physics Publishing, 2002); and L. H. Monsein, "Primer on Medical Device Regulation Part II: Regulation of Medical Devices by the U.S. Food and Drug Administration," *Radiology* 205, no. 1 (1997): 10–18.

61. To achieve consistency with the Uruguay Round of trade negotiations, Congress in 1994 enacted legislation that changed the term of patents in the United States to run for twenty years from the date of filing (P.L. 103–465). Patent terms had previously run for seventeen years from the date of approval.

62. R. Levy, "The Pharmaceutical Industry: A Discussion of Competitive and Antitrust Issues in an Environment of Change," Federal Trade Commission, March 1999, http://www.ftc.gov/reports/pharmaceutical/drugrep.pdf: p. 11 (7 October 2005).

63. *United States v. Generix Drug Corporation,* 460 U.S. 453 (1983).

64. P.L. 98–417, 1984 Stat. 1538 (codified as amended in scattered sections of 21 and 35 U.S.C.).

65. Levy, "Pharmaceutical Industry."

66. P.L. 100–670.

67. Pharmaceutical Research and Manufacturers Association of America, *PhRMA: Opportunities and Challenges for Pharmaceutical Innovation. Industry Profile, 1996* (Washington, DC: PhRMA, 1996).

68. Levy, "Pharmaceutical Industry."

69. The nature of patents is described by the U.S. Patent and Trademark Office at "Patents: The Collection for All Reasons," 15 March 2005, http://www.uspto.gov/go/ptdl/patreaso .htm (7 November 2005).

70. These conditions are listed in the congressional findings in support of the Orphan Drug Act, 21 U.S.C. §§ 360aa et seq. (1983), available at http://www.fda.gov/orphan/oda.htm.

71. Orphan Drug Act, 21 U.S.C. §§ 360aa et seq. (1983).

72. 21 U.S.C. § 360bb (1985).

73. J. Henkel, "Orphan Products: New Hope for People with Rare Disorders," FDA Consumer Special Report, January 1995, http://www.fda.gov/fdac/special/newdrug/orphan .html (7 October 2005).

74. Prescription Drug Marketing Act of 1987, 21 U.S.C. §§ 331, 333, 353, 381 (1988).

75. Nutrition Labeling and Education Act of 1990, 21 U.S.C. §§ 343 et seq., 350. (1990).

76. Safe Medical Devices Act of 1990, 21 U.S.C. §§ 360c et seq. (1990).

77. Federal Food, Drug, and Cosmetic Act, 21 U.S.C. § 321 (g)(1).

78. Dietary Supplement Health and Education Act of 1994, 21 U.S.C. §§ 321, 343 et seq., 350, 42 U.S.C. § 287c-11.

79. The lack of a requirement for premarket approval in DSHEA has engendered concern regarding substances such as ephedra that have been found to cause harm only after reaching the market. See P. B. Fontanarosa and D. Rennie, "The Need for Regulation of Dietary Supplements—Lessons from Ephedra," *Journal of the American Medical Association* 289, no. 12 (2003): 1568–1570.

80. D. M. Marcus and A. P. Grollman, "Botanical Medicines—The Need for New Regulations," *New England Journal of Medicine* 347, no. 25 (2002): 2073–2076.

81. Hilts, *Protecting America's Health,* 289.

82. Research indicates that most users of dietary supplements support increased government regulation of them, including requirements for premarket review and approval. See R. J. Blendon et al., "American's Views on the Use and Regulation of Dietary Supplements," *Archives of Internal Medicine* 161, no. 6 (2001): 805–810.

83. P.L. 102–571.

84. The effects of PDUFA on approval times for new drugs are described at U.S. Food

and Drug Administration, "Overview FY 2004 Performance Report to Congress," http:// www.fda.gov/ope/pdufa/report2004/overview.html (25 October 2005).

85. U.S. General Accounting Office, "Food and Drug Administration: Effect of User Fees on Drug Approval Times, Withdrawals and Other Agency Activities," Report No. GAO-02–958, 17 September 2002.

86. There is some question as to whether the reduction in FDA approval times for new drugs that was experienced after PDUFA's enactment was due to the user fee mechanism embodied in the law or to an increase in FDA staff during the five years prior to its passage. See D. Carpenter, M. Chernew, D. G. Smith, and A. M. Fendrick, "Approval Times for New Drugs: Does the Source of Funding for FDA Staff Matter?" *Health Affairs*, Web Exclusive, W3 (17 December 2003): W618–W624.

87. The challenge faced by the FDA in regulating new kinds of drug promotional efforts is described in D. A. Kessler and W. L. Pines, "The Federal Regulation of Prescription Drug Advertising and Promotion," *Journal of the American Medical Association* 264, no. 18 (1990): 2409–2415.

88. See A. R. Zappacosta, "Reversal of Baldness in Patient Receiving Minoxidil for Hypertension," *New England Journal of Medicine* 303, no. 25 (1980): 1480–1481.

89. *Washington Legal Foundation v. Shalala,* 13 F.Supp. 2d 51 (D.D.C. 1998).

90. 50 *Federal Register* 36677 (1999).

91. 64 *Federal Register* 43197 (1999).

92. Ibid.

93. This second guidance was published as a draft, and issuance of a final version was still pending as of late 2005, although it is likely to be quite similar.

94. U.S. National Institutes of Health, ClinicalTrials.gov, June 2004, http://clinicaltrials .gov (7 October 2005).

95. P.L. 105–115, § 112.

96. P.L. 105–115, § 113.

97. See R. E. Kauffman, "Scientific Issues in Biomedical Research with Children," in M. A. Grodin and L. H. Glantz, eds., *Children as Research Subjects* (New York: Oxford University Press, 1994), 29–80.

98. 21 U.S.C. § 355a (2005).

99. Modernization of the Food and Drug Administration, Testimony of Jane E. Henney, M.D., Commissioner of Food and Drug Administration before the Committee on Health, Education, Labor, and Pensions United States Senate, 21 October 1999, http:// www.fda.gov/ola/1999/modernization.html (25 October 2005).

100. 63 *Federal Register* 66632–72 (1998).

101. The long-term status of the Pediatric Rule is somewhat uncertain. A legal challenge is pending to its validity contending that it exceeds the FDA's authority, but a congressional proposal would codify it through statute.

102. R. Steinbrook, "Testing Medications in Children," *New England Journal of Medicine* 347, no. 18 (2002): 1462–1470.

103. Centers for Disease Control and Prevention, National Center for Health Statistics, "Therapeutic Drug Use," 1 August 2005, http://www.cdc.gov/nchs/fastats/drugs.htm (7 October 2005).

104. Alliance for Health Reform, "Chapter 7: Prescription Drugs," *Covering Health Issues 2002–2003: A Sourcebook for Journalists,* January 2003, http://www.allhealth.org/sourcebook2002/ch7_3.html (25 October 2005).

105. P.L. 108–173.

106. See A. S. Adams, S. B. Soumerai, and D. Ross-Degnan, "The Case for a Medicare Drug Coverage Benefit: A Critical Review of Empirical Evidence," *Annual Review of Public Health* 22 (2001): 49–61.

107. Prescription Drug Marketing Act of 1987, 21 U.S.C. §§ 331, 333, 353, 381 (1988).

108. Medicine Equity and Drug Safety Act, 21 U.S.C. § 384 (2000).

109. Medicare Prescription Drug, Improvement, and Modernization Act of 2003, Title XI.

110. Swann, "Food and Drug Administration," 250; see also Hilts, *Protecting America's Health.*

111. Hilts, *Protecting America's Health,* xiv.

112. Ibid., xv.

113. Professional and Occupational Licenses, N.M. Stat. Ann. § 61–9–17.1.

114. R. D. Miller and R. C. Hutton, *Problems in Health Care Law* (Gaithersburg, MD: Aspen, 2000), 78.

115. Federal Trade Commission Act, 15 U.S.C. § 45, 21 U.S.C. § 334.

116. Federal Alcohol Administration Act, 27 U.S.C. §§ 201, 202, 203, 204, 205.

117. Consumer Product Safety Act, 15 U.S.C. §§ 1261, 1262.

118. 21 U.S.C. §§ 451, 601, 604, 606, 671, 679c.

119. U.S. Drug Enforcement Administration, "DEA History," 17 September 2005, http://www.dea.gov/history.htm (7 October 2005).

120. Political challenges in FDA regulation are discussed in R. I. Field. "Political Realities," in M. I. Smith, A. I. Wertheimer, and J. E. Finchman, eds., *Pharmacy and the U.S. Health Care System* (Binghamton, NY: Pharmaceutical Products Press, 2005).

121. U. E. Reinhardt, "Perspectives on the Pharmaceutical Industry," *Health Affairs* 20, no. 5 (2001): 136–149.

122. L. Noah and B. A. Noah, *Law, Medicine and Medical Technology* (New York: Foundation Press, 2002), 6.

123. See Field, "Political Realities," 63.

Chapter 6

1. U.S. Department of Health and Human Services, "Public Health in America," 14 December 1999, http://www.hhs.gov/phfunctions/public.htm (15 May 2006).

2. P. Starr, *The Social Transformation of American Medicine* (New York: Basic Books, 1982), 185.

3. Ibid., 190.

4. P. A. Torrens and L. Breslow, "The Evolution of Public Health: A Joint Public-Private Responsibility," in S. J. Williams and P. A. Torrens, eds., *Introduction to Health Services,* 5th ed. (Albany, NY: Delmar, 1999), 207–225.

5. E. Fee and T. M. Brown, "The Unfulfilled Promise of Public Health: Déjà Vu All Over Again," *Health Affairs* 21, no. 6 (2002): 31–43.

6. G. Rosen, *A History of Public Health* (New York: MD Publications, 1958), 246.

7. Fee and Brown, "Unfulfilled Promise of Public Health," 31–43.

8. Starr, *Social Transformation of American Medicine,* 184.

9. Ibid., 185.

10. B. J. Turnock and B. Atchison, "Governmental Public Health in the United States: The Implications of Federalism," *Health Affairs* 21, no. 6 (2002): 68–78.

11. F. Mullan, *Plagues and Politics: The Story of the United States Public Health Service* (New York: Basic Books, 1989), 56.

12. Ibid.

13. Ibid., 31.

14. Ibid., 53.

15. U. Sinclair, *The Jungle* (New York: Viking, 1946).

16. Centers for Disease Control and Prevention, "Achievements in Public Health, 1900–1999: Safer and Healthier Foods," *Morbidity and Mortality Weekly Report* 48, no. 40 (1999): 905–913.

17. U.S. Department of Agriculture, "1999 Agriculture Fact Book," http://www.usda .gov/news/pubs/fbook99/sections/milestones.pdf (25 October 2005).

18. U.S. Department of Agriculture, Food and Nutrition Service, "Nutrition Connections: People, Programs, and Science; Conference Highlights and Proceedings," February 2003, http://www.fns.usda.gov/oane/menu/NNEC/2003NNEC/Files/proceedingspt1.pdf, (18 October 2005), p. 17.

19. J. L. Parascandola, "Public Health Service," in G. T. Kurian, ed., *A Historical Guide to the U.S. Government* (New York: Oxford University Press, 1998), 487–493.

20. Mullan, *Plagues and Politics.*

21. Centers for Disease Control and Prevention, "About CDC—Our Story," http:// www .cdc.gov/about/ourstory.htm (25 October 2005).

22. Parascandola, "Public Health Service."

23. U.S. Department of Health, Education, and Welfare, *Smoking and Health: Report of the Advisory Committee to the Surgeon General of the Public Health Service,* Public Health Service Publication No. 1103. (Washington, DC: U.S. Government Printing Office, 1964).

24. For background on CDC activities with regard to chronic diseases, see Centers for Disease Control and Prevention, *The Burden of Chronic Diseases and Their Risk Factors: National and State Perspectives 2004,* 19 May 2005, http://www.cdc.gov/nccdphp/burdenbook2004 (25 October 2005). The Epidemiology Branch, now know as the Epidemiology Program Office, is described at 18 March 2003, http://www.cdc.gov/epo/aboutepo.htm (25 October 2005).

25. P. Cotton, "CDC Nears Close of First Half-Century," *Journal of the American Medical Association* 263, no. 19 (1990): 2579–2580.

26. Centers for Disease Control and Prevention, "Office of Communication Media Relations," 22 October 2001, http://www.cdc.gov/od/oc/media/timeline.htm (25 October 2005).

27. As an example of this concern, in 1990, Congress passed the Nutrition Labeling and Education Act, P.L. 101-535, which regulates packaging information on food content and health

claims. Nutrition programs at CDC are described at http://www.cdc.gov/nccdphp/dnpa/about_ us/index .htm (7 November 2005), and at USDA at http://www.nutrition.gov/ (7 November 2005).

28. National Environmental Protection Act of 1969, P.L. 91-190, codified at 42 U.S.C. §§ 4321-4347 (1 January 1970).

29. Federal Water Pollution Control Act of 1977, commonly known as the Clean Water Act of 1977, P.L. 95-217, codified at 33 U.S.C. §§ 1251 et seq. The law was originally enacted as the Federal Water Pollution Control Act Amendments of 1972, P.L. 92-500, and became known as the Clean Water Act when it was amended in 1977.

30. Clean Air Act of 1970, P.L. 91-604, 84 Stat. 1678, codified at 42 U.S.C. §§ 7401 et seq. (31 December 1970). The history of the law is discussed in E. S. Muskie, "NEPA to CERCLA—The Clean Air Act: A Commitment to Public Health," *Environmental Forum,* January/February 1990, http://www.cleanairtrust.org/nepa2cercla.html (25 October 2005).

31. Resource Conservation and Recovery Act of 1976, P.L. 94-580, codified at 42 U.S.C. §§ 6901 et seq.

32. Comprehensive Environmental Response, Compensation and Liability Act of 1980, P.L. 96-510, 94 Stat. 2767 (11 December 1980), codified at 42 U.S.C. §§ 9601 et seq.

33. Ibid.

34. Agency for Toxic Substances and Disease Registry, "About ATSDR," http://www .atsdr.cdc .gov/about.html (3 November 2005).

35. An example of a state environmental regulatory agency is the Pennsylvania Department of Environment Protection, which administers programs related to air pollution, water pollution, land use including waste disposal, and energy use and production. See Department of Environmental Protection, Commonwealth of Pennsylvania, http://www .depweb.state.pa.us/dep/site/default.asp (7 November 2005).

36. P.L. 91-596, 84 Stat. 1590 (29 December 1970).

37. See, for example, S. P. Wolff, "Correlation between Car Ownership and Leukemia: Is Non-Occupational Exposure to Benzene from Petrol and Motor Vehicle Exhaust a Causative Factor in Leukemia and Lymphoma?" *Cellular and Molecular Life Sciences* 48, no. 3 (1992): 301–304.

38. The history of mental health care is discussed in G. N. Grob, *The Mad among Us: A History of the Care of America's Mentally Ill* (New York: Free Press, 1994).

39. See A. H. C. Wong and H. H. M. Van Tol, "Schizophrenia: From Phronmenology to Neurobiology," *Neuroscience and Behavioral Reviews* 27, no. 3 (2003): 269–306.

40. Advances in scientific understanding of mental illness and issues in its treatment are discussed in G. Norquist and S. E. Hyman, "Advances in Understanding and Treating Mental Illness: Implications for Policy," *Health Affairs* 18, no. 5 (1999): 32–47.

41. S. S. Sharfstein, A. M. Stoline and L. M. Moran, "Mental Health Services," in A. R. Kovner and S. Jonas, eds., *Health Care Delivery in the United States,* 6th ed. (New York: Springer, 1999), 243–278.

42. Ibid., 253.

43. P.L. 88-164.

44. M. Richardson and S. Shiu-Thornton, "Mental Health Service," in S. J. Williams and P.R. Torrens, eds., *Introduction to Health Services,* 5th ed. (Albany, NY: Delmar, 1999), 357–359.

45. P.L. 102-321.

46. U.S. Department of Health and Human Services, The Substance Abuse and Mental Health Services Administration, "Agent Overview," February 2004, http://alt.samhsa.gov/about/backround.htm (7 October 2005).

47. J. K. Igelhart, "The Mental Health Maze and the Call for Transformation," *New England Journal of Medicine* 350, no. 5 (2004): 508.

48. Ibid., 510.

49. Centers for Disease Control and Prevention, "Achievements in Public Health, 1900–1999."

50. Turnock and Atchinson, "Governmental Public Health in the United States."

51. Centers for Disease Control and Prevention, "CDC Mission," http://www.cdc.gov/about/mission.htm (7 November 2005).

52. Centers for Disease Control and Prevention, "About CDC," http://www.cdc.gov/about/cio.htm (14 October 2005).

53. E. W. Etheridge, *Sentinel for Health: A History of the Centers for Disease Control* (Berkeley: University of California Press, 1992), 67.

54. For background on polio and its eradication, see D. M. Oshinsky, *Polio: An American Story* (New York: Oxford University Press, 2005); and J. Kluger, *Splendid Solution: Jonas Salk and the Conquest of Polio* (New York: Penguin Group, 2004).

55. Cotton, "CDC Nears Close of First Half-Century," 2579–2580.

56. The early history of the AIDS epidemic is chronicled in R. Shilts, *And the Band Played On: Politics, People and the AIDS Epidemic* (New York: St. Martin's Press, 1987).

57. Starr, *Social Transformation of American Medicine*, 182.

58. Mullan, *Plagues and Politics*, 185.

59. Ibid., 187.

60. Ibid.

61. National Health Service Corps, "About NHSC," 30 May 2003, http://nhsc.bhpr.hrsa.gov/about (7 October 2005).

62. U.S. Department of Health and Human Services, "HRSA Strategic Plan FY 2005–2010," http://www.hrsa.gov/about/strategicplan05–10.htm (7 November 2005).

63. Ibid.

64. Economic Research Service, "Home," http://www.ers.usda.gov (3 November 2005).

65. Food Safety and Inspection Service, "Home," http://www.fsis.usda.gov (3 November 2005).

66. 21 U.S.C. §§ 601 et seq. and 21 U.S.C. §§ 451 et seq.

67. Food and Nutrition Service, "Home," http://www.fns.usda.gov/fns/default.htm (3 November 2005).

68. Center for Nutrition Policy and Promotion, "Homepage," 21 October 2005, http://www.cnpp.usda.gov (11 November 2005).

69. The U.S. Department of Agriculture's food pyramid combines several elements of nutrition advice and is available at http://www.mypyramid.gov (7 November 2005).

70. U.S. Department of Homeland Security, "Emergency and Diseases—Preparing America," http://www.dhs.gov/dhspublic/theme_home2.jsp (3 August 2005).

71. Ibid.

72. Fee and Brown, "Unfulfilled Promise of Public Health," 31–43.

73. J. Lewis, "The Birth of EPA," *EPA Journal* (November 1985), 13 December 2004, http://www.epa.gov/history/topics/epa/15c.htm (7 November 2005).

74. Federal Insecticide, Fungicide and Rodenticide Act, 21 U.S.C. § 321.

75. Water Pollution Control Act, 42 U.S.C. §§ 300g-2, et seq.; Air Pollution Control Act, 42 U.S.C. § 7671, et seq.; Shoreline Erosion Protection Act, P.L. 89-298, § 310b, 79 Stat. 1095; Solid Waste Disposal Act, 42 U.S.C. §§ 6901 et seq.

76. National Environmental Policy Act of 1969, 42 U.S.C. §§ 4321, 4331, 4368b.

77. Lewis, "Birth of EPA."

78. U.S. Environmental Protection Agency, "EPA History—Topics," 13 December 2004, http://www.epa.gov/history/topics/index.htm (7 November 2005).

79. Ibid.

80. See, for example, *Chevron U.S.A. v. Natural Resources Defense Council*, 467 U.S. 837 (1984), in which the Supreme Court upheld the EPA's regulatory definition of a "source" of pollution under the federal Clean Air Act; and *Alaska Department of Environmental Conservation v. Environmental Protection Agency*, 540 U.S. 461 (2004), in which the Supreme Court upheld the EPA's decision to overrule a permit granted by the state of Alaska to a private company to operate a zinc concentrate mine.

81. U.S. Environmental Protection Agency, "Allowance Trading Basics," 12 May 2005, http://www.epa.gov/airmarkets/trading/basics (16 October 2005). Background on the pollution allowance trading mechanism is discussed in R. Rico, "The U.S. Allowance Trading System for Sulfur Dioxide: An Update on Market Experience," *Environmental and Resource Economics* 5, no. 2 (1995): 115–129.

82. U. S. Environmental Protection Agency, "Allowance Trading Basics."

83. U. S. Department of Health and Human Services, Agency for Toxic Substances and Disease Registry, "About ATSDR," http://www.atsdr.cdc.gov/about.html (25 October 2005).

84. Ibid.

85. Occupational Safety and Health Administration, "OSHA 30–Year Milestones," http://www.osha.gov/as/opa/osha30yearmilestones.html (7 November 2005).

86. U.S. Department of Labor, Occupational Safety and Health Administration, "OSHA's Mission," http://www.osha.gov/oshinfo/mission.html (25 October 2005).

87. P.L. 91-596, 84 Stat. 1590, codified at 29 U.S.C. §§ 651 et seq.

88. Occupational Health and Safety Act of 1970, 29 U.S.C. §§ 651, 653, 654, 655, 659, 666, 667. See also G. A. Rosier, "We Benefit from Fewer OSHA regulations, Not More," *Occupational Health and Safety* 70, no. 6 (2001): 10.

89. Centers for Disease Control and Prevention, National Institute of Occupational Safety and Health, "About NIOSH," http://www.cdc.gov/niosh/about.html (25 October 2005).

90. Occupational Safety and Health Administration, "OSHA Facts—December 2004," 25 January 2005, http://www.osha.gov/as/opa/oshafacts.html (7 November 2005).

91. See, for example, D. Byren et al., "Mortality and Cancer Morbidity in a Group of Swedish VCM and PCV Production Workers," *Environmental Health Perspective* 17 (October 1976): 167–170; P. F. Infante, J. K. Wagoner, and R. J. Waxweiler. "Carcinogenic, Mutagenic and Teratogenic Risks Associated with Vinyl Chloride," *Mutation Research* 41

(November 1976): 131–141; and P. F. Infante, "Benzene: An Historical Perspective on the American and European Occupational Setting," in D. Gee et al., eds., *Late Lessons from Early Warnings: The Precautionary Principle 1896–2000* (Luxembourg: Office for Official Publications of the European Communities, 2001), 38–15.

92. *Marshall v. Whirlpool,* 445 U.S. 1 (1980).

93. Biological monitoring of workers was required in the OSHA standard for exposure to lead, which is published at 29 C.F.R. § 1910.1025. The provisions on biological monitoring are included in section 1910.1025(j)(2).

94. The rule on repetitive stress injuries was originally published at 29 C.F.R. § 1910.900 (14 November 2000). The original proposal was published at 64 *Federal Register* 65768–66078 (23 November 1999) and is available at http://www.osha.gov/pls/oshaweb/owadisp.show_ document?p_table=FEDERAL_REGISTER&p_id=16305 (16 October 2005). Guidelines that replaced these rules are available at http://www.osha.gov/SLTC/ergonomics/four-pronged_ factsheet.html (16 October 2005).

95. U.S. Department of Labor, Occupational Safety and Health Administration, "Part 1910 Occupational Safety and Health Standards—Bloodborne Pathogens (1910.1030)," 18 January 2001, http://www.osha.gov/pls/oshaweb/owadisp.show_document?p_table= STANDARDS&p_id=10051 (25 October 2005).

96. P. Torrens and L. Breslow, "The Evolution of Public Health: A Joint Public-Private Responsibility," in S. J. Williams and P. R. Torrens, eds., *Introduction to Health Services,* 5th ed. (Albany, NY: Delmar, 1999), 212–213.

97. The public health systems in thirteen states are described in S. Wall, "Transformations in Public Health Systems," *Health Affairs* 17, no. 3 (1998): 64–80.

98. Ibid.

99. Ibid.

100. Welcome to California: The Official State Site, "Department of Health Services—Medical Care Services," 2004, http://www.dhs.ca.gov/mcs/medi-calhome/default .htm (14 October 2005).

101. Torrens and Breslow, "Evolution of Public Health," 171–203.

102. Ibid.

103. Wall, "Transformations in Public Health Systems," 73–80.

104. PA Department of Health, "You and Your Family's Health," 2005, http://www.dsf .health.state.pa.us/health/site/default.asp (14 October 2005).

105. New York State Association of County Health Officials, "About Us," 5 October 2005, http://www.nysacho.org/About_Us/about_us.html (14 October 2005).

106. New York State Department of Health, "Directory Services: N.Y.S. County Health Departments," February 2005, http://www.health.state.ny.us/nysdoh/lhu/map.htm (14 October 2005).

107. Welcome to California: The Official State Site, "Organizational Structure of CDHS," 2004, http://www.dhs.ca.gov/home/aboutcdhs/structure.htm (14 October 2005).

108. A. de Tocqueville, *Democracy in America* (New York: Penguin Putnam, 1984), 62–71. See also the discussion of de Tocqueville's observations on American federalism in P. J. Watson and R. J. Morris, "Individualist and Collective Values: Hypotheses Suggested by Alexis de Tocqueville," *Journal of Psychology* 136, no. 3 (2002): 263–271.

109. U.S. Const., Amend. X.

110. Torrens and Breslow, "Evolution of Public Health."

111. United Health Foundation, "America's Health: State Health Rankings 2004, Percent of Health Dollars for Public Health," 2005, http://www.unitedhealthfoundation.org/shr2004/components/percentph.html (14 October 2005).

112. Recent changes in the structure of Medicaid coverage for the poor may be accelerating a trend toward greater emphasis by public health agencies on population-based prevention and less on the direct provision of services through primary care clinics. See Wall, "Transformations in Public Health Systems," 73–80.

113. M. Wei and P. Wei, "Occupational Risk Factors for Selected Cancers," *American Journal of Public Health* 94, no. 7 (2004): 1078.

114. Starr, *Social Transformation of American Medicine*, 182.

Chapter 7

1. National Coalition on Health Care, "Health Insurance Cost," 2004, http://www.nchc.org/facts/cost.shtml (14 October 2005).

2. P.L. 107-204, 116 Stat. 746.

3. J. J. Sokolov, "Will MD Solo Practice Survive? No," *Hospitals and Health Networks* 68, no. 11 (1994): 10.

4. Federal Trade Commission, "90th Anniversary Symposium Program," September 2004, http://www.ftc.gov/ftc/history/90thAnniv_Program.pdf (14 October 2005).

5. Ibid.

6. Federal Trade Commission Improvement Act of 1975, 15 U.S.C. §§ 2301–45, 46, 57a, 58.

7. Hart-Scott-Rodino Antitrust Improvements Act of 1976, 15 U.S.C. §§ 1, 1311, 6204.

8. *Goldfarb v. Virginia State Bar*, 421 U.S. 773 (1975).

9. 15 U.S.C. §1 et seq.

10. Clayton Act, 15 U.S.C. § 18.

11. Federal Trade Commission Act, 15 U.S.C. § 45.

12. See discussion in T. H. Stanton, "Fraud-and-Abuse Enforcement in Medicare: Finding Middle Ground," *Health Affairs* 20, no. 4 (2001): 28–42.

13. P.L. 95-142, 91 Stat. 1183 (1977), codified at 42 U.S.C. § 1320a–7b.

14. 42 U.S.C. § 1320a–7b.

15. IRC § 501(c)3.

16. Health Insurance Portability and Accountability Act of 1996, 42 U.S.C. §§ 300gg-1, et seq.

17. See K. Fonkych and R. Taylor, *The State and Pattern of Health Information Technology Adoption* (Santa Monica, CA: Rand Corporation, 2005), 1.

18. See discussion of health care antitrust in W. A. Zelman, *The Changing Health Care Marketplace* (San Francisco: Jossey-Bass, 1996), 171–195.

19. 15 U.S.C. §§ 1 et seq.

20. For background on the consolidation of much of American industry at the time, see N. Lamoreaux, *The Great Merger Movement in American Business, 1895–1904* (New York: Cambridge University Press, 1985).

21. Hospital Survey and Construction Act of 1946 (Hill-Burton Act), P.L. 79–725.

22. For a discussion of the range of applications of antitrust law to health care, see D. Haas-Wilson, *Managed Care and Monopoly Power: The Antitrust Challenge* (Cambridge, MA: Harvard University Press, 2003), 66–80.

23. This was the finding of the Supreme Court in *Arizona v. Maricopa Country Medical Society,* 457 U.S. 332 (1982).

24. The consolidation of several teaching hospitals during the 1990s is discussed in J. A. Kastor, *Mergers of Teaching Hospitals in Boston, New York, and Northern California* (Ann Arbor: University of Michigan Press, 2001).

25. See *Hospital Corporation of America,* 3 Trade Reg. Rep. (CCH) 22,301 (FTC 25 October 1985).

26. U.S. Department of Justice and Federal Trade Commission, "Statements of Antitrust Enforcement Policy in Health Care," 4 Trade Reg. Rep. (CCH) ¶13,153 (18 August 1996).

27. See discussion of the safety zones in Haas-Wilson, *Managed Care and Monopoly Power,* 84–86.

28. For a discussion of antitrust liability engendered by physician boycotts, see P. J. Hammer and W. M. Sage, "Antitrust, Health Care Quality, and the Courts," *Columbia Law Review* 102 (April 2002): 545–649.

29. JCAHO accreditation rules are described at Joint Commission on Accreditation of Healthcare Organizations, "Facts about Hospital Accreditation," 2004, http://www.jcaho.org/htba/hospitals/facts.htm (7 November 2005).

30. See discussion in Haas-Wilson, *Managed Care and Monopoly Power,* 65–66.

31. See discussion of private antitrust enforcement in T. L. Greaney, "Whither Antitrust? The Uncertain Future of Competition Law in Health Care," *Health Affairs* 21, no. 2 (2002): 190.

32. U.S. Federal Trade Commission, "Guide to the Federal Trade Commission," March 2004, http://www.ftc.gov/bcp/conline/pubs/general/guidetoftc.htm (7 November 2005).

33. Ibid.

34. Information on the organization and structure of the U.S. Department of Justice is available at 17 March 2005, http://www.usdoj.gov/jmd/mps/mission.htm (7 November 2005).

35. U.S. Department of Justice, "Overview: Antitrust Division," http://www.usdoj.gov/atr/overview.html (14 October 2005).

36. *United States v. Greber,* 760 F.2d 68 (3rd Cir. 1985).

37. J. F. Blumstein, "The Fraud and Abuse Statute in an Evolving Health Care Marketplace: Life in the Health Care Speakeasy," *American Journal of Law and Medicine* 22, no. 2 (1996): 213.

38. See discussion in Stanton, "Fraud-and-Abuse Enforcement in Medicare," 29–30.

39. Ibid., 219.

40. 42 C.F.R. § 101.952.

41. Ibid.

42. Ibid.

43. Blumstein, "Fraud and Abuse Statute in an Evolving Health Care Marketplace," 209.

44. U.S. Department of Health and Human Services, Office of Inspector General, *Financial Arrangements between Physicians and Health Care Business: Report to Congress* (Washington, DC: U.S. Government Printing Office, 1989).

45. Medicare Amendments, 42 U.S.C. § 1395nn.

46. 42 C.F.R. Subpart J, §§ 350 et seq.

47. T. S. Jost and S. L. Davies, "The Empire Strikes Back: A Critique of the Backlash against Fraud and Abuse Enforcement," *Alabama Law Review* 51, no. 1 (1999): 239–309.

48. See discussion in Blumstein, "Fraud and Abuse Statute in an Evolving Health Care Marketplace," 210–211.

49. Zelman, *Changing Health Care Marketplace*, 259–260.

50. 42 U.S.C. § 1395nn.

51. Centers for Medicare and Medicaid Services, "Program Information on Medicare, Medicaid, SCHIP, and Other Programs of the Centers for Medicare and Medicaid Services," June 2002, http://www.cms.hhs.gov/charts/series/sec2.pdf (14 October 2005).

52. U.S. Health and Human Services, Office of Inspector General, "Fraud Prevention and Detection," http://www.oig.hhs.gov/fraud.html (14 October 2005).

53. B. R. Furrow et al. *Health Law,* 5th ed. (St. Paul, MN: West, 2004), 1010.

54. 31 U.S.C. § 3730.

55. U.S. Department of Health and Human Services, Office of Inspector General, "Fraud Prevention and Detection: Advisory Opinions," 16 August 2005, http://www.oig.hhs.gov/fraud/advisoryopinions/opinions.html (14 October 2005).

56. U. S. Department of Health and Human Services, Office of Inspector General, "Publication of OIG Special Fraud Alerts," 19 December 1994, http://www.oig.hhs.gov/fraud/docs/alertsandbulletins/121994.html (30 May 2006).

57. 65 *Federal Register* 9274–9277 (24 February 2000).

58. Office of Inspector General, "Publication of OIG Special Fraud Alerts."

59. U.S. Department of Health and Human Services, Office of Inspector General, "Hospital Discounts Offered to Patients Who Cannot Afford To Pay Their Hospital Bills," 19 February 2004, http://www.oig.hhs.gov/fraud/docs/alertsandbulletins/2004/FA021904 hospitaldiscounts.pdf (14 October 2005).

60. The structure of the Office of Inspector General is described at 69 *Federal Register* no. 127 (2 July 2004): 40386–40391, http://oig.hhs.gov/organization/oigorgstatement 070204 .pdf (25 October 2005). See also http://oig.hhs.gov/organization.html (25 October 2005).

61. See D. M. Thornton, "Perspectives on Current Enforcement: 'Sentinel Effect' Shows Fraud Control Works," *Journal of Health Law,* 32, no. 4 (1999): 493–502.

62. See J. Krauss, "The Role of the States in Combating Managed Care Fraud and Abuse," *Annals of Health Law* 8 (1999): 179.

63. P. Starr, *The Social Transformation of American Medicine* (New York: Basic Books, 1982).

64. Ibid., 170.

65. R. Stevens, *In Sickness and in Wealth: American Hospitals in the Twentieth Century* (New York: Basic Books, 1989).

66. W. L. Dowling, "Hospitals and Health Systems," in S. J. Williams and P. R. Torrens, *Introduction to Health Services,* 5th ed. (Albany, NY: Delmar, 1999), 271.

67. See discussion in U. E. Reinhardt, "The Economics of For-Profit and Not-for-Profit Hospitals," *Health Affairs* 19, no. 6 (2000): 178–186.

68. For a discussion of the amount of uncompensated care rendered by nonprofit and for-profit hospitals, see U.S. General Accounting Office, *Nonprofit Hospitals: Better Standards Needed for an Exemption,* Report GAO-HRD-90–84, 30 May 1990.

69. *Parrino v. FHP,* 146 F.3d 699 (9th Cir. 1998).

70. Ibid.

71. Internal Revenue Service, Internal Revenue Manual, 7.25.41.4, "Insurance Activities: Blue Cross/Blue Shield," http://www.irs.gov/irm/part7/ch10s29 .html #d0e97487 (20 October 2005).

72. See Furrow et al., *Health Law,* 869.

73. See, for example, *City of Washington v. Board of Assessment,* 500 Pa. 175, 704 A.2d 120 (1997).

74. The Pennsylvania Supreme Court laid out a five-part test for determining whether a nonprofit hospital qualifies for state tax-exempt status that includes indicia of charitable purpose in the case of *Hospital Utilization Project v. Commonwealth of Pennsylvania,* 507 Pa. 1, 487 A.2d 1306 (1985).

75. See J. E. Karns, "Justifying the Nonprofit Hospital Tax Exemption in a Competitive Market Environment," *Widener Law Journal* 13, no. 2 (2004): 399.

76. 26 U.S.C. § 501(c).

77. 26 U.S.C. § 501(c)(3).

78. Internal Revenue Service, "Exemption Requirements," http://www.irs.gov/charities/charitable/article/0,,id=96099,00.html (14 October 2005).

79. 26 U.S.C. §§ 1 et seq.

80. IRS Rev. Ruling 69–545.

81. Ibid.

82. See Zelman, *Changing Health Care Marketplace,* 261.

83. For a discussion of the use of fair market value in an IRS ruling, see M. I. Sanders, "Health Care and Tax Exemption: The Push and Pull of Tax Exemption Law on the Organization and Delivery of Health Care Services: Health Care Joint Ventures between Tax-Exempt Organizations and For-Profit Entities," *Health Matrix* 15 (Winter 2005): 112. For a ruling in which fair market value was considered, see IRS Private Ruling 9636026, 11 June 1996.

84. IRS filing requirements for charitable organizations to demonstrate ongoing compliance with tax exemption requirements are described at http://www.irs.gov/charities/article/0,,id=96103,00.html (25 October 2005).

85. Internal Revenue Service, "Exempt Organizations—Potential Examination Consequences," 2005, http://www.irs.gov/charities/charitable/article/0,,id=123408,00.html (14 October 2005).

86. Internal Revenue Service, "Unrelated Business Income Tax," http://www.irs.gov/charities/charitable/article/0,,id=123293,00.html (14 October 2005).

87. *Geisinger Health Plan v. Commissioner of Internal Revenue Service,* 30 F.3d 494 (3rd Cir. 1994).

88. See R. V. Pattison, and H. M. Katz, "Investor-Owned and Not-for-Profit Hospitals: A Comparison Based on California Data," *New England Journal of Medicine* 309, no. 6 (1983), 347–353.

89. For background on nonprofit corporations, see D. R. Young and L. M. Salamon, "Commercialization, Social Ventures and For-Profit Competition," in L. M. Salamon, ed., *The State of Nonprofit America* (Washington, DC: Brookings Institution, 2002), 423–446.

90. For background on the role of the Securities and Exchange Commission, see "The Investors Advocate: How the SEC Protects Investors and Maintains Market Integrity," 26 October 2005, http://www.sec.gov/about/whatwedo.shtml (7 November 2005).

91. For general background on the antitrust laws, see J. E. Rubin, *General Overview of United States Antitrust Law,* Congressional Research Service, The Library of Congress, CRS Report to Congress, Order Code RL31026, 18 June 2001, available at http://www.cnie.org/nle/crsreports/risk/rsk-62.pdf (25 October 2005).

92. See discussion in Zelman, *Changing Health Care Marketplace,* 292–301.

93. For a discussion of differences in the performance of for-profit and nonprofit hospitals, see A. R. Kovner, "Governance and Management," in A. R. Kovner and S. Jonas, eds., *Health Care Delivery in the United States,* 6th ed. (New York: Springer, 1999), 349–350.

94. Internal Revenue Service, "IRS History and Structure," http://www.irs.gov/irs/article/0,,id=98142.00.html (14 October 2005).

95. U.S. Const., Amend. XVI.

96. Internal Revenue Service Restructuring and Reform Act of 1998, 26 U.S.C. §§ 6015, 6621.

97. Internal Revenue Service, "At a Glance: IRS Divisions and Principal Offices," http://www.irs.gov/irs/article/0,,id=149199,00.html (20 October 2005).

98. Internal Revenue Service, "Tax Exempt and Government Entities Division at-a-Glance," http://www.irs.gov/irs/article/0,,id=100971,00.html (14 October 2005).

99. Internal Revenue Service, "The Agency, Its Mission and Statutory Authority," http://www.irs.gov/irs/article/0,,id=98141,00.html (14 October 2005).

100. The Hippocratic oath is commonly recited by graduates of American medical schools at commencement. The text can be found in L. Edelstein, "The Hippocratic Oath: Text, Translation and Interpretation," in O. Temkin and C. L. Temkin, eds., *Ancient Medicine: Selected Papers of Ludwig Edelstein* (Baltimore: Johns Hopkins University Press, 1967), 3–64, 65. For background on the Hippocratic oath, see the discussion in H. Markel, "Becoming a Physician: 'I Swear by Apollo'—On Taking the Hippocratic Oath," *New England Journal of Medicine* 350, no. 20 (2004): 2026–2029.

101. See A. Etzioni, *The Limits of Privacy* (New York: Basic Books, 1999), 144–148.

102. See P. Starr, "Health and the Right to Privacy," *American Journal of Law and Medicine* 25, no. 2 (1999): 193–210.

103. See L. C. Burton, G. F. Anderson, and I. W. Kues, "Using Electronic Health Records to Help Coordinate Care," *Millbank Quarterly* 82, no. 3 (2004): 457–481. See also Etzioni, *Limits of Privacy,* 150–155.

104. For a discussion of the potential uses of computerized patient records, see Committee on Improving the Patient Record, Institute of Medicine, *The Computer-Based Patient Record: An Essential Technology for Health Care,* rev. ed. (Washington, DC: National Academy Press, 1997), 74–99.

105. P.L. 104–191.

106. National Committee on Vital Health Statistics, *Introduction to the NCVHS,* 14 June 2004, http://www.ncvhs.hhs.gov/intro.htm (7 November 2005).

107. For a discussion of HIPAA's privacy provisions, see G. J. Annas, "HIPAA Regulations: A New Era of Medical-Record Privacy?" *New England Journal of Medicine* 348, no. 15 (2003): 1486–1490.

108. 45 C.F.R. § 160.203.

109. L. Gostin et al., *Legislative Survey of State Confidentiality Laws, with Specific Emphasis on HIV and Immunization,* Report to the United States Centers for Disease Control and Prevention, 1996.

110. See, for example, Code of George §33–54–2, and California Civil Code §56.17.

111. 45 C.F.R. Part 164.

112. Ibid.

113. Ibid.

114. See Starr, "Health and the Right to Privacy," 198–201.

115. 45 C.F.R. Part 164.

116. See discussion in Annas, "HIPAA Regulations," 1488.

117. 45 C.F.R. Part 164.

118. Annas, "HIPAA Regulations," 1490.

119. U.S. Department of Health and Human Services, Office for Civil Rights, "HIPAA," 19 July 2005, http://www.hhs.gov/ocr/hipaa (18 October 2005).

120. U.S. Department of Health and Human Services, Office for Civil Rights, "Budget Request FY 2005," http://www.hhs.gov/ocr/fy2005.pdf (25 October 2005).

121. U.S. Department of Health and Human Services, Office for Civil Rights, "Welcome," 7 October 2005, http://www.hhs.gov/ocr/ (18 October 2005).

122. For an economic explanation of asymmetry of information, see S. Folland, A. C. Goodman, and M. Stano, *The Economics of Health and Health Care* (Upper Saddle River, NJ: Prentice Hall, 2004), 187–193.

123. Ibid., 35–36.

124. Ibid., 155–159.

125. See discussion in Etzioni, *Limits of Privacy,* 155–182.

126. For a discussion of the notion of consumer-driven health care, see R. E. Hertzlinger, *Consumer-Driven Health Care: Implications for Providers, Payers, and Policymakers* (San Francisco: Jossey-Bass, 2004).

127. J. Kendall. "Why Is Healthcare Tied to the Workplace?" *Boston Globe,* 16 October 2005.

Chapter 8

1. A. Kornberg, "The NIH Did It," *Science* 278, no. 5345 (1997): 1863.

2. National Institutes of Health, "The NIH Almanac—Appropriations," 20 January 2005, http://www.nih.gov/about/almanac/appropriations/index.htm (18 October 2005).

3. L. Thomas, as quoted in S. Wolfe, "A Commentary on the Evolution of NIH: What's In, What's Out, What's Hot, What's Not," *Integrative and Behavioral Science* 33, no. 2 (1998): 115.

4. V. A. Harden, National Institute of Health Office of NIH History, "A Short History of the National Institutes of Health," http://history.nih.gov/exhibits/history/index.html (18 October 2005).

5. Ibid.

6. Ibid.

7. V. A. Harden, *Inventing the NIH: Federal Biomedical Research Policy, 1887–1937* (Baltimore: Johns Hopkins University Press, 1986), 3.

8. V. A. Harden, "A Short History of the National Institutes of Health: WWI and the Ransdell Act of 1930," http://history .nih.gov/exhibits/history/docs/page_04.html (18 October 2005).

9. Ransdell Act, P.L. 71–251, 46 Stat. 379 (1930).

10. J. Cohen, "Conflicting Agendas Shape NIH," *Science* 261, no. 5129 (1993): 1674–1679.

11. National Institutes of Health, *The NIH Almanac—Historical Data,* available at http://www.nih.gov/about/almanac/historical/chronology_of_events.htm (25 October 2005).

12. C. Garnett, "Last of 'Treetops,' Bldg. 15K Is Refurbished," http://www.nih.gov/news/NIH-Record/05_29_2001/story01.htm (25 October 2005).

13. F. D. Roosevelt, "The Dedication of the National Institutes of Health," *Clinical Research* 36, no. 1 (1988): 1–2.

14. J. C. Robinson, *Noble Conspirators: Florence S. Mahoney and the Rise of the National Institutes of Health* (Washington, DC: Francis Press, 2001), 59.

15. Ibid.

16. J. A. Shannon, "The Advancement of Medical Research: A Twenty-Year View of the Role of the National Institutes of Health," *Journal of Medical Education* 42, no. 2 (1967): 97–108.

17. Ibid., 99.

18. Public Health Service Act, 42 U.S.C. §§ 201 et seq.

19. National Institutes of Health, *The NIH Almanac—Appropriations,* available at http://www.nih.gov/about/almanac/appropriations/index.htm (25 October 2005).

20. National Institutes of Health, *About NIH,* available at http://www.nih.gov/about/NIHoverview.html (25 October 2005).

21. V. A. Harden, "A Short History of the National Institutes of Health: WWII Research and the Grants Program," http://history.nih.gov/exhibits/history/docs/page_06.html (18 October 2005).

22. Shannon, "Advancement of Medical Research," 103.

23. Harden, "A Short History of the National Institutes of Health."

24. Robinson, *Noble Conspirators,* 114.

25. R. A. Rettig, "The Politics of Sciences," *Health Affairs* 21, no. 3 (2002): 274–276.

26. J. B. Wyngaarden, "The National Institutes of Health in Its Centennial Year," *Science* 237, no. 4817 (1987): 869–874.

27. V. A. Harden, "A Short History of the National Institutes of Health: NIH's Centers," http://history.nih.gov/exhibits/history/docs/page_10.html (5 November 2005).

28. National Cancer Act of 1971, 42 U.S.C. § 201.

29. National Heart, Blood Vessel, Lung, and Blood Act, 42 U.S.C. § 201.

30. The history of the AIDS epidemic is chronicled in R. Shilts, *And the Band Played On: Politics, People and the AIDS Epidemic* (New York: St. Martin's Press, 1987).

31. Committee to Study Strategies to Strengthen the Scientific Excellence of the National Institutes of Health Intramural Research Program, Institute of Medicine, *Report of a Study: A Healthy NIH Intramural Program: Structural Change or Administrative Remedies?* (Washington, DC: National Academy Press, 1988).

32. D. S. Greenberg, *Science, Money, and Politics* (Chicago: University of Chicago Press, 2001), 447.

33. Committee to Study Strategies to Strengthen the Scientific Excellence of the National Institutes of Health Intramural Research Program, *Report of a Study.*

34. The National Center for Complementary and Alternative Medicine is described at http://www.nih.gov/about/almanac/organization/NCCAM.htm (25 October 2005) and the National Center on Minority Health and Health Disparities at http://www.nih.gov/about/almanac/organization/NCMHD.htm (25 October 2005).

35. For discussions of controversies surrounding stem cell research, see D. C. Wertz, "Embryo and Stem Cell Research in the United States: History and Politics," *Gene Therapy* 9, no. 11 (June 2002), 674–678; and G. J. Annas, A. Caplan, and S. Elias, "Stem Cell Politics, Ethics and Medical Progress," *Nature Medicine* 5 (1999): 1339–1341. For a discussion in the general press of the controversy surrounding stem cell research, see E. Berger. "Research Avenue Adds Fuel to Stem Cell Controversy," CNN.com/Health (18 July 2001), available at http://archives.cnn.com/2001/HEALTH/07/11/stem.cell.fact/ (25 October 2005).

36. The White House, Office of the Press Secretary, "Remarks by the President on Stem Cell Research," 21 August 2001, http://www.whitehouse.gov/news/releases/2001/08/20010809-2.html (18 October 2005).

37. State laws regarding stem cell research are discussed in National Conference of State Legislatures, State Embryonic and Fetal Research Laws, 2005, available at http://www.ncsl.org/programs/health/genetics/embfet.htm (25 October 2005).

38. Bayh-Dole Act, 35 U.S.C. §§ 202, 210.

39. Ibid.

40. A. Bar-Shalom and R. Cook-Deegan, "Patents and Innovation in Cancer Therapeutics: Lessons from CellPro," *Millbank Quarterly* 80, no. 4 (2002): 637–676.

41. A. Schofield, "The Demise of Bayh-Dole Protections against the Pharmaceutical Industry's Abuses of Government-Funded Inventions," *Journal of Law, Medicine and Ethics* 32, no. 4 (suppl.) (2004): 777–783.

42. National Science Foundation Act of 1950, P.L. 507, 64 Stat. 149, codified at 42 U.S.C. §§ 1861 et seq.

43. National Science Foundation, *First Annual Report,* 1950–1951 (Washington, DC: National Science Foundation, 1951), quoted at National Science Foundation, "NSF History —50th Anniversary," 31 March 2006, http://www.nsf.gov/about/history/50thanni.jsp (5 November 2005).

44. National Science Foundation, "NSF Congressional Highlight: Congress Reduces NSF Budget to $5.47 Billion," 23 November 2004, http://www.nsf.gov/about/congress/108/highlights/cu04_1123.jsp (5 November 2005).

45. Greenberg, *Science, Money, and Politics,* 41.

46. V. Bush, *Science: The Endless Frontier* (Washington, DC: National Science Foundation, 1990).

47. National Science Board, *Science and Engineering Indicators* (Arlington, VA: National Science Foundation, 1998).

48. National Science Foundation, "Important Historical Dates," http://www.nsf.gov/about/history/important-dates.jsp (6 November 2005).

49. National Science Foundation, "Agency Profile and Goals," http://www.nsf.gov/pubs/2001/nsf0186/nsf0186_1.pdf (6 November 2005).

50. For a review of abuses of subjects in research involving children, see S. E. Laderer and M. A. Grodin, "Historical Overview: Pediatric Experimentation," in M. A. Grodin and L. H. Glantz, eds., *Children as Research Subjects: Science, Ethics, and Law* (New York: Oxford University Press, 1994), 3–21.

51. V. A. Harden, "A Short History of the National Institutes of Health: The Clinical Center," http://www.history.nih.gov/exhibits/history/docs/page_08.html (5 November 2005).

52. L. H. Glantz, "The Law of Human Experimentation with Children," in M. A. Grodin and L. H. Glantz, eds., *Children as Research Subjects: Science, Ethics, and Law* (New York: Oxford University Press, 1994), 103.

53. For background on Nazi medical experiments, see R. J. Lifton, *The Nazi Doctors: Medical Killing and the Psychology of Genocide* (New York: Basic Books, 1986).

54. National Institutes of Health, Office of Human Subjects Research, "Regulations and Ethical Guidelines," http://www.nihtraining.com/ohsrsite/guidelines/graybook.html (6 November 2005).

55. Centers for Disease Control and Prevention, "The Tuskegee Study: A Hard Lesson Learned," 23 May 2005, http://www.cdc.gov/nchstp/od/tuskegee/time.htm (18 October 2005).

56. National Research Act, 42 U.S.C. §§ 201, 218.

57. For a discussion of the operation of institutional review boards, see Glantz, "Law of Human Experimentation with Children," 121–127.

58. NIH regulations for institutional review boards are published at 45 C.F.R. Part 46; FDA regulations are published at 21 C.F.R. Part 56.

59. Critics contend that many IRBs are overburdened and unable to perform reviews that are as thorough as are necessary to fully protect human research subjects. See Committee on Assessing the System for Protecting Human Research Subjects, Institute of Medicine, *Responsible Research: A Systems Approach to Protecting Research Participants* (Washington, DC: National Academies Press, 2002).

60. See NIH regulations published at 45 C.F.R. Part 46, and FDA regulations published at 21 C.F.R. Part 56.

61. U.S. Department of Health and Human Services, National Commission for the Protection of Human Subjects of Biomedical and Behavioral Research, *The Belmont Report*, 18 April 1979, http://www.hhs.gov/ohrp/humansubjects/guidance/belmont.htm (18 October 2005).

62. Pharmaceutical Research and Manufacturers Association of America, "Newsroom/ Press Releases: PhRMA Companies Committed to Finding New Medicines to Treat HIV/ AIDS," 14 June 2005, http://www.phrma.org/mediaroom/press/releases/14.06.2005.1178 .cfm (18 October 2005).

63. 21 U.S.C. §§ 301 et seq.

64. Aggregate research spending by the pharmaceutical industry is larger than that of NIH or any other research sponsor. I. M. Cockburn, "The Changing Structure of the Pharmaceutical Industry," *Health Affairs* 23, no.1 (2004): 10–22.

65. Background on FDA regulation of institutional review boards is presented at http:/ /www.fda.gov/oc/ohrt/irbs/operations.html.

66. FDA regulations governing the operations of IRBs are published at 21 C.F.R. Part 56.

67. 21 C.F.R. § 50.20.

68. Robert Wood Johnson Foundation, "Assessment of the First Decade of the Agency for Health Care and Policy Research," March 2002, http://www.rwjf.org/reports/grr/037565 .htm (18 October 2005).

69. J. J. Clinton and G. Hernandez, "AHCPR Background and History," *Decubitus* 4, no. 2 (1991): 22–26.

70. Clinical practice guidelines developed under the auspices of federal agencies are published through the National Guideline Clearinghouse and are available at http://www .guidelines.gov/.

71. Clinton and Hernandez, "AHCPR Background and History."

72. B. H. Gray, M. K. Gusmano, and S. R. Collins, "AHCPR and the Changing Politics of Health Services Research," *Health Affairs*, Web Exclusive, W3, (25 June 2003): W283–W307.

73. Committee on Quality of Health Care in America, Institute of Medicine, *To Err Is Human* (Washington, DC: National Academy Press, 2000).

74. Agency for Healthcare Research and Quality, *Quality Research for Quality Health Care*, AHRQ Publication No. 01-0018, March 2001, http://www.ahrq.gov/about/qualres.pdf (18 October 2005).

75. Agency for Healthcare Research and Quality, "AHRQ Fiscal Year 2003 Budget in Brief," February 2002, http://www.ahrq.gov/about/cj2003/budbrf03.htm (18 October 2005).

76. The discovery of DNA is described in R. Olby, *The Path to the Double Helix: The Discovery of DNA* (London: Macmillan, 1974).

77. Background on the process of developing recombinant DNA is discussed in M. Zoller, J. Watson, M. Gilman, and J. Witkowski, *Recombinant DNA* (New York: Freeman, 1992). NIH maintains guidelines for research involving recombinant DNA, which were first published at *Federal Register* 59 (5 July 1994): 34496, and have been amended several times.

78. The Human Genome Project of the U.S. Department of Energy, Office of Science, "Human Genome Project Information: History of the Human Genome Project," 24 August

2005, http://www.ornl.gov/sci/techresources/Human_Genome/project/hgp.shtml (18 October 2005).

79. Ibid.

80. Greenberg, *Science, Money, and Politics,* 26.

81. The Human Genome Project of the U.S. Department of Energy, Office of Science, "Human Genome Project Information: Ethical, Legal, and Social Issues," 16 September 2004, http://www.ornl.gov/sci/techresources/Human_Genome/elsi/elsi.shtml (18 October 2005).

82. Executive Order 13145, 8 February 2000. See also H. T. Greely, "Banning Genetic Discrimination," *New England Journal of Medicine* 353, no. 9 (1 Sep 2005): 865–867; and M. A. Rothstein, "Genetic Privacy and Confidentiality: Why They Are So Hard to Protect," *Journal of Law, Medicine and Ethics* 26, no. 3 (1998): 198–204.

83. U.S. Department of Veteran Affairs, "Facts about the Department of Veterans Affairs," 20 September 2005, http://www1.va.gov/opa/fact/vafacts.html (18 October 2005).

84. Ibid.

85. U.S. Department of Health and Human Services, Health Resources and Services Administration, "About HRSA," http://www.hrsa.gov/about/htm (18 October 2005).

86. Ibid.

87. Centers for Medicare and Medicaid Services, "Research Projects," 12 October 2005, http://www.cms.hhs.gov/researchers/projects/default.asp (18 October 2005).

88. Centers for Disease Control and Prevention, "National Center for Health Statistics," 13 October 2005, http://www.cdc.gov/nchs (18 October 2005).

89. U.S. Department of Agriculture, "Agencies, Services, & Programs," 18 March 2005, http://www.usda.gov/wps/portal/!ut/p/_s.7_0_A/7_0_10B?navtype=MA&navid=AGENCIES_OFFICES (18 October 2005).

90. The U.S. Department of Agriculture's food pyramid is available at http://www.mypyramid.gov.

91. U.S. Department of Health and Human Services, National Institutes of Health, "About NIH," 23 June 2006. http://www.nih.gov/about/ (3 August 2006).

92. U.S. Department of Health and Human Services, National Institutes of Health, "An Overview," 17 May 2004, http://www.nih.gov/about/NIHoverview.html. (18 October 2005).

93. Ibid.

94. R01 grants are described at http://grants2.nih.gov/grants/funding/r01.htm, and R03 grants at http://grants2.nih.gov/grants/funding/r03.htm.

95. U.S. Department of Health and Human Services, National Institutes of Health, "An Introduction to Extramural Research at NIH," 4 April 2005, http://grants.nih.gov/grants/intro2oer.htm (5 November 2005).

96. U. S. Department of Health and Human Services, National Institutes of Health, "The NIH Almanac—Nobel Laureates," 10 May 2006, http://www.nih.gov/about/almanac/nobel/index.htm (30 May 2006).

97. Ibid.

98. National Science Foundation, "About the National Science Foundation," 28 February 2005, http://www.nsf.gov/about/ (5 November 2005).

99. Ibid.

100. Food and Drug Administration, "Guidance for Institutional Review Boards and

Clinical Investigators—1998 Update," 19 December 2001, http://www.fda.gov/oc/ohrt/irbsl (18 October 2005).

101. Ibid.

102. Ibid.

103. U. S. Department of Veterans Affairs, "VA Research and Development," 7 April 2006, http://www1.va.gov/resdev/ (3 August 2006).

104. See Health Resources and Services Administration, About HRSA, http://www.hrsa.gov/about/default.htm (5 November 2005).

105. Ibid.

106. H. Moses et al., "Financial Anatomy of Biomedical Research," *Journal of the American Medical Association* 294, no. 11 (2005): 1333–1342.

107. See discussion in R. I. Field et al., "Towards a Policy Agenda on Medicaid Research Funding: Results of a Symposium," *Health Affairs* 22, no. 3 (2003): 224–230.

108. Harden, "A Short History of the National Institutes of Health."

109. Committee on the NIH Research Priority-Setting Process, Institute of Medicine, *Scientific Opportunities and Public Needs: Improving Priority Setting and Public Input at NIH* (Washington, DC: National Academy Press, 1998).

110. For background on ethical issues in genetics, see M. J. Reiss and R. Straughan, *Improving Nature? The Science and Ethics of Genetic Engineering* (New York: Cambridge University Press, 1996).

Chapter 9

1. P. Starr, *The Social Transformation of American Medicine* (New York: Basic Books, 1982), 4.

2. Kaiser Family Foundation, "Health Insurance/Costs," http://www.kff.org/insurance/index.cfm (27 September 2005).

3. See Kaiser Family Foundation, *Medicare Chart Book* (Washington, DC: Kaiser Family Foundation, 2005), 55, available at http://www.kff.org/medicare/7284.cfm (12 October 2005). See also Kaiser Family Foundation, "Key Medicare and Medicaid Statistics," 2005, http://www.kff.org/medicaid/upload/Key%20Medicare%20and%20Medicaid%20Statistics.pdf (12 October 2005).

4. World Health Organization, *Health Systems: Improving Performance* (Geneva: World Health Organization, 2000).

5. G. F. Anderson, "In Search of Value: An International Comparison of Cost, Access, and Outcomes," *Health Affairs* 16, no. 6 (1997): 163–171.

6. Committee on Quality of Health Care in America, Institute of Medicine, *To Err Is Human* (Washington, DC: National Academy Press, 2000).

7. Kaiser Commission on Medicaid and the Uninsured, *Health Insurance Coverage in America, 2003 Update* (Washington, DC: Henry J. Kaiser Family Foundation, 2004), 7.

8. Kaiser Family Foundation, "Health Insurance/Costs," http://www.kff.org/insurance/index.cfm (27 September 2005).

9. See discussion in B. B. Longest, *Health Policymaking in the United States* (Chicago: Health Administration Press, 1998), 20–27.

10. See W. A. Zelman, *The Changing Health Care Marketplace* (San Francisco: Jossey-Bass, 1996), 222–226.

11. H. A. Sultz and K. M. Young, *Health Care USA: Understanding Its Organization and Delivery* (Gaithersburg, MD: Aspen, 2001), 399. See also A. Etzioni, *The Limits of Privacy* (New York: Basic Books, 1999), 150–155.

12. J. E. Wennberg and M. M. Cooper, eds., *The Quality of Medical Care in the United States—A Report on the Medicare Program, The Dartmouth Atlas of Health Care 1999* (Chicago: American Hospital Association, 1999).

13. See P. Spath, *Provider Report Cards: A Guide for Promoting Health Care Quality to the Public* (San Francisco: Jossey-Bass, 1999). For a description of provider report cards, see Rand Health, "Report Cards for Health Care—Is Anyone Checking Them?" RB-4544 (2002), http://www.rand.org/publications/RB/RB4544/ (25 October 2005).

14. S. P. Westphal, "Test Predicts Response to Cancer Drugs," *Wall Street Journal* (27 September 2005), D1.

15. R. Field, "The Frontiers of Genetics and the Transformation of Medicine and Business," in I. Farquhar, K. Summers, and A. Sorkin, eds., *Investing in Health: The Social and Economic Benefits of Health Care Innovation* (New York: Elsevier Science, 2001), 1–21.

16. E. A. Zerhouni, "US Biomedical Research," *Journal of the American Medical Association* 294, no. 11 (2005): 1352–1358.

17. D. P. Goldman et. al., "Consequences of Health Trends and Medical Innovation for the Future Elderly," *Health Affairs,* Web Exclusive W5 (26 September 2005): W5–W17.

18. P.L. 104–191.

19. For background on the Office of the National Technology Coordinator for Health Information Technology, see U.S. Department of Health and Human Services, "Office of the National Coordinator for Health Information Technology (ONC)," 4 November 2005, http://www.hhs.gov/healthit/ (7 November 2005).

20. L. O. Gostin, Z. Lazzarini, and K. M. Flaherty, "Legislative Survey of State Confidentiality Laws, with Specific Emphasis on HIV and Immunization," 1996, http://www.epic.org/privacy/medical/cdc_survey.html (7 September 2005).

21. P. Killbridge, "The Cost of HIPAA Compliance," *New England Journal of Medicine* 348, no. 15 (2003): 1423–1424.

22. See Etzioni, *Limits of Privacy*, 152–154.

23. Pennsylvania Act 13, 2002, 40 P.S. § 1303.303 (2002).

24. An example of a Web site containing report cards on physicians, hospitals, and nursing homes is one maintained by Health Grades, a private company, at http://www.healthgrades.com/.

25. A. Milstein et al., "Improving the Safety of Health Care: The Leapfrog Initiative," *Effective Clinical Practice* 3, no. 6 (2000): 313–316.

26. See Centers for Medicare & Medicaid Services, "Fact Sheet: Medicare 'Pay For Performance (P4P)' Initiatives," 31 January 2005, available at http://www.cms.hhs.gov/media/press/release.asp?Counter=1343 (25 October 2005).

27. U.S. Department of Health and Human Services, "Hospital Compare: A Tool for

Adults, Including People with Medicare," 1 September 2005, http://www.hospitalcompare
.hhs.gov (12 October 2005).

28. This mechanism is described in R. E. Hertzlinger, *Consumer-Driven Health Care: Implications for Providers, Payers and Policy-Makers* (San Francisco: Jossey-Bass, 2004).

29. Medical savings accounts were authorized in the Balanced Budget Act of 1997, P.L. 105-33, and were reauthorized as health savings accounts in the Medicare Prescription Drug, Improvement, and Modernization Act of 2003, P.L. 108-173.

30. See V. G. Rodwin, "Comparative Analysis of Health Systems: An International Perspective," in A. R. Kovner and S. Jonas, eds., *Health Care Delivery in the United States*, 6th ed. (New York: Springer, 1999), 133.

31. S. Woolhandler and D. U. Himmelstein, "Paying for National Health Insurance—and Not Getting It," *Health Affairs* 21, no. 4 (2002): 88–98.

32. S. Wall, "Transformations in Public Health Systems," *Health Affairs* 17, no. 3 (1998): 64–80.

33. E. Fee and T. M. Brown, "The Unfulfilled Promise of Public Health: Déjà Vu All over Again," *Health Affairs* 21, no. 6 (2002): 31–43.

34. See P. R. Torrens and L. Breslow, "The Evolution of Public Health: A Joint Public-Private Responsibility," in S. J. Williams and P. A. Torrens, eds., *Introduction to Health Services*, 5th ed. (Albany, NY: Delmar, 1999), 222–224.

35. See Longest, *Health Policymaking in the United States*, 37–52.

36. B. J. Turnock and C. Atchison, "Government Public Health in the United States: The Implications of Federalism," *Health Affairs* 21, no. 6 (2002): 68–78.

37. See discussion of policy modification in Longest, *Health Policymaking in the United States*, 212–231.

38. Starr, *Social Transformation of American Medicine*, 363–378.

39. R. A. Culbertson and P. R. Lee, "Medicare and Physician Autonomy," *Health Care Financing Review* 18, no. 2 (1996): 115–130.

40. Kaiser Family Foundation. *Medicare Chart Book*, 55.

41. G. C. Pope and J. E. Schneider, "Trends in Physician Income," *Health Affairs* 11, no. 1 (1992): 181–193.

42. P.L. 102–571.

43. For a description of the basis for this estimate of the cost to develop a new drug, see J. A. DiMasi, R. W. Hansen, and H. G. Grabowski, "The Price of Innovation: New Estimates of Drug Development Costs," *Journal of Health Economics* 22, no. 2 (2003): 151–185.

44. Committee to Study the Role of Allied Health Personnel, Institute of Medicine, *Allied Health Services: Avoiding Crises* (Washington, DC: National Academy Press, 1989).

45. Liaison Committee on Medical Education, "Overview: Accreditation and the LCME," 7 July 2004, http://www.lcme.org/overview.htm (12 August 2005).

46. Committee to Study the Role of Allied Health Personnel, *Allied Health Services*.

47. U.S. Government Accountability, *Medicare: CMS Needs Additional Authority to Adequately Oversee Patient Safety in Hospitals*, Report No. GAO-05–850, 20 July 2004.

48. See Longest, *Health Policymaking in the United States*, 20–27.

Selected Bibliography

Publications in Print

Adams, A. S., S. B. Soumerai, and D. Ross-Degnan. "The Case for a Medicare Drug Coverage Benefit: A Critical Review of Empirical Evidence." *Annual Review of Public Health* 22 (2001): 49–61.

American Medical Association. *State Medical Licensure Requirements and Statistics.* Chicago: American Medical Association, 1999.

Anderson, G. F. "In Search of Value: An International Comparison of Cost, Access, and Outcomes." *Health Affairs* 16, no. 6 (1997): 163–71.

Anderson, G. F., P. S. Hussey, B. K. Frogner, and H. R. Waters. "Health Spending in the United States and the Rest of the Industrialized World." *Health Affairs* 24, no. 4 (2005): 903–14.

Annas, G. J. "HIPAA Regulations—A New Era of Medical-Record Privacy?" *New England Journal of Medicine* 348, no. 15 (2003): 1486–90.

Baker, J. J. "Medicare Payment System for Hospital Inpatients: Diagnosis-Related Groups." *Journal of Health Care Finance* 28, no. 3 (2002): 1–13.

Baker, L. C. and L. S. Baker. "Excess Cost of Emergency Department Visits for Nonurgent Care." *Health Affairs* 13, no. 5 (1994): 162–71.

Ballentine, C. "Taste of Raspberries, Taste of Death: The 1938 Elixir Sulfanilamide Incident." *FDA Consumer* 31, no. 6 (1981): 18–21.

Bar-Shalom, A., and R. Cook-Deegan. "Patents and Innovation in Cancer Therapeutics: Lessons from CellPro." *Millbank Quarterly* 80, no. 4 (2002): 637–76.

Bass, R. R. P. S. Gainer, and A. R. Carlini. "Update on Trauma System Development in the United States." *Journal of Trauma* 47, no. 3 (1999): supplement 15–21.

Bazzoli, G. J., K. J. Madura, G. F. Cooper, E. J. MacKenzie, and R. V. Maier. "Progress in the Development of Trauma Systems in the United States: Results of a National Survey." *Journal of the American Medical Association* 273, no. 5 (1995): 395–401.

Bhatia, A. J., S. Blackstock, R. Nelson, and T. S. Ng. "Evolution of Quality Review Programs for Medicare: Quality Assurance to Quality Improvement." *Health Care Financing Review* 22, no. 1 (2000): 69–75.

Blendon, R. J., C. M. DesRoches, J. M. Benson, M. Brodie, and D. E. Altman. "American's Views on the Use and Regulation of Dietary Supplements." *Archives of Internal Medicine* 161, no. 6 (2001): 805–10.

Blumstein, J. F. "The Fraud and Abuse Statute in an Evolving Health Care Marketplace: Life in the Health Care Speakeasy." *American Journal of Law and Medicine* 22, no. 2 (1996): 205–31.

Bodenheimer, T. S., and K. Grumbach. *Understanding Health Policy: A Clinical Approach.* New York: Lange Medical Books/McGraw-Hill, 2002.

Brennan, T. A., R. I. Horowitz, F. D. Duffy, C. K. Cassel, L. D. Goode, and A. S. Lipner. "The Role of Physician Specialty Board Certification Status in the Quality Movement." *Journal of the American Medical Association* 292, no. 9 (2004): 1038–43.

Brown, L. D. "Political Evolution of Federal Health Care Regulation." *Health Affairs* 11, no. 4 (1992): 17–37.

Burton, L. C., G. F. Anderson, and I. W. Kues. "Using Electronic Health Records to Help Coordinate Care." *Millbank Quarterly* 82, no. 3 (2004): 457–81.

Bush, V. *Science: The Endless Frontier.* Washington, DC: National Science Foundation, 1990.

Byren, D., G. Engholm, A. Englund, and P. Westerholm. "Mortality and Cancer Morbidity in a Group of Swedish VCM and PCV Production Workers." *Environmental Health Perspectives* 17 (1976): 167–70.

Carroll, A., and J. M. Ambrose. "Any-Willing-Provider Laws: Their Financial Effect on HMOs." *Journal of Health Politics, Policy and Law* 27, no. 6 (2002): 927–45.

Clinton, J. J., and G. Hernandez. "AHCPR Background and History." *Decubitus* 4, no. 2 (1991): 22–26.

Cohen, J. "Conflicting Agendas Shape NIH." *Science* 261, no. 5129 (1993): 1674–79.

Committee on Assessing the System for Protecting Human Research Subjects, Institute of Medicine. *Responsible Research: A Systems Approach to Protecting Research Participants.* Washington, DC: National Academy Press, 2002.

Committee on Quality of Health Care in America, Institute of Medicine. *Crossing the Quality Chasm: A New Health System for the Twenty-first Century.* Washington, DC: National Academy Press, 2001.

———. *To Err Is Human.* Washington, DC: National Academy Press, 2000.

Committee on the NIH Research Priority-Setting Process, Institute of Medicine. *Scientific Opportunities and Public Needs: Improving Priority Setting and Public Input at NIH.* Washington, DC: National Academy Press, 1998.

Committee to Study the Role of Allied Health Personnel, Institute of Medicine. *Allied Health Services: Avoiding a Crisis.* Washington DC: National Academy Press, 1989.

Connor, J. T. H. *Doing Good: The Life of Toronto's General Hospital.* Toronto: University of Toronto Press, 2000.

Cotton, P. "CDC Nears Close of First Half-Century." *Journal of the American Medical Association* 263, no. 19 (1990): 2579–80.

Crossen, C. "How Elixir Deaths Led U.S. to Require Proof of New Drugs' Safety." *Wall Street Journal*, 3 October 2005, B1.

Culbertson, R. A., and P. R. Lee. "Medicare and Physician Autonomy." *Health Care Financing Review* 18, no. 2 (1996): 115–30.

Cunningham, R., and R. M. Cunningham. *The Blues: A History of the Blue Cross and Blue Shield System*. DeKalb, IL: Northern Illinois University Press, 1997.

Derbyshire, R. C. *Medical Licensure and Discipline in the United States*. Westport, CT: Greenwood, 1978.

DiMasi, J. A. R. W. Hansen, and H. G. Grabowski. "The Price of Innovation: New Estimates of Drug Development Costs." *Journal of Health Economics* 22, no. 2 (2003): 151–85.

Dobson, A., D. Moran, and G. Young. "The Role of Federal Waivers in the Health Policy Process." *Health Affairs* 11, no. 4 (1992): 72–94.

Donabedian, A. "The Quality of Care: How Can It Be Assessed?" *Journal of the American Medical Association* 260, no. 12 (1998): 1743–58.

Duff, S. "Drop in the Bucket: Newly Seen Surplus Not Encouraging." *Modern Healthcare* 32, no. 10 (2002): 16.

Etheridge, E. W. *Sentinel for Health: A History of the Centers for Disease Control*. Berkeley: University of California Press, 1992.

Etzioni, A. *The Limits of Privacy*. New York: Basic Books, 1999.

Farquhar, I., K. Summers, and A. Sorkin, eds. *Investing in Health: The Social and Economic Benefits of Health Care Innovation*. New York: Elsevier Science, 2001.

Fee, E., and T. M. Brown. "The Unfulfilled Promise of Public Health: Déjà Vu All Over Again." *Health Affairs* 21, no. 6 (2002): 31–43.

Field, R. I., B. J. Plager, R. A. Baranowski, M. A. Healy, and M. L. Longacre. "Towards a Policy Agenda on Medicaid Research Funding: Results of a Symposium." *Health Affairs* 22, no. 3 (2003): 224–30.

Fleming, K. C., J. M. Evans, and D. S. Chutka. "A Cultural and Economic History of Old Age in America." *Mayo Clinic Proceedings* 78, no. 10 (2003): 914–21.

Flexner, A. *Medical Education in the United States and Canada: A Report to the Carnegie Foundation for the Advancement of Teaching*. New York: Carnegie Foundation for the Advancement of Teaching, 1910.

Folland, S., A. C. Goodman, and M. Stano. *The Economics of Health and Health Care*. Upper Saddle River, NJ: Prentice Hall, 2004.

Fonkych, K., and R. Taylor. *The State and Pattern of Health Information Technology Adoption*. Santa Monica, CA: Rand Corporation, 2005.

Fontanarosa, P. B., D. Rennie, and C. D. DeAngelis. "Postmarketing Surveillance—Lack of Vigilance, Lack of Trust." *Journal of the American Medical Association* 292, no. 21 (2004): 2647–50.

Furrow, B. R. "Regulating Patient Safety: Toward a Federal Model of Medical Error Reduction." *Widener Law Review* 12, no. 1 (2006): 1–38.

Furrow. B. R., T. L. Greaney, S. H. Johnson, T. S. Jost, and R. L. Schwartz. *Health Law*. 5th ed. St. Paul, MN: West, 2004.

Gee, D., P. Harremoes, J. Keys, M. MacGarvin, A. Stirling, S. Vaz, and B. Wynne, eds. *Late Lessons from Early Warnings: The Precautionary Principle 1896–2000.* Luxembourg: Office for Official Publications of the European Communities, 2001.

Gevitz, N. *The DOs: Osteopathic Medicine in America.* Baltimore: Johns Hopkins University Press, 2004.

Gold, M. "Medicare+Choice: An Interim Report Card." *Health Affairs* 20, no. 4 (2001): 120–38.

Greaney, T. L. "Whither Antitrust? The Uncertain Future of Competition Law in Health Care." *Health Affairs* 21, no. 2 (2002): 186–96.

Greely, H. T. "Banning Genetic Discrimination." *New England Journal of Medicine* 353, no. 9 (2005): 865–67.

Greenberg, D. S. *Science, Money, and Politics.* Chicago: University of Chicago Press, 2001.

Grob, G. N. *The Mad Among Us: A History of the Care of America's Mentally Ill.* New York: Free Press, 1994.

Haas-Wilson, D. *Managed Care and Monopoly Power: The Antitrust Challenge.* Cambridge, MA: Harvard University Press, 2003.

Hackey, R., and D. Rochefort. *The New Politics of State Health Policy.* Lawrence, KS: University Press of Kansas, 1994.

Halpern, S. D., P. A. Ubal, and A. L. Caplan. "Solid-Organ Transplantation in HIV-Infected Patients." *New England Journal of Medicine* 347, no. 4 (2002): 284–87.

Ham, C. "Retracing the Oregon Trail: The Experience of Rationing and the Oregon Health Plan." *British Medical Journal* 316, no. 7149 (1998): 1965–69.

Hammer, P. J., and W. M. Sage. "Antitrust, Health Care Quality, and the Courts." *Columbia Law Review* 102 (April 2002): 545–649.

Harden, V. A. *Inventing the NIH: Federal Biomedical Research Policy, 1887—1937.* Baltimore: Johns Hopkins University Press, 1986.

Harrington, C., S. Anzaldo, A. Burdin, M. Kitchener, and N. Miller. "Trends in State Certificate of Need and Moratoria Programs for Long-Term Care Providers." *Journal of Health and Social Policy* 19, no. 2 (2004): 31–58.

Hayes, H. A. "Food and Drug Regulation after 75 Years." *Journal of the American Medical Association* 246, no. 11 (1981): 1223–26.

Heath, W. J. "America's First Drug Regulation Regime: The Rise and Fall of the Import Drug Act of 1848." *Food Drug Law Journal* 59, no. 1 (2004): 169–99.

Heller, W. M. "The United States Pharmacopeia: Its Value to the Professions." *Journal of the American Medical Association* 213, no. 4 (1970): 576–79.

Hertzlinger, R. E. *Consumer-Driven Health Care: Implications for Providers, Payers, and Policy-Makers.* San Francisco: Jossey-Bass, 2004.

Hilts, P. *Protecting America's Health: The FDA, Business, and One Hundred Years of Regulation.* New York: Knopf, 2003.

Hoffman, E. D., B. S. Klees, and C. A. Curtis. "Overview of the Medicare and Medicaid Programs." *Health Care Financing Review* 22, no. 1 (2000): 175–93.

Holahan, J., S. Zuckerman, A. Evans, and S. Rangarajan. "Medicaid Managed Care in Thirteen States." *Health Affairs* 17, no. 3 (1998): 43–63.

Hsiao, W. C., M. S. Harvey, D. L. Dunn, and S. L. Weiner. "Lessons of the New Jersey DRG Payment System." *Health Affairs* 5, no. 2 (1986): 32–45.

Hutt, P. B. "The Transformation of United States Food and Drug Law." *Journal of the Association of Food and Drug Officials* 68, no. 3 (1996): 1.

Hutt, P. B., and P. B. Hutt II. "A History of Government Regulation of Adulteration and Misbranding of Food." *Food, Drug, and Cosmetic Law Journal* 39 (1984): 2–73.

Igelhart, J. K. "Congress Moves to Bolster Peer Review: The Health Care Quality Improvement Act of 1986." *New England Journal of Medicine* 316, no. 15 (1987): 960–64.

———. "The American Health Care System—Community Hospitals." *New England Journal of Medicine* 329, no. 5 (1993): 372–76.

———. "The American Health Care System—Teaching Hospitals." *New England Journal of Medicine* 329, no. 14 (1993): 1052–56.

———. "The End-Stage Renal Disease Program." *New England Journal of Medicine* 328, no. 5 (1993): 366–71.

———. "The American Health Care System—Medicare." *New England Journal of Medicine* 340, no. 4 (1999): 317–32.

———. "The Centers for Medicare and Medicaid Services." *New England Journal of Medicine* 345, no. 26 (2001): 1920–24.

———. "Medicare's Declining Payments to Physicians." *New England Journal of Medicine* 346, no. 24 (2002): 1924–30.

———. "The Mental Health Maze and the Call for Transformation." *New England Journal of Medicine* 350, no. 5 (2004): 507–14.

Infante, P. F., J. K. Wagoner, and R. J. Waxmeiler. "Carcinogenic, Mutagenic and Teratogenic Risks Associated with Vinyl Chloride." *Mutation Research* 41 (1976): 131–41.

Janssen, W. "The Story of the Laws behind the Labels." *FDA Consumer* 15, no. 5 (June 1981): 32–45.

Jost, T. S. "Oversight of the Quality of Medical Care: Regulation, Management, or the Market?" *Arizona Law Review* 37 (Fall 1995): 825–68.

Jost, T. S., and S. L. Davies. "The Empire Strikes Back: A Critique of the Backlash against Fraud and Abuse Enforcement." *Alabama Law Review* 51, no. 1 (1999): 239–309.

Jost, T. S., L. Mulcahy, S. Strasser, and L. A. Sachs. "Consumers, Complaints and Professional Discipline: A Look at Medical Licensure Boards." *Health Matrix* 3 (1993): 309–38.

Kaiser Commission on Medicaid and the Uninsured. *The Medicaid Resource Book*. Washington, DC: The Henry J. Kaiser Family Foundation, 2002.

———. *Health Insurance Coverage in America 2003 Data Update*. Washington, DC: The Henry J. Kaiser Family Foundation, 2004.

Kaplan, A. H. "Fifty Years of Drug Amendments Revisited in Easy-to-Swallow Capsule Form." *Food and Drug Law Journal* 50, no. 5 (1995): 179–97.

Karns, J. E. "Justifying the Nonprofit Hospital Tax Exemption in a Competitive Market Environment." *Widener Law Journal* 13, no. 2 (2004): 383–561.

Kastor, J. A. *Mergers of Teaching Hospitals in Boston, New York, and Northern California*. Ann Arbor: University of Michigan Press, 2001.

Kazis, L. E., X. S. Ren, A. Lee, K. Skinner, W. Rogers, J. Clark, and D. R. Miller. "Health Status in VA Patients: Results from the Veterans Health Study." *American Journal of Medical Quality* 14, no. 1 (1999): 28–38.

Keough, L. L. "DSH Adjustment Controversies Continue." *Healthcare Financial Management* 56, no. 11 (2002): 84–86.

Kessler, D. A., and W. L. Pines. "The Federal Regulation of Prescription Drug Advertising and Promotion." *Journal of the American Medical Association* 264, no. 18 (1990): 2409–15.

Khuri, S. F., J. Daley, W. Henderson, et al. "The Department of Veterans Affairs' NSQIP: The First National, Validated, Outcome-Based, Risk-Adjusted, and Peer-Controlled Program for the Measurement and Enhancement of the Quality of Surgical Care." *Annals of Surgery* 228, no. 4 (1998): 491–507.

Killbridge, P. "The Cost of HIPAA Compliance." *New England Journal of Medicine* 348, no. 15 (2003): 1423–24.

Kissick, W. *Medicine's Dilemmas.* New Haven, CT: Yale University Press, 1994.

Kluger, J. *Splendid Solution: Jonas Salk and the Conquest of Polio.* New York: Penguin Group, 2004.

Kovner, A. R., and S. Jonas, eds. *Health Care Delivery in the United States.* 6th ed. New York: Springer, 1999.

Kurian, G. T., ed. *A Historical Guide to the U.S. Government.* New York: Oxford University Press, 1998.

Kuttner, R. "The American Health Care System: Health Insurance Coverage." *New England Journal of Medicine* 340, no. 2 (1999): 163–68.

Lamoreaux, N. *The Great Merger Movement in American Business, 1895–1904.* New York: Cambridge University Press, 1985.

Lepkowski, W. "The Saccharin Debate: Regulation and the Public Taste." *Hastings Center Report* 7, no. 6 (1977): 5–7.

Lifton, R. J. *The Nazi Doctors: Medical Killing and the Psychology of Genocide.* New York: Basic Books, 1986.

Light, D. W., and M. Widman. *Regulating Prospective Payment: An Analysis of the New Jersey Hospital Rate Setting Commission.* Ann Arbor, MI: Health Administration Press, 1988.

Longest, B. B. *Health Policymaking in the United States.* Chicago: Health Administration Press, 1998.

Lubbers, J. S. *A Guide to Federal Agency Rulemaking.* 3rd ed. Chicago: ABA Books, 1998.

Mant, J. "Process versus Outcome Indicators in Assessment of Quality of Health Care." *International Journal for Quality in Health Care* 13, no. 6 (2001): 475–80.

Markel, H. "Becoming a Physician: 'I Swear by Apollo'—On Taking the Hippocratic Oath." *New England Journal of Medicine* 350, no. 20 (2004): 2026–29.

Mathieu, M. *New Drug Development: A Regulatory Overview.* Waltham, MA: Parexel International, 1994.

McArdle, F. P. "Opening Up the Federal Employee Benefits Program." *Health Affairs* 14, no. 2 (1995): 40–50.

McDonough, J. E. "Tracking the Demise of State Hospital Rate Setting." *Health Affairs* 16, no. 1 (1997): 142–49.

Mechanic, D. "A Balanced Framework for Change." *Journal of Health Politics, Policy and Law* 24, no. 5 (1999):1107–14.

Melling, J. "An Inspector Calls: Perspectives on the History of Occupational Diseases and Accident Compensation in the United Kingdom." *Medical History* 49, no. 1 (2005): 102–6.

Miller, R. D., and R. C. Hutton. *Problems in Health Care Law.* Gaithersburg, MD: Aspen, 2000.

Milstein, A., R. S. Galvin, S. F. Delbanco, F. Salber, and C. R. Buck Jr. "Improving the Safety of Health Care: The Leapfrog Initiative." *Effective Clinical Practice* 3, no. 6 (2000): 313–16.

Morreim, E. E. *Holding Health Care Accountable.* New York: Oxford University Press, 2001.

Moses, H., E. R. Dorsey, D. H. M. Matheson, and S. O. Thier. "Financial Anatomy of Biomedical Research." *Journal of the American Medical Association* 294, no. 11 (2005): 1333–42.

Mullan, F. *Plagues and Politics: The Story of the United States Public Health Service.* New York: Basic Books, 1989.

Nissenson, A. R., and R. A. Rattig. "Renal Disease Program: Current Status and Future Prospects." *Health Affairs* 18, no. 1 (1999): 161–79.

Noah, L., and B. A. Noah. *Law, Medicine and Medical Technology.* New York: Foundation Press, 2002.

Office of Inspector General, U.S. Department of Health and Human Services. *Financial Arrangements between Physicians and Health Care Business: Report to Congress.* Washington, DC: U.S. Government Printing Office, 1989.

Olby, R. *The Path to the Double Helix: The Discovery of DNA.* London: Macmillan, 1974.

Oliver, T. R., P. R. Lee, and H. L. Lipton. "A Political History of Medicare and Prescription Drug Coverage." *Milbank Quarterly* 82, no. 2 (2004): 283–354.

Oshinsky, D. M. *Polio: An American Story.* New York: Oxford University Press, 2005.

Palmisano, D. J., D. W. Emmons, and G. D. Wozniak. "Expanding Insurance Coverage through Tax Credits, Consumer Choice, and Market Enhancements: The American Medical Association Proposal for Health Insurance Reform." *Journal of the American Medical Association* 291, no. 18 (2004): 2237–42.

Patterson, C. H. "Joint Commission on Accreditation of Healthcare Organizations." *Infection Control and Hospital Epidemiology* 16, no. 1 (1995): 36–42.

Pope, G. C., and J. E. Schneider. "Trends in Physician Income." *Health Affairs* 11, no. 1 (1992): 181–93.

Reinhardt, U. E. "The Economics of For-Profit and Not-for-Profit Hospitals." *Health Affairs* 19, no. 6 (2000): 178–86.

———. "Perspectives on the Pharmaceutical Industry." *Health Affairs* 20, no. 5 (2001): 136–49.

Rettig, R. A. "The Politics of Sciences." *Health Affairs* 21, no. 3 (2002): 274–76.

Risse, G. *Mending Bodies, Saving Souls: A History of Hospitals.* New York: Oxford University Press, 1999.

Robinson, J. *Noble Conspirator: Florence S. Mahoney and the Rise of the National Institutes of Health.* Washington, DC: Francis Press, 2001.

Robinson, J. C. *The Corporate Practice of Medicine.* Berkeley: University of California Press, 1999.

Rosen, G. *A History of Public Health.* New York: MD Publications, 1958.

Rosenberg, C. E. *The Care of Strangers: The Rise of America's Hospital System.* Baltimore: Johns Hopkins University Press, 1995.

Rosoff, A. J. "The Business of Medicine: Problems with the Corporate Practice Doctrine." *Specialty Law Digest—Health Care Monthly* 9, no. 14 (1988): 7–25.

Rothstein, M. A. "Genetic Privacy and Confidentiality: Why They Are So Hard to Protect." *Journal of Law, Medicine and Ethics* 26, no. 3 (1998): 198–204.

Rowland, D., and R. Garfield. "Health Care for the Poor: Medicaid at 35." *Health Care Financing Review* 22, no. 1 (2000): 23–34.

Samkoff, J. S., and R. W. McDermott. "Recognizing Physician Impairment." *Pennsylvania Medicine* 91, no. 4 (1988): 36–38.

Sanders, M. I. "Health Care and Tax Exemption: The Push and Pull of Tax Exemption Law on the Organization and Delivery of Health Care Services: Health Care Joint Ventures between Tax-Exempt Organizations and For-Profit Entities." *Health Matrix* 15 (Winter 2005): 83–123.

Schactman, D. "Specialty Hospitals, Ambulatory Surgery Centers, and General Hospitals: Charting a Wise Public Policy Course." *Health Affairs* 24, no. 3 (2005): 868–73.

Schiff, R. L., D. A. Ansell, J. E. Schlosser, A. H. Idris, A. Morrison, and S. Whitman. "Transfers to a Public Hospital." *New England Journal of Medicine* 314, no. 9 (1986): 552.

Schofield, A. "The Demise of Bayh-Dole Protections against the Pharmaceutical Industry's Abuses of Government-Funded Inventions." *Journal of Law, Medicine and Ethics,* 32:4 (supp.), 777–783, 2004.

Shannon, J. A. "The Advancement of Medical Research: A Twenty-Year View of the Role of the National Institutes of Health." *Journal of Medical Education* 42, no. 2 (1967): 97–108.

Shilts, R. *And the Band Played On: Politics, People and the AIDS Epidemic.* New York: St. Martin's Press, 1987.

Sinclair, U. *The Jungle.* New York: Viking Press, 1946.

Smith, M. I., A. I. Wertheimer, and J. E. Finchman, eds. *Pharmacy and the U.S. Health Care System.* Binghamton, NY: Pharmaceutical Products Press, 2005.

Snoe, J. A. *American Health Care Delivery Systems.* St. Paul, MN: West Group, 1998.

Snyder, C., and G. Anderson. "Do Quality Improvement Organizations Improve the Quality of Hospital Care for Medicare Beneficiaries?" *Journal of the American Medical Association* 293, no. 23 (2005): 2900–2907.

Stanton, T. H. "Fraud-and-Abuse Enforcement in Medicare: Finding Middle Ground." *Health Affairs* 20, no. 4 (2001): 28–42.

Starr, P. *The Social Transformation of American Medicine.* New York: Basic Books, 1982.

Steinbrook, R. "Testing Medications in Children." *New England Journal of Medicine* 347, no. 18 (2002): 1462–70.

Stephens, T. D. *Dark Remedy: The Impact of Thalidomide and Its Revival as a Vital Medicine.* Cambridge, MA: Perseus, 2001.

Stevens, R. *In Sickness and in Wealth: American Hospitals in the Twentieth Century.* New York: Basic Books, 1989.

Sultz, H. A., and K. M. Young. *Health Care USA: Understanding Its Organization and Delivery.* Gaithersberg, MD: Aspen, 2001.

Suthummanon, S., and V. K. Omachonu. "DRG-Based Cost Minimization Models: Applications in a Hospital Environment." *Health Care Management Science* 7, no. 3 (2004): 197–205.

Tannenwald, R. "Implications for the Balanced Budget Act of 1997 for the 'Devolution Revolution.'" *Publius* 28, no. 1 (1998): 23–28.

Temkin, O., and C. L. Temkin, eds. *Ancient Medicine: Selected Papers of Ludwig Edelstein.* Baltimore: Johns Hopkins University Press, 1967.

Thornton, D. M. "Perspectives on Current Enforcement: 'Sentinel Effect' Shows Fraud Control Works." *Journal of Health Law,* 32, no. 4 (1999): 493–502.

Tolley, M. C. "Judicial Review of Agency Interpretation of Statutes: Deference Doctrines in Comparative Perspective." *Policy Studies Journal* 31, no. 3 (2003): 421–40.

Turnock, B. J., and C. Atchison. "Governmental Public Health in the United States: The Implications of Federalism." *Health Affairs* 21, no. 6 (2002): 68–78.

Van Amerongen, D. "Physician Credentialing in a Consumer-Centric World." *Health Affairs* 21, no. 5 (2002): 152–56.

Wall, W. "Transformations in Public Health Systems." *Health Affairs* 17, no. 3 (1998): 64–80.

Watson, P. J., and R. J. Morris. "Individualist and Collective Values: Hypotheses Suggested by Alexis de Tocqueville." *Journal of Psychology* 136, no. 3 (2002): 263–71.

Wei, M., and P. Wei. "Occupational Risk Factors for Selected Cancers." *American Journal of Public Health* 94, no. 7 (2004): 1078.

Weil, A. "Chipping Away at the Uninsured." *Health Affairs* 23, no. 5 (2004): 153–54.

Weissert, C. S., and W. G. Weissert. *Governing Health: The Politics of Health Policy.* Baltimore: Johns Hopkins University Press, 2002.

Wennberg, D. E. "Variation in the Delivery of Health Care: The Stakes Are High." *Annals of Internal Medicine* 128, no. 10 (1998): 866–68.

Wennberg, J. E., and M. M. Cooper, eds. *The Quality of Medical Care in the United States: A Report on the Medicare Program—The Dartmouth Atlas of Health Care 1999.* Chicago: American Hospital Association, 1999.

Whitcomb, M. "Correcting the Oversupply of Specialists by Limiting Residencies for Graduates of Foreign Medical Schools." *New England Journal of Medicine* 333, no. 7 (1995): 454–56.

White, C. "Rehabilitation Therapy in Skilled Nursing Facilities: Effects of Medicare's New Prospective Payment System." *Health Affairs* 22, no. 3 (2003): 214–23.

Whitnah, D. R., ed. *Government Agencies.* Westport, CT: Greenwood Press, 1983.

Williams, S. J., and P. R. Torrens. *Introduction to the Health Services.* 5th ed. Albany, NY: Delmar, 2002.

Wilson, N. J., and K. W. Kizer. "The VA Health Care System: An Unrecognized National Safety Net." *Health Affairs* 16, no. 4 (1997): 200–204.

Woolhandler, S., and D. U. Himmelstein. "Paying for National Health Insurance—and Not Getting It." *Health Affairs* 21, no. 4 (2002): 88–98.

World Health Organization. *Health Systems: Improving Performance.* Geneva: World Health Organization, 2000.

Wyngaarden, J. B. "The National Institutes of Health in Its Centennial Year." *Science* 237 no. 4817 (1987): 869–74.

Wynia, M. K., S. R. Latham, A. C. Kao, J. W. Berg, and L. L. Emanuel. "Medical Professionalism in Society." *New England Journal of Medicine* 341, no. 21 (1999): 1612–17.

Yohn, K. C. "The History and Role of the Federation of State Medical Boards of the United States." *Federation Bulletin* 75, no. 9 (1988): 275–77.

Young, J. H. *Pure Food: Securing the Federal Food and Drugs Act of 1906.* Princeton, NJ: Princeton University Press, 1989.

Zelman, W. A. *The Changing Health Care Marketplace.* San Francisco: Jossey-Bass, 1996.

Zerhouni, E. A. "U.S. Biomedical Research." *Journal of the American Medical Association* 294, no. 11 (2005): 1352–58.

Resources On the Internet

Agency for Healthcare Research and Quality. http://www.ahrq.gov/.

Agency for Toxic Substances and Disease Registry. http://www.atsdr.cdc.gov/.

Alliance for Health Reform. http://www.allhealth.org.

American Association of Retired Persons. http://www.aarp.org/.

American Board of Internal Medicine. http://www.abim.org/.

American Board of Medical Specialties. http://www.abms.org

American Health Planning Association. http://ahpanet.org.

American Medical Association, http://www.ama-assn.org/.

American Osteopathic Association. http://www.osteopathic.org/index.cfm.

American Pharmacists Association. http://www.aphanet.org.

American Society of Health-System Pharmacists. http://www.ashp.org/.

Center for Health System Change. http://hschange.org/.

Center for Medicare & Medicaid Services. http://www.cms.hhs.gov/.

The Clean Air Trust. http://www.cleanairtrust.org/index.html.

Council on Graduate Medical Education. http://www.cogme.gov/.

Educational Commission for Foreign Medical Graduates. http://www.ecfmg.org/.

ElderWeb. http://www.elderweb.com/.

Federal Trade Commission. http://www.ftc.gov.

Federation of State Medical Boards. http://www.fsmb.org/.

Food and Drug Administration. http://www.fda.gov/.

Government Accountability Office. http://www.gao.gov.

Health Grades. http://www.healthgrades.com.

Health Resources and Services Administration. http://www.hrsa.gov/.

Human Genome Project Information. http://www.ornl.gov/sci/techresources/Human_Genome/home.shtml.

Indian Health Services. http://www.ihs.gov/.

Joint Commission on Accreditation of Healthcare Organizations. http://www.jcaho.org

Kaiser Family Foundation, http://www.kff.org/.

Liaison Committee on Medical Education. http://www.lcme.org/start.htm.

National Academy for State Health Policy. http://nashp.org.

National Board of Medical Examiners. http://www.nbme.org.

National Community Pharmacists Association. http://www.ncpanet.org/

National Health Service Corps. http://nhsc.bhpr.hrsa.gov/about.

National Institutes of Health. http://www.nih.gov/.

Occupational Health and Safety Administration. http://www.osha.gov/index.html.

Public Citizen's Health Research Group. http://www.citizen.org/

The Robert Wood Johnson Foundation. http://rwjf.org/index.jsp.

TRICARE: U.S. Department of Defense, Military Health System. http://www.tricare.osd.mil.

United Health Foundation. http://www.unitedhealthfoundation.org.

United Network for Organ Sharing. http://www.unos.org/.

U.S. Department of Health and Human Services. http://www.hhs.gov/.

U.S. Department of Health and Human Services, Hospital Compare. http://www .hospitalcompare .hhs.gov.

U.S. Department of Health and Human Services, Office of Inspector General. http://oig.hhs .gov/.

U.S. Department of Justice, Antitrust Division. http://www.usdoj.gov/atr/index.html.

U.S. Department of Labor, Bureau of Labor Statistics. http://www.bls.gov/.

U.S. Department of Veterans Affairs. http://www.va.gov/index.htm.

U.S. Drug Enforcement Administration. http://www.dea.gov/index.htm.

U.S. Equal Employment Opportunity Commission. http://www.eeoc.gov/.

Index

Page numbers in bold indicate tables.

Lightning Source UK Ltd.
Milton Keynes UK
UKOW06n2258040915